- 426

PUBLICATIONS OF
THE WELLCOME INSTITUTE OF THE HISTORY OF MEDICINE

General Editor : F. N. L. Poynter, Ph.D., D.Litt., Hon.M.D.(Kiel)

New Series, Volume XIX

ENGLAND'S FIRST STATE HOSPITALS AND THE METROPOLITAN ASYLUMS BOARD

1867-1930

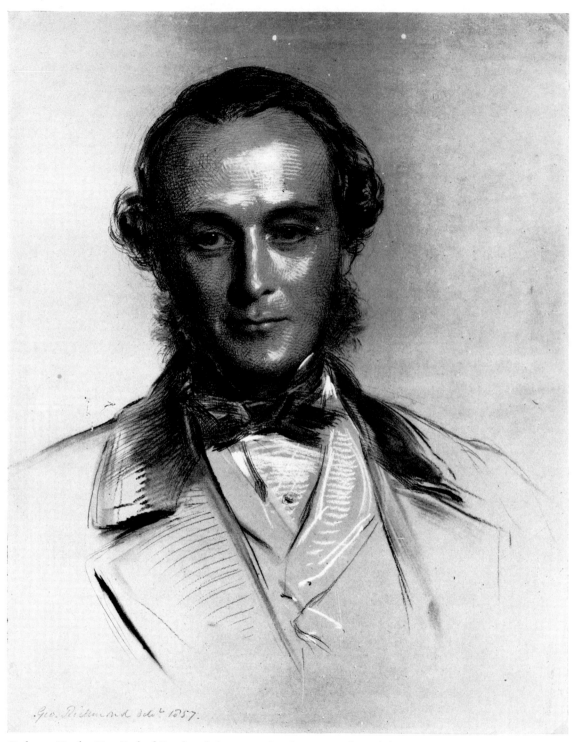

Geo. Richmond delt 1857.

Gathorne Hardy, First Earl of Cranbrook (1814–1906), who, as President of the Poor Law Board, introduced the Metropolitan Poor Bill, 1867, to establish State Hospitals in London.

From a portrait by George Richmond, 1857: by kind permission of the Fourth Earl of Cranbrook and the National Portrait Gallery, London.

ENGLAND'S FIRST STATE HOSPITALS
AND THE
METROPOLITAN ASYLUMS BOARD
1867–1930

by

GWENDOLINE M. AYERS

LONDON

WELLCOME INSTITUTE OF THE HISTORY OF MEDICINE

1971

This work is based on a thesis approved by the Senate of the University of London for the award of the degree of Doctor of Philosophy.

Made and printed in Great Britain by
William Clowes and Sons, Limited, London, Beccles and Colchester

TO
THOSE WHO
DID NOT PASS BY

Preface

CHANGES in the status of our hospitals and in the administration of medical care arising out of the National Health Service Act of 1946 challenged our limited historical knowledge of the elements which had been welded together to form the new national hospital service. These deficiencies were remedied in large measure by such works as *The National Health Service in Great Britain*, by James Stirling Ross, 1952; *Hospitals and the State*, by the Acton Society Trust, 1955–59; *The Evolution of Hospitals in Britain*, edited by F. N. L. Poynter, 1964; *The Hospitals, 1800–1948*, by Brian Abel-Smith, 1964; and *The Origins of the National Health Service: The Medical Services of the New Poor Law, 1834–71*, by Ruth G. Hodgkinson, 1967. At the same time, these studies uncovered fields which called for further research.

This work attempts to penetrate a hitherto neglected area of English social administration—our nineteenth-century State hospital system. It is basically a case study of the Metropolitan Asylums Board and its medical services. But, as an investigation of the creation and functions of England's first regional hospital board demanded wider research into the extent of State intervention on behalf of the destitute sick, and into the causes and outcome of changes in poor law philosophies and practice, it came to reflect significant facets of the developing 'administrative State' during the century following the 1834 Poor Law Amendment Act. At the same time, evidence of the dynamic of the human spirit as a vital element in progress is articulate in the unfolding of this episode of social change.

The tensions and events which led to legislation in 1867 for governing the provision and administration of special poor law hospitals in London are discussed in the Introduction. The main part of the study is devoted to the period 1867 to 1930, the life-span of the statutory authority created to establish and manage the new institutions—the Metropolitan Asylums Board. Although this name suggests that the sole function of the new body was the care of the mentally ill, this was not the case. It was called upon, initially, to erect and administer fever and smallpox hospitals, as well as mental institutions. Part One, covering the Board's first three decades, deals with its work for the chronic insane and the fever-stricken in the face of persistent epidemics, public hostility and acrimonious conflicts with an obscurantist bureaucracy. The development of the Board's hospital and ambulance services for infectious patients is discussed in some detail, as it illustrates the lineal descent of our modern health and welfare services from the original poor law service. Part Two examines the organizational structure of the Asylums Board, its institutional administration, staff and finance. The history of the hospitals is resumed in Part Three. Instead of a continuous narrative chronologically interweaving all aspects of the

Board's expanding empire during the latter half of its term of administration from 1900 to 1930, this period is covered by a series of studies devoted to the separate services of the Metropolitan Asylums system, since each originated in different circumstances and evolved along independent lines. In this way, it is hoped that the results of this research will be more readily available to specialist workers who may be interested in the part played by the Metropolitan Asylums Board in such fields as the care of the mentally disordered; medical education and research; the control of epidemic diseases, tuberculosis and venereal disease; child care in experimental hospital-schools; or in the Board's extra-medical services for youthful offenders, vagrants and war-time refugees. The Epilogue traces the fluctuating fortunes of the Board during the decade of reconstruction following World War I. After discussing the Board's dissolution and the transfer of its 24,000-bed hospital system to the London County Council in 1930, the study concludes with a brief survey of the repercussions and 'lessons' of the State's initial incursion into the field of institutional medical care.

The story of this pioneering venture has been built up largely from the official records of the Metropolitan Asylums Board, supplemented by the reports of relevant government departments, royal commissions and departmental committees of enquiry.[1] The Asylums Board conferred fortnightly in plenary session for 63 years from June 1867. The minutes of these meetings, bleakly succinct but complete, have provided the factual skeleton around which the biography of this body has been moulded. For some twenty years following its creation, records of the Board's deliberations received only a very limited circulation. Although it received periodical reports from its medical superintendents and management committees, the Board published no annual record of its work before 1886. An outstanding feature of the annual reports which were made generally available thereafter was the supplement produced by the Board's special statistical committee. From 1890, spot maps showing notifications and hospital admissions of acute infectious diseases were included, presenting for the first time a comprehensive picture of the incidence of pestilence in the metropolitan area. The Board's arsenal of statistical records has been selectively drawn upon, and most of the resulting tables are set out in appendices to this study in order to relieve the text of congesting detail. Background material has been drawn from specialist literature and journals of the period and from the works of medical historians, biographers and epidemiologists. Acknowledgment to these scholars has been made in footnotes to the text.

In the course of this research, I have been grateful for the co-operation of numerous library assistants. In particular, I should like to thank Mr. E. W. P. Rhoades, of the British Library of Political and Economic Science; and Mr. Sidney H. Watkins, of the Wellcome Institute's photographic unit, whose willing help and expertise have been immensely valuable, especially in the production of the illustrations to this work.

To Sir Harry Verney I should like to offer my warmest thanks for so kindly giving me

[1] For the long loan of many of these official papers I would like to record my grateful thanks to the British Library of Political and Economic Science.

viii

access to the Nightingale papers at Claydon House and for regaling me with reminiscences of his venerated great-aunt.

In the field of social administration, I am especially indebted to Professor Brian Abel-Smith. This study owes much to his guidance, constructive criticism and encouragement. I am also very grateful to Professor Richard M. Titmuss for his penetrating observations during the early stages of the work, and for his kindness and wise counsel at all times. The comments of Professor David Marsh, Mr. Robert Pinker and Dr. S. R. Speller have likewise been very stimulating and much appreciated.

In the medical world, my very special thanks are due to Dr. H. Stanley Banks and Dr. Alexander Walk. Dr. Banks has been kind enough to advise on the epidemiological aspects of the study and generously given time to assess the completed text; while Dr. Walk has gone to much trouble to give me the benefit of his wide clinical experience and historical knowledge of the care of the mentally disordered. I should also like to thank Dr. Ian Brown, Dr. Arthur D. Morris and Dr. Michael M. Palmer for their encouraging interest in the project.

While gratefully acknowledging this helpful co-operation, I must emphasize that the shortcomings which remain are the fault of no one but myself.

Without the generous financial support of the Wellcome Trust, this work would not have been possible. I am extremely grateful to the Trustees for giving me this opportunity to explore a little-known area of hospital history and so to contribute in some small measure to our knowledge of the aims, errors and achievements of the past. I must also include my appreciation of the consideration shown to me by Dr. P. O. Williams, Secretary to the Trust. Finally, I would like to record my grateful thanks to Dr. Noël Poynter for publishing this work. His helpful suggestions and those of Dr. Ruth G. Hodgkinson, Assistant Editor, have been most valuable.

Willingdon, Sussex   Gwen Ayers
May 1969

CONTENTS

Prevention Metropolis Act, 1883: removal of pauper stigma from patients in M A B isolation hospitals—Smallpox epidemic of 1884–85: conditions at the Darenth hospital encampment; relaxation by the M A B of admission regulations in advance of legislation—Expansion and reorganization of the Board's services for infectious patients.

PART TWO:
ANATOMY OF THE M A B HOSPITAL SYSTEM

PART THREE:
THE M A B—1900 to 1930: THREE DECADES OF
TWENTIETH-CENTURY DEVELOPMENT

xiv

the statutory exclusion of the M A B from sanatorium provision—The National Insurance Act, 1913, waiving the poor law status of the M A B and empowering it to provide residential accommodation for insured tuberculosis patients—The Public Health (Prevention and Treatment of Diseases) Act, 1913, and the inclusion in the London prevention scheme of residential provision by the M A B for both insured and uninsured tuberculosis patients—The role of the M A B in wartime and post-war arrangements—Cessation of 'sanatorium benefit' under the National Insurance Act of 1920, and the transfer of responsibility to local authorities under the Public Health (Tuberculosis) Act, 1921—Proposed annexation of the M A B by the LCC—Development of the tuberculosis branch of the M A B hospital empire.

TABLES APPENDED TO CHAPTERS

Appendices

TABLES, EXPLANATORY NOTES, CHARTS, MAPS and BIBLIOGRAPHIES

Appendix III *M A B Mental Institutions*

Appendix IV *M A B Finance*

CONTENTS

List of Illustrations

Thanks are due to the following for permission to reproduce illustrations: The Earl of Cranbrook; the Greater London Council; The National Portrait Gallery; *Illustrated London News*; and the Wellcome Trustees. The source of each illustration is given on the page where it is reproduced.

Abbreviations

A M O	Assistant Medical Officer
B M A	British Medical Association
B M J	British Medical Journal
B P P	British Parliamentary Papers
E S N	educationally subnormal
G L C	Greater London Council
H/C	House of Commons
H/L	House of Lords
L C C	London County Council
L G B	Local Government Board
M A B*	Metropolitan Asylums Board
M A B *Mins*	Minutes of the Metropolitan Asylums Board in plenary session
M C P F	Metropolitan Common Poor Fund
M O	Medical Officer (hospital)
M O H	Medical Officer of Health
My. of H	Ministry of Health
N A P S S	National Association for the Promotion of Social Science
P L B	Poor Law Board
W H O	World Health Organization

* The Metropolitan Asylums Board is abbreviated to 'M A B' throughout the text from the beginning of Part One.

INTRODUCTION

Origins of the Metropolitan Asylums Board

'The origin of the English Social Services of modern times is to be found mainly in the fixed and ancient laws of England; and partly in the beneficent devices of voluntary social aspirations and mutual good-will. It is a strange medley of State regulation and humanitarian endeavour.'

Sir George Newman, *English Social Services* (1941).

CHAPTER 1

The Destitute Sick and the Pursuit of a Policy

STATE direction in the sphere of medical care in modern England[1] may be traced from 1867, when the Metropolitan Poor Act of that year led to the founding of special hospitals for the indigent sick of London. For some sixty years, these institutions were managed by a statutory authority confusingly known as the Metropolitan Asylums Board. This study seeks to define the forces which influenced the creation of this body and to follow its development as a link between the nineteenth-century poor law and the twentieth-century welfare revolution.

The advent of the Metropolitan Asylums Board was closely bound up with the hapless lot of ailing paupers during the middle nineteenth century. Before 1867, no statutory provision existed for the destitute sick who needed institutional care. The Royal Commission of 1832–34, which studied the administration of the poor laws, was concerned mainly with the problem of able-bodied destitution. The one positive recommendation that can be extracted from its report concerning other categories of the poor was the repeated demand that, where they required indoor relief, they should not be placed in a single 'mixed' institution but in separate buildings under quite independent management. It was suggested that distinct institutions should be provided for 'at least four classes—the aged and impotent, the children, the able-bodied females and the able-bodied males'.[2] But the report contained no clarification of the term 'impotent' and offered no clear alternative to the current practice of providing the sick poor with outdoor relief. Notwithstanding the emphatic recommendations of the 1834 Report and their statutory endorsement by the Poor Law Amendment Act of 1834,[3] general mixed workhouses were allowed to persist by the Poor Law Commissioners of 1834–47 and by the Poor Law Board which succeeded them.

---

[1] Public provision for the care of the sick and needy was universal throughout the countries of Greece and Rome. In his Linacre lecture, 1914, on 'Public Medical Service and the Growth of Hospitals', Sir T. Clifford Allbutt produced evidence of Roman municipal hospitals staffed by salaried doctors; of publicly financed *iatreia* where doctors received patients; and of the management of these services by regional health committees. (Sir T. Clifford Allbutt, *Greek Medicine in Rome* (1921), pp. 443–71).

[2] *Report from His Majesty's Commissioners for Inquiring into the Administration and Practical Operation of the Poor Laws*, 1834 (Fellowes: 1905 reprint), p. 306.

[3] 4 & 5 Wm. IV c. 76 'for the amendment and better administration of the laws relating to the poor of England and Wales'.

The purpose of the 1834 Act was not so much to create a new system of poor laws as to restore the scope and intention of the Elizabethan statute of 1601 by establishing a two-tier administrative structure for controlling the dispensation of poor relief and thereby remedying the abuses which had resulted in the rapid growth of the poor rate. In each parish, or union of parishes, all classes of the needy were placed under a single local authority known as a 'board of guardians of the poor'. The function of these elective bodies was to administer relief in accordance with rules laid down by the three Commissioners appointed under the Act as representatives of the central government.

As the guardians were dependent for their position on their ratepaying electorates, they were more concerned to save the ratepayers' money than to provide for the separate needs of the poor. One institution was as much as most boards were prepared to maintain. In many rural areas, the number of the poor in each class would have been too small in any case to justify the expense of separate buildings. All categories of the poor thus came to be accommodated together under one roof. The Assistant Commissioners (responsible for the twenty-one districts into which the country was divided under the 1834 Act), finding these establishments easier to inspect than several buildings under separate management, converted their official superiors to the practical nature of these institutions.[1] The general mixed workhouse thus became established with all its attendant evils. As an instrument for testing destitution, it was administered with the object of making life inside less tolerable than employment in field or factory—the principle of 'less eligibility', as it was called. While this policy might deter the work-shy, it inflicted undeserved hardship upon sick and aged inmates, since no alternative system was provided by law for regulating their relief according to their special needs. The following indictment by a learned lawyer in 1852 embodied the essence of much that has been written concerning the effects of this drift in poor law administration.[2]

> ... I have visited many prisons and lunatic asylums, not only in England, but in France and Germany. A single English workhouse contains more that justly calls for condemnation ... than is found in the very worst prisons or public lunatic asylums that I have seen. The workhouse, as now organised, is a reproach and disgrace to England; nothing corresponding to it is found throughout the whole continent of Europe. In France, the medical patients of our workhouses would be found in 'hôpitaux'; the infirm aged poor would be in 'hospices'; and the blind, the idiot, the lunatic, the bastard child and the vagrant would similarly be placed in an appropriate but separate establishment. With us, a common *malebolge* is provided for them all. ... It is at once shocking to every principle of reason and every feeling of humanity that all these varied forms of

[1] The Assistant Commissioners were told in their first instructions that 'the sick must have separate wards or rooms appropriate for them' (unpublished minute dated 4 November 1834, cited by S. and B. Webb, *English Local Government: English Poor Law History—The Last Hundred Years* (1929), p. 135 n.).

[2] See appended Bibliography, Section X, Relief of the Poor. For a detailed account of the problems discussed in this chapter see Ruth G. Hodgkinson, *The Origins of the National Health Service: The Medical Services of the New Poor Law, 1834–71*.

wretchedness should thus be crowded together into one common abode; that no attempt should be made by law . . . to provide appropriate places for the relief of each.[1]

There were, however, some exceptions to the general absence of discrimination in the treatment of the unfit. A few parochial boards provided separate wards where the sick and insane were tolerably well treated,[2] while others subscribed to the voluntary hospitals in order to secure admission for their infectious and surgical cases.

It took more than thirty years to convince the central authority that it had made a mistake in merging the sick in the general mixed workhouse. Meantime, the numbers in receipt of poor relief continued to increase, particularly in urban areas, where the pressure of population growth was aggravated by the influx from the country. This provoked the guardians to maintain even more rigorously the 'less eligibility' principle. They economized to the utmost and spent the minimum on medical and nursing services.

The post of workhouse medical officer was normally a part-time appointment. Sometimes one practitioner combined the duties of workhouse and district medical officer, as was the case in sixteen of the forty London unions. Only a few of the largest institutions employed resident medical officers. Four of these were in London. Emoluments varied considerably. By the middle 'sixties, they ranged from £50 p.a. in some rural areas to the exceptional rate of £950 p.a. at the St. Marylebone workhouse. Medical officers personally bore the cost of drugs out of their salaries and sometimes paid for an assistant or dispenser. The position of the workhouse medical officer was rendered even more untenable by the fact that he was subordinate in status to the lay workhouse master, who was usually of a lower social class.[3] Most of the nursing was done by elderly and illiterate pauper inmates of the 'Sairey Gamp' type. By 1866, some 21,000 sick and aged patients in the London workhouses were being attended by only 142 paid non-pauper nurses, very few of whom had received any hospital training.[4] Most of the provincial institutions suffered from similar deficiencies.

With the general improvement in economic conditions which had set in during the

---

[1] Cited by S. and B. Webb, *The Break-Up of the Poor Law*, p. 15.

[2] In the Sheffield and Eccleshall workhouses, separate wards were provided after 1834 for the sick and insane, with special accommodation for infectious cases and lunatics. (*The Sheffield Hospitals*, published by the Sheffield City Libraries, 1959.) In Chorlton, the guardians established a model infirmary in the early 1860s where the nursing was supervised by Anglican nuns. In London, not all the workhouses were mismanaged. At the Islington institution, the system worked reasonably well. (B. Abel-Smith, *A History of the Nursing Profession* (1960), p. 13.) At the vast City of London workhouse, 'a great deal appeared satisfactory' to one Poor Law Board President on a visit in 1866. 'The wards were, in my judgment, well ventilated,' he reported, 'and the imbeciles, especially, carefully tended.' (A. E. Gathorne-Hardy (ed.), *Gathorne-Hardy, First Earl of Cranbrook—a Memoir* (1910), pp. 192–3.)

[3] *Report of Dr. Edward Smith, MO to the PLB, on the Sufficiency of the existing Arrangements for the Care and Treatment of the Sick Poor in Forty-eight Provincial Workhouses in England and Wales* (BPP, 1867–68, vol. lx (H/C 4), Appendix, pp. 26, 40, 66 and 92; and *Report of Dr. Edward Smith . . . on the Metropolitan Workhouse Infirmaries and Sick Wards*, dated 19 June 1866 (BPP, 1866, vol. lxi (H/C 372) 171), Appendix, pp. 77–8 and pp. 65–6. See also B. Abel-Smith, *The Hospitals, 1800–1948*, chapter 4, passim.

[4] *Report of Dr. Edward Smith on Metropolitan Workhouse Infirmaries*, op cit., pp. 6, 24; and *Report of Dr. Edward Smith on Provincial Workhouses*, op. cit., p. 13.

late 1840s, more of the able-bodied poor found employment, and the proportion of the sick and aged in workhouses began to increase. In some cases, they were so numerous that they occupied the greater part of the institution.[1] By 1863, some 50,000 sick paupers throughout the country were receiving indoor relief, but no coherent policy had been formulated by the central authority concerning the care of these helpless dependants of the State. At times, the Poor Law Board positively discouraged progressive guardians from introducing medical improvements. In 1850, for instance, it forbade the Croydon board to employ additional nurses in its infirmary.

> . . . Three at least of the paid servants in this hospital must be discontinued [wrote the PLB]. In the greater number of country unions there is no paid nurse and in none, it is believed, more than one. In pronouncing upon this point, the Poor Law Board attach more weight to the results of experience than to the opinion of the medical officer of the Croydon Workhouse, though supported by that of three of his professional friends. If, for instance, the infirmary of the Wandsworth and Clapham union workhouse can be, as it is, perfectly well managed under one paid nurse, why should the medical officers say that five paid nurses are required in the much smaller infirmary of the Croydon workhouse?[2]

Although the Poor Law Board was fully entitled, in legal theory, to issue such dictatorial edicts to local boards, it was unable to enforce its will on reluctant guardians. The 1834 Act had endowed it with legal power but had provided it with no effective instrument of control. In the metropolis, the Act applied only in limited measure to a number of poor law authorities (incorporations) which had been established previously under special Local Acts.

The 'new' Poor Law had never lacked critics. Many of them had directed their attacks particularly to the general absence of suitable provision for the indigent sick. By the late 1850s, when the spate of protesting publications[3] had failed to arouse the central authority from its complacency, concerted action was organized. An effective rostrum was provided by the National Association for the Promotion of Social Science (NAPSS), which included on its Council some progressive members of the aristocracy. At its inaugural conference in 1857, a paper on pauperism was read by Miss Louisa Twining, daughter of an Anglican clergyman. She disclosed the unsatisfactory state of the Strand Workhouse and other poor law institutions, which she and her friends had visited during the previous

---

[1] In the City of London workhouse, Mr. Gathorne Hardy observed in 1866 that 'Almost all the sick are aged . . . and of really able-bodied there are hardly any.' A. E. Gathorne-Hardy, op. cit., p. 193.

[2] Letter from the PLB to the Croydon Board of Guardians, 11 February 1850, cited by Mr. Gathorne Hardy (*Hansard*, vol. clxxxv (third series), 1867, col. 158).

[3] These publications included: J. Yelloly, *Observations on the Arrangements connected with the Relief of the Sick Poor* (1837); F. J. Charles Lord, *Letter to . . . Charles Buller on the Position and Remuneration of the Poor Law Medical Staff* (1848); H. W. Rumsey, *Essays on State Medicine* (1856); H. Bence Jones, *Report on the Accommodation in St. Pancras Workhouse* (1856); S. J. Burt, *West London Union (Report on Complaints)* (1856); Edmund Lloyd, *The Requirements and Resources of the Sick Poor* (1858); *The Poor Laws unmasked, being a general exposition of our workhouse institutions*, by a late Relieving Officer (1859).

4

four years.[1] Her revelations led to the formation the following year of the Workhouse Visiting Society under the auspices of the NAPSS. The Visiting Society grew; well over one hundred of its members penetrated the workhouses of the metropolis and the provinces; and individual members published their impressions, with demands for the release of the sick from penal conditions appropriate to the able-bodied, work-shy pauper.[2]

The Health Section of the NAPSS became a centre where poor law medical officers voiced their own grievances[3] and pleaded the cause of their pauper patients. Dr. Richard Griffin, medical officer of the Weymouth union, in particular, read papers at sectional meetings, wrote letters to the medical journals, and founded a provincial Poor Law Medical Reform Association. The improvements he advocated included the establishment of pauper dispensaries, a parliamentary grant for the provision of medicine, and the appointment of medical men to the Poor Law inspectorate.[4]

The hostility and suspicion with which the public and guardians alike had regarded the central authority since its inception in 1834 reached a climax in the severe winter of 1860–61, when widespread unemployment and distress overtaxed the already crowded workhouses. The guardians received no directive from the Poor Law Board to aid them in their unprecedented difficulties. Instead, they were plagued, they alleged, by vexatious regulations which hampered their attempts to make effective arrangements for the relief of the destitute. The general impression prevailed that the poor law had broken down. Demands were made that the Poor Law Board should be shorn of its powers or discontinued altogether.

This led in 1861 to the appointment of a Select Committee of the House of Commons to study the question of poor relief throughout the country. Charles Pelham Villiers, Liberal President of the Poor Law Board since 1859, was appointed chairman.[5] In 1864, the Committee presented its final report.[6] Despite the evidence of such witnesses as Miss Twining and Dr. Griffin, it concluded that 'there are not sufficient grounds for materially interfering with the present system of medical relief... which appears to be administered with general advantage'.[7] The Committee did recommend, however, that 'cod liver oil, quinine and other expensive medicines' should be provided at the expense of the guardians and not, as previously, by the medical officers.[8] This, the only improvement in

---

[1] *Trans. of the NAPSS*, 1857, pp. 571–74.

[2] Louisa Twining, 'The objects and aims of the Workhouse Visiting Society', *Trans. of the NAPSS*, 1858, p. 666; 'Workhouse Inmates', ibid., 1860, I, 834; *The Sick in Workhouses and how they are treated* (1861); Frances Power Cobbe, 'Workhouse Sketches', *Macmillan's Magazine*, II (April 1861), p. 448; 'The Sick Poor in Workhouses', *Journal of the Workhouse Visiting Society*, p. 487 et seq.; *The Workhouse as Hospital* (1861).

[3] The predicament of poor law medical officers during this period is described by Ruth G. Hodgkinson in 'Poor Law Medical Officers in England, 1834–1871', *J. Hist. Med. All. Sci.*, vol. xi, 1956, pp. 299–338.

[4] Richard Griffin, *The Grievances of the Poor Law Medical Officers*, 1858.

[5] This appointment illustrates the changed place and function of a central government department in local affairs.

[6] *Final Report of the Select Committee on Poor Relief*, 1864: BPP, 1864, vol. ix (349) 187.

[7] Ibid., p. 51.   [8] Ibid.

3

regard to medical relief, resulted from the testimony of Dr. Joseph Rogers, the persistent and courageous medical officer of the Strand Union.[1] The Committee conceded that in many cases the union workhouses were 'insufficient for the purpose of the proper classification of the inmates', and voiced the opinion that 'wider powers should be given to the Central Board . . . to require the guardians to make adequate arrangements for such classification.[2]

In December 1864, a few months following the publication of this report, a pauper—an Irish navvy named Timothy Daly—died in the Holborn Workhouse. The inquest revealed that death had resulted from gross neglect. *The Times* printed the inquest proceedings in full and led the attack on the whole structure of poor law medical relief.[3] Some weeks later, in February 1865, another pauper, named Gibson, died in the St. Giles Workhouse in similar circumstances. Deplorable as these deaths were, they proved to be not in vain. For the poor law critics, they provided fresh ammunition. For Miss Florence Nightingale, in particular, they served to strengthen her plea for nursing reforms.

During the greater part of 1864, Miss Nightingale had been engaged in organizing the introduction of trained nurses into the Brownlow Hill Infirmary in Liverpool. In January 1864, William Rathbone, the Liverpool philanthropist, renewed his contact with her. Three years before, she had collaborated with him in establishing in Liverpool a training school for District Nurses. Now, concerned at the wretchedness of the twelve hundred sick paupers in the Liverpool workhouse, he had offered to recruit and finance a staff of trained nurses to attend them. To Miss Nightingale he appealed for help in organizing the scheme. A year of battling with the local authorities in Liverpool had convinced her of the impossibility of correcting workhouse abuses by piecemeal methods. An entirely new system of finance and administration was needed, and this would require fresh legislation.[4]

Immediately after Daly's death, Miss Nightingale wrote to Mr. Villiers at the Poor Law Board. She knew that there was nothing as effective as a death on a departmental doorstep to galvanize Whitehall into action. Emphasizing the overwhelming need for nursing reform in workhouse infirmaries, which the Daly case had so patently proved, she invited Mr. Villiers to visit her, ostensibly to describe the nursing experiment in Liverpool. He came away from his talk with Miss Nightingale in January 1865 convinced of the necessity for instituting a full-scale enquiry into the treatment of the sick poor. 'I was so much obliged to that poor man for dying', she wrote to a friend a month later.[5]

---

[1] The efforts of Dr. Joseph Rogers to improve conditions for the sick poor, including the founding of a Metropolitan Poor Law Medical Officers' Association in 1866, are described in *Joseph Rogers, MD, Reminiscences of a Workhouse Medical Officer*, edited by his brother, Professor J. E. Thorold Rogers (1889).

[2] *Report of the Select Committee on Poor Relief*, 1864, op. cit., pp. 47–48.

[3] *The Times*, 24, 28 and 29 December 1864.

[4] This and subsequent references to Florence Nightingale are drawn mainly from Mrs. Cecil Woodham-Smith's *Florence Nightingale, 1820–1910* (Constable, 1951; Penguin Books, 1955) and from private correspondence with Sir Harry Verney, grandson of Florence Nightingale's brother-in-law of the same name.

[5] Letter from Florence Nightingale to Sir John McNeil, dated 7 February 1865 (cited by Mrs. Woodham-Smith, op. cit., p. 348).

Early in February 1865, Mr. Villiers sent Mr. H. B. Farnall to see her. He was Poor Law Inspector for the Metropolitan District. The outcome of the interview was a draft 'Form of Enquiry' drawn up by Miss Nightingale and Mr. Farnall for use in an investigation of every workhouse infirmary and sick ward in London. Mr. Villiers approved and the questionnaires were sent out at the end of February. In the course of the next few weeks, Mr. Villiers directed that a circular should be sent to all metropolitan boards of guardians calling on them to appoint trained nurses and to discontinue the employment of untrained inmates for attending the sick.[1] As this was not in the nature of an Order, it had little immediate effect, but it served to suggest to an angry public and an impatient Miss Nightingale that an official awakening might be expected.

Other forces entered the lists for reform. In July 1865, at the instigation of Dr. Ernest Hart, a physician attached to the staff of the *Lancet*, its radical proprietor, Dr. James Wakley, appointed a special commission to investigate all the unions of the metropolis. Consisting of Drs. Hart, Anstie and Carr,[2] the commission visited and reported on every workhouse in the London area. Week after week in the *Lancet*, for the greater part of a year and a half, the detailed accounts appeared, with demands for poor law medical reform.[3] They revealed a bleak and ugly picture of insanitary conditions, inadequate nursing, defective appliances, insufficient ventilation and overcrowding. Concerning the sick wards, the Commission declared that 'these accidental excrescences of the workhouse are not, and never can be, either in government, arrangement or service, fully used as hospitals—nevertheless, they are great hospitals—*the* great hospitals of London.[4]

When the allegations of two former workhouse nurses were investigated the following year by Poor Law Board inspectors, the *Lancet* Commission's findings were substantiated in horrifying detail.[5] At its 1865 annual conference, the British Medical Association sup-

[1] PLB circular to the metropolitan boards of guardians, dated 5 May 1865 (BPP, 1966, vol. lxi (469), p. 457).

[2] Dr. Ernest Hart, DCL, was also on the staff of St. Mary's Hospital and later became editor of the BMJ; Dr. Anstie was on the staff of the Westminster Hospital; and Dr. Carr was a poor law medical officer in Blackheath.

[3] *Lancet*, 1865, I, pp. 71, 410, 547, 666; 1865, II, pp. 14, 71–72, 73, 131, 184, 240, 296, 355, 513, 575, 711; 1866, I, pp. 104, 178, 376, 639; 1866, II, pp. 45, 169, 214, 234, 242, 343, 361, 446.

[4] *Lancet*, 1866, II, p. 234.

[5] Charges made by Nurse Matilda Beeton concerning the Rotherhithe Workhouse Infirmary included: the absence of night nurses; 'many sick patients were dirty, their bodies crawling with vermin'; 'no waterproof sheets, no air cushions, no bed-rests, no night-stools and but one bed pan . . .'; sheets changed once in three weeks—'soiled sheets had to be washed in the infirmary at night'; 'a bad supply of towels used for every clean and dirty purpose'; beds of flock—'maggots would crawl from them by hundreds'; 'sick diet was a mockery—milk was not heard of'; 'patients were allowed to wear their own nightdresses if they could afford to pay for the washing of them and they often had to sell their nourishment to do this . . .' (Report by Mr. Farnall, PLB Inspector, of 5 July 1866, BPP, 1866, vol. lxi (H/C 518) 523, p. 21). This enquiry was conducted after two deputations to the PLB by the Workhouse Visiting Society. Similar allegations were made by Nurse Beeton of the Strand Union Workhouse (Report by Mr. R. B. Cane, PLB Inspector, of 4–6 June 1866, BPP, 1866, vol. lxi (H/C 362) 557) and by Nurse Jane Bateman concerning the Paddington Workhouse (Report by Mr. Farnall, BPP, 1866, vol. lxi (H/C 517) 495).

ported the initiative of the *Lancet* and followed with another committee of enquiry, which included Drs. Anstie and Griffin.[1]

In January 1866, Drs. Hart, Anstie and Rogers met to plan a means of mobilizing public support for their reform campaign. They convened an open meeting on 3 March 1866, with the Earl of Carnarvon in the chair. Supporters, rallied by the convenors, included eminent men of both political parties and such well-known figures as Charles Dickens and John Stuart Mill. 'The Association for the Improvement of the Infirmaries of London Workhouses' was formally established and the reforms at which it aimed were discussed. These had been outlined already by Dr. Hart in an article published in the *Fortnightly Review* in December 1865.[2] They included the provision of six Poor Law hospitals in London of one thousand beds each; the re-classification and re-housing of the workhouse population; and the grouping of all the metropolitan poor law districts into one hospital region which would collectively bear the cost of the sick poor. The meeting finally resolved that a deputation be sent to the President of the Poor Law Board to determine his willingness to introduce a suitable Bill. If he resisted, it was recommended that the Association should 'take independent means to bring forward an appropriate measure in Parliament during the present session'.[3] Dr. Hart elaborated the London reform scheme in a further article in the *Fortnightly Review*[4] and, as part of the campaign, published the collected *Lancet* reports in one volume.[5] Appended, was a brief statement over the names of seven leading medical men, including the President of the Royal College of Physicians, Sir Thomas Watson. Drafted by Hart and Anstie, who had solicited the signatures, this recapitulated the reforms already advocated, in particular, 'consolidated infirmaries', with trained nurses, resident medical officers, and medicines financed from the rates.[6]

Meantime, Miss Nightingale had been working on similar lines. She was intent on pressing for immediate legislation for the fundamental reorganization of workhouse administration. Dubious concerning Mr. Villiers' capacity to carry it through, she approached the Prime Minister, Lord Palmerston, family friend of her early days. He promised that, if she would draft a Bill, he would use his influence to get it through the Cabinet. She discussed her scheme with Dr. John Sutherland, old associate of the Crimean Sanitary Commission,[7] and began to work with Mr. Farnall. But before she was able to submit her plan to Lord Palmerston he become ill, and in October 1865 he died. This was a cruel blow. Up to now, her hopes had been rising, as replies to the questionnaires coming in from the workhouse authorities consistently revealed deficiencies which even the Poor Law Board could not ignore. 'So long,' she wrote, 'as a sick man, woman or child is

---

[1] *BMJ*, 1865, I, p. 601; 1865, II, pp. 158–59, 486–88.

[2] Ernest Hart, 'The Condition of our State Hospitals', *Fortnightly Review*, III (Dec. 1865), pp. 218–21.

[3] *The Times*, 5 March 1866, p. 7.

[4] Ernest Hart, 'Metropolitan Infirmaries for the Pauper Sick', *Fortnightly Review*, IV (April 1866), pp. 460–62.

[5] *Report of the Lancet Sanitary Commission for Investigating the State of the Infirmaries of Workhouses, 1866.*

[6] *BMJ*, 1867, I, p. 175.

[7] Sir Edward Cook, *The Life of Florence Nightingale* (1913), vol. II, pp. 133–34.

considered administratively to be a pauper, to be repressed and not a fellow creature to be nursed into health, so long will these shameful disclosures have to be made. The sick, infirm or mad pauper ceases to be a pauper when so afflicted.'[1] Miss Nightingale, utterly opposed to 'poor law-mindedness' in the treatment of the destitute sick, was determined that reorganization should be based on her personal philosophy that suffering was sufficient claim to raise the sick individual beyond the realm of normal values, moral judgments and social class.

She completed the draft of her recommendations and sent it to Mr. Villiers in December 1865. This 'A B C of Workhouse Reform'—as she called it—was based on three main principles: (A) the sick, insane, incurable and children should be dealt with separately in appropriate institutions; (B) the 'medical relief of London' should be under one central management; and (C) the system should be financed by 'consolidation and a general rate' and not out of parochial rates. 'The care and government of the *sick* poor is a thing totally different from the government of paupers', she emphasized. 'Once acknowledge this principle and you must have suitable establishments for the care of the sick and infirm.' On receiving her communication, Mr. Villiers agreed at once to press for a new London Poor Law Bill.[2]

Miss Nightingale's proposals were basically similar to those outlined by Dr. Hart in the article which had just appeared in the December issue of the *Fortnightly Review*. It is probable that she was in touch with Dr. Hart and his associates—possibly through Mr. Farnall. Nevertheless, it would seem that she had given them no hint of Mr. Villiers' promising attitude. From the wording of the March resolution of the Association for the Improvement of London Infirmaries and the weight of the deputation which it sent to Mr. Villiers in April 1866, it is obvious that opposition was anticipated. The petitioners included the Earls of Carnarvon and Shaftesbury, the Archbishop of York and Drs. Hart and Rogers. Mr. Villiers received them cordially, however, and promised that their proposals would be given 'favourable consideration'. In a letter of 2 May to Harriet Martineau, Florence Nightingale identified herself with the Association by describing how 'we' have been sending 'our Earls, Archbishops and MPs to storm him [Villiers] in his den'.[3]

Immediately following the April deputation from the Infirmaries Association, Mr. Villiers instituted an enquiry into the arrangements for the care of the sick in the metropolitan workhouses. For this task, he deputed his poor law Inspectors, Mr. Farnall and Dr. Edward Smith. The latter had been appointed the previous year and was the first physician to hold the office of Inspector.[4] Mr. Villiers' attempts to institute improvements,

---

[1] Woodham-Smith, op. cit., p. 351.   [2] Ibid., p. 352.

[3] Cook, op. cit., vol. I, p. 105.

[4] 'According to all that I heard in after years from Dr. Smith on the subject of his office', wrote Sir John Simon, 'the old secretarial belief as to the best way of dealing with matters of medical administration had vigorously survived the fact of his appointment as Medical Officer of the Board; and I understood that he, in relation to such matters, was not expected to advise in any general, or any initiative sense, but only to answer in particular cases on such particular points as might be referred to him.' (Sir J. Simon, *English Sanitary Institutions* (1890), p. 352.)

however, were short-lived. By the late spring of 1866, the Whig Government was tottering. Mr. Villiers was afraid to introduce so controversial a subject as workhouse infirmary reform. On 18 June 1866, the Government fell and with it the reformers' hopes of the new infirmary Bill.

Although ill during most of the summer, Miss Nightingale persevered with her scheme. She sent a copy of her 'A B C' to John Stuart Mill, who was then sitting on the Select Committee of the House of Commons on the Local Government of the Metropolis. At his suggestion, she sent another copy to Edwin Chadwick, the only surviving member of the 1832–34 Poor Law Commission. In so doing, she successfully resuscitated a powerful voice in the cause of the sick pauper. A few weeks later, *Fraser's Magazine* published an article by Edwin Chadwick on 'The Administration of Medical Relief to the Destitute Sick in the Metropolis'. If not a concerted effort, it had all the signs of being Nightingale-inspired. Chadwick confirmed that the current evils concerning medical relief in London were condemned at the time of the 1832–34 inquiry and had continued in contravention of the 1834 Act. 'The leading administrative principle made out by our enquiry as specially applicable to the metropolis', he wrote, 'was that of making the largest *aggregation* of cases practicable for the purpose . . . of *segregation*, or the most full and complete classification for distinct and appropriate treatment in separate houses. . . .' Chadwick, the one-time vigorous champion of central administration on the model of France, went on to emphasize 'the great advantages derived from the unity of local administration of Paris in having all the public hospitals under one direction with a central *bureau d'admission*', and urged its applicability to the administration of medical relief in the metropolis.[1]

Determined to recover the infirmary Bill, which twice had been so nearly within her grasp, Miss Nightingale watched her opportunity with the new Tory administration. In July 1866, Lord Derby appointed Mr. Gathorne Hardy to succeed Mr. Villiers at the Poor Law Board. Known as 'an admirable House of Commons man', Mr. Gathorne Hardy hitherto had held only one junior ministerial post. Recently, he had won a seat for Oxford University in an exciting election contest against Mr. Gladstone. In Lord Derby's judgment, Gathorne Hardy was 'one of the fittest men in Her Majesty's dominions to put things straight'.[2]

After only a few days in office, the new President of the Poor Law Board received a long and urgent letter from Miss Nightingale, enclosing her scheme of reform which she offered to expound personally. He suspected that, in the heat of her crusading fervour, she regarded God and Ministers of State alike as her private secretaries. An ambitious man, Gathorne Hardy intended to 'put things straight' in his own way. He had no wish to add the finishing touches to a project begun by his Liberal predecessor. His gracious reply to Miss Nightingale some three weeks later 'hastened' to assure her that he would bear in mind the offer she had made and in all probability avail himself of it to the full.[3] He never

---

[1] *Fraser's Magazine for Town and Country*, vol. lxxiv, no. ccccxli (September 1866), pp. 353–65.
[2] J. E. Thorold Rogers, op. cit., p. 57.
[3] Woodham-Smith, op. cit., p. 353.

did. Miss Nightingale was shut out of the Poor Law Board. A post in Yorkshire was found for Mr. Farnall.

The results of Miss Nightingale's labours, however, had been insinuated into the archives of the Board. The reports of Mr. Farnall and his medical colleague, Dr. Edward Smith, had been completed before Mr. Gathorne Hardy took office, but no action had been taken on them. When questioned in the House of Commons on his first appearance as President of the Poor Law Board, Mr Gathorne Hardy seemed confident that he could deal with the workhouse evils 'under the powers . . . now possessed by the Poor Law Board', which he believed to be 'sufficient in the main'.[1] He thereupon set about discovering the extent of these powers. From Mr. Farnall's report, he learned that his Board had 'no power to compel boards of guardians to build infirmaries for the sick poor, or to oblige guardians to elect and pay resident medical officers, or to enforce the paying for drugs out of the rates.' The report strongly urged that the Poor Law Board should acquire legal powers to enable it to order guardians to provide sufficient wards for the sick poor and to require these to be adequately staffed with resident officers and trained nurses, and supplied with drugs and medical appliances. 'Hospitals', the report insisted, 'should be built wholly apart from the metropolitan workhouses . . . and the cost of building and maintenance be defrayed by a common rating of the metropolis.'[2] For a number of years, Mr. Farnall's routine reports on the London workhouses had been such as to occasion no concern. It is, therefore, not unsafe to assume that Miss Nightingale was behind his expansive recommendations. Some of the more insistent and synoptical passages of his report displayed a curiously apt imitation of her style and embodied themes already elaborated in her *Notes on Hospitals*.[3]

Dr. Edward Smith's report pointed to the numerous causes of defective workhouse management, which by now had become familiar reading. In particular, he suggested that certain categories of inmates should be warded separately. These were: scarlet fever and smallpox cases; 'the noisy and dangerous lunatics who were admitted on occasion when the county asylums refused to receive them'; and the 'far too many children too young to be removed to the district schools'.[4]

These reports, based largely on subjective evaluation, suggested to Mr. Gathorne Hardy the need for quantitative data. Clearly, overcrowding was a basic cause of the evils to be eradicated; but what constituted overcrowding, he wished to know; and if, as was obvious, some classes of the sick had to be removed, how much accommodation would they require, and what space should be allowed for the inmates who remained? On these matters the reports were conflicting and confusing. Mr. Gathorne Hardy decided to make a fresh start and appointed two new Inspectors to the metropolitan area, Dr. W. O.

[1] *Hansard*, 1866, vol. clxxxiv, 17 July, col. 939.

[2] *Report of Mr. H. B. Farnall, Poor Law Inspector, on the Infirmary Wards of the several Metropolitan Workhouses . . .*' 12 June 1866, BPP, 1866, vol. lxi (H/C 387) 389, p. 8.

[3] Florence Nightingale, *Notes on Hospitals*, 1863.

[4] *Report of Dr. Edward Smith . . . on the Metropolitan Infirmaries and Sick Wards*, 19 June 1866, BPP, 1866, vol. lxi (H/C 327) 171, pp. 35–37.

Markham, formerly editor of the *British Medical Journal* and a sympathetic advocate of poor law medical reform, and Mr. Uvedale Corbett, 'an inspector of much experience'. In September 1866, the President instructed them to visit the London workhouses with a view to procuring information which might assist him in drafting new legislation for the reform of workhouse infirmaries. Their report, which included statistical studies of the diseases and accommodation of the non-able-bodied, strongly urged the establishment of separate hospitals for the sick who would be removed from the workhouse, and dispensaries for the outdoor poor.[1]

The system of out-patient clinics, or dispensaries, where the poor were attended by qualified medical practitioners, was already in operation in Paris and Ireland.[2] To Ireland, then, Gathorne Hardy sent John Lambert,[3] a senior civil servant at the Poor Law Board, with instructions to report on how the system worked.

As for the new hospitals which his advisers and the leading reformers had advocated, Gathorne Hardy was not yet fully convinced of their need. He consulted the President of the Royal College of Physicians, Sir Thomas Watson, who immediately convened a committee of eminent medical and sanitary experts[4] to examine the London workhouses and their provision for the sick. Early in February 1867, the Watson Committee presented an extensive report,[5] which included recommendations on the construction of infirmary wards, ventilation and the amount of space for different classes of inmate. One of the report's numerous appendices was a lengthy contribution on nursing, which Florence Nightingale had persuaded the committee to include. In this, she restated her case for the complete reform of workhouse administration.[6] Undeterred by his apparent indifference to her suggestions, she sent a copy urgently to Gathorne Hardy and followed this by numerous letters. He refrained from giving her any hint of his intentions.

The Watson Committee, like Gathorne Hardy's other advisers, urged that the workhouse sick should be provided with separate accommodation and special care; and, in particular, that those suffering from infectious fevers and smallpox, and the insane, should be removed from the workhouses and treated in specially erected hospitals.

At this time, isolation accommodation in the metropolis was limited to 182 beds in the London Fever Hospital in Islington (opened in 1802) and about one hundred beds in the

---

[1] *Report of W. O. Markham and U. Corbett to the President of the PLB on the Metropolitan Workhouses*, 18 January 1867, BPP, 1867, vol. lx (H/C 18), 119.

[2] *Hansard*, 1867, vol. clxxxv (third series), col. 166.

[3] John Lambert had been on the staff of the PLB since 1856. Among other special assignments, he had assisted the former President, C. P. Villiers, with measures for the relief of distress caused by the Lancashire cotton famine in 1863.

[4] In addition to Sir Thomas Watson, the committee included: Dr. Henry W. Acland, FRS; Dr. Francis Sibson, FRS; Mr. T. Holmes, FRCS; and Captain Douglas Galton.

[5] *Report of the Committee appointed to consider the cubic space of Metropolitan Workhouses* (the Watson Committee), 7 February 1867, BPP, 1867, vol. lx (H/C 185), 3786.

[6] Ibid., Appendix XVI: Florence Nightingale, 'Suggestions on the subject of providing, training and organizing Nurses for the Sick Poor in Workhouse Infirmaries', section III on the 'Relation of Hospital Management to Efficient Nursing'.

Smallpox Hospital in Highgate (founded in 1746). These two establishments were supported mainly by voluntary contributions and intended primarily for paying patients but when beds were available, poor law patients were sometimes admitted.[1] The guardians, like the general hospitals, were becoming increasingly reluctant to admit infectious cases to their institutions. Of London's twelve leading voluntary hospitals—providing some 3,300 beds[2]—none treated smallpox; and, while eight claimed to admit fever patients, they actually received very few.[3] These were scattered among non-infectious cases in the general wards,[4] for, although the germ-theory was already well founded, it was not yet fully understood.

For the mentally disordered, London was served by a number of institutions with varying standards of care. Some 300 charitable beds were provided by the Bethlehem Royal Hospital (Bethlem), of monastic origin, and a similar number by St. Luke's, founded by voluntary subscription in 1751. Guy's Hospital also admitted the mentally afflicted into its 'lunatic ward'. Of the thirty-nine privately owned licensed houses functioning in the London area at this time, three (each with over 400 beds) entered into contracts with the parochial authorities for the reception of poor law patients. Hanwell (now St. Bernard's Hospital) and Colney Hatch (now Friern Hospital)—the 2,000-bed county 'lunatic asylums' of Middlesex—were also available to the metropolitan community. These public asylums had not escaped the censure which the lunacy authority at this period levelled at a number of private, charitable and other mental institutions. Although private patients were subsequently admitted to the county asylums by arrangement with the visiting committees, they were intended originally for destitute persons who were severely disturbed, dangerous, or suffering from the more curable mental disorders—'pauper lunatics', as they were called. Congenital mental defectives—idiots and imbeciles—and other harmless 'incurables' were, therefore, not strictly eligible for admission. Consequently, the vast majority of this preponderant section of the mentally disordered became the responsibility of the poor law authorities. Some were given relief in their own

[1] The fee at the London Fever Hospital was two guineas, and admission was usually by a subscriber's or a governor's letter. For pauper patients, the charge was 1/– a day, but there was always uncertainty concerning their admission.

[2] See Table 1 at end of chapter for details concerning the voluntary hospitals of London at this time. In addition to the general hospitals, thirty special institutions provided the capital with 3,000 beds limited to particular classes of patients and specific diseases.

[3] During the middle 1860s, infectious fever cases represented about 4 per cent of the total admissions at St. Bartholomew's Hospital and about 2 per cent at Guy's Hospital. Other general hospitals in London received an even smaller proportion of infectious cases (see Report of the Watson Committee of 7 February 1867, op. cit., Appendix XIII on the 'Character of Diseases in Infirmaries and Hospitals', by Dr. Francis Sibson). Sir John Simon, Medical Officer of the Privy Council, was particularly censorious of this discrimination against infectious patients. (Sixth Report of the MO to the Privy Council, 1863, pp. 73–74). In the Scottish hospitals, every disease was admitted and the system of separate wards or blocks for fever and smallpox was universal. Many Scottish hospitals admitted a very large proportion of fever cases. (Bristowe-Holmes *Report on United Kingdom Hospitals*, appended to the Sixth Report of the MO to the Privy Council, op. cit., p. 470, et seq.).

[4] Bristowe-Holmes *Report on United Kingdom Hospitals*, op. cit., p. 473.

homes or were boarded out, but many were kept in the union workhouses.[1] The distribution of mental cases between the asylums and the workhouses was, however, largely haphazard. As the poor law institutions were neither equipped nor staffed for the care of the mentally ill and subnormal, the 'harmless chronics' existed for the most part in wretched conditions, often deprived of adequate facilities, food and medical care.[2] Furthermore, they aggravated the pressing problem of overcrowding.

Following Daly's death in the Holborn workhouse, demands for poor law medical reform had become increasingly focused on London, and most of the investigations—both independent and official—had been centred on the metropolitan institutions.[3] Miss Nightingale and Dr. Hart had formulated their schemes for immediate application to London. It was obvious that sweeping reforms could not be absorbed at once throughout the country. If first established in the capital, it was confidently anticipated that improvements would spread, sooner or later, to the provinces. Legislation for the metropolis was, therefore, the reformers' immediate goal.

The reform movement had been motivated partly by humanitarian concern for the helpless poor, partly by the professional self-interest of poor law medical officers, and partly by Miss Nightingale's crusade for improved workhouse nursing. These forces, however, were inevitably allied to the ever-present menace of disease and death in Victorian London. The ultimate arbiter of State intervention was fear lest the infectious destitute sick in crowded workhouses and insanitary dwellings should suscitate the uncontrolled dissemination of disease, with its toll of human life and economic dislocation.

Progenitor of State medicine in the past, fear of pestilence[4] was now moving the Government towards a new area of social responsibility. Early in 1867, Gathorne Hardy and his assistant, John Lambert, embarked on the draft of a new poor law Bill. It was clear that a break with the past was essential; that the Poor Law Board must acknowledge and define its responsibilities towards the destitute sick; that the principle of 'less eligibility' must be revised; and that the central authority must acquire fresh powers for implementing a new policy. On 6 February 1867, in the Speech from the Throne, the Government announced its intention of introducing a measure 'for improving the management of sick and other poor in the metropolis'.[5]

[1] Table 2 at the end of this chapter shows the size and classification of London's workhouse population in the mid-1860s.

[2] A comprehensive account of the problems of lunacy and pauperism at this period is given by Ruth G. Hodgkinson in her article 'Provision for Pauper Lunatics, 1834–71', *Medical History*, vol. x, no. 2, April 1966. Provision for the subnormal is discussed further in Chapters 4 and 14 following.

[3] Official investigations were subsequently extended to a number of provincial workhouses. (Report of Dr. Edward Smith on the *Sufficiency of the existing Arrangements for the Care and Treatment of the Sick in Forty-eight Provincial Workhouses in England and Wales*, 1867–68, op. cit.)

[4] Fear of disease had led, for example, to the Quarantine Acts, which dated from the Great Plague; the first consultative Board of Health, appointed under the presidency of Sir Henry Halford in 1831; its successor, the General Board of Health, in 1832, and the 'cholera legislation' of 1832; the first Vaccination Act of 1840; the first Public Health Act of 1848; and the Diseases Prevention Act of 1855.

[5] *Hansard*, vol. clxxxv (1867), col. 7.

TABLE 1

London Voluntary Hospitals, 1863

Bed Complement, Annual Admissions and Case Fatality Rates

Hospital	No. of beds	Patients per annum	Death Rates per cent
(i) General			
F St. Bartholomew's[1] (founded 1123)	632	5,389	11·2
Charing Cross[4]	118	950	7·8
F St. George's[3]	345	3,713	8·8
F Guy's[1,3]	574	4,888	9·6
F King's College[4]	147	1,332	10·7
London[3]	457	4,164	7·6
F St. Mary's[4]	155	1,715	10·2
F Middlesex[3]	293	2,278	11·6
F St. Thomas'[1,2] (founded 1200)	207	1,846	10·3
University College[4]	115	Not known	12·1
F Westminster[3]	191	1,828	10·4
Royal Free[4]	84	1,254	7·2
(ii) Special Infectious			
F London Fever Hospital (founded 1802)	182	2,656	17·7
F Smallpox Hospital (founded 1746)	100	Not known	19·9

Notes:

[1] The three endowed hospitals of London.

[2] St. Thomas' had been recently dispossessed of the site on which, for more than six centuries, it had stood at the south end of London Bridge. Before its removal it made up to 520 beds.

[3] These five hospitals were founded during the first half of the eighteenth century.

[4] These five hospitals were founded between 1818 and 1856.

'F' indicates the hospitals which admitted fever cases.

Source: J. S. Bristowe and T. Holmes: 'Report on the Hospitals of the United Kingdom', *Sixth Report of the Medical Officer to the Privy Council*, 1863, Appendix 15, pp. 569–70.

TABLE 2

Population of London's Forty-three Workhouses at the end of 1866

Able-bodied		Temporarily Disabled		Old and Infirm		Children	
Men	868	Men	3,014	Men	6,068	Aged 2–16	2,150
Women	2,031	Women	4,032	Women	7,617	Infants (under 2 years)	1,015
Total	2,899	Total	7,046[1]	Total	13,685[2]	Total	3,165[3]

Total Population of all 43 Metropolitan Workhouses: 26,795
(estimated population of London, mid-1866: 3,040,761)

Notes:

[1] Of the 'temporarily disabled', those suffering from infectious fevers numbered 212 at a census in February and 328 in August 1866.

[2] Of the 'old and infirm', 1,977 were classed as 'insane' at the end of 1866.

[3] Of the children, 51 were classed as 'insane' at the end of 1866.

In addition, 6,800 metropolitan paupers were accommodated in county lunatic asylums and licensed houses.

Source: Report of W. O. Markham and U. Corbett (Inspectors of the PLB) on the Metropolitan Workhouses, 18 January 1867 (BPP, 1867, vol. lx (H/C 18) 119).

CHAPTER 2

'Gathorne Hardy's Act' and the Birth of the Metropolitan Asylums Board

ON 8 February 1867, Mr. Gathorne Hardy introduced his Metropolitan Poor Bill.[1] In broad terms, its purpose was to extend the 1834 Poor Law Amendment Act, so far as the metropolis was concerned, by providing for the separate management of certain categories of the non-able-bodied poor, for whom the deterrent principle was inappropriate. A system of medical care was to be inaugurated by the creation of hospitals and dispensaries; and for this purpose the unit of administration and finance was to be extended beyond the existing parishes and unions. In order to implement its new policy, the Poor Law Board asked for wider and more specific powers of control.

This proposed legislation amounted to an explicit acknowledgment of the State's responsibility for the destitute sick as a class, entirely separate from the able-bodied poor; and, as such, it introduced a fundamental variant of traditional poor law practice. For Gathorne Hardy, head of an impermanent ministry and member of a party without a straight majority, this was not an easy measure to steer through the House of Commons. While his own right wing might curb advances it considered revolutionary, the radical opposition would insist that he was insufficiently progressive. The Bill was skilfully drafted for Gathorne Hardy's immediate purposes, even though later developments were to disclose technical flaws concerning its implementation.[2] It provided a flexible framework in which a smaller or larger number of projects could be initiated, on a lesser or greater scale, with varying degrees of local participation and central control.

Gathorne Hardy began his introductory speech with a dispassionate account of the evils which the measure was designed to eradicate. He reported the unpalatable facts with disarming frankness, and submitted his solution with impressive sincerity and confidence. Sedulously, he abstained from attributing blame. 'The office of a guardian is one of great difficulty and delicacy', he observed, speaking with first-hand experience as an *ex officio* member of a Kentish board of guardians. It was expedient for Gathorne Hardy to respect the sensitivity of the parochial mind on the subject of local self-government. It was also

---

[1] For a summary of the 1867 Metropolitan Poor Act (30 & 31 Vict. c. 6), see Appendix I, Document II. The Bill reached the Statute Book almost unchanged.

[2] See Chapter 6.

necessary to win the confidence of the radical opposition, particularly that of his predecessor in office, Mr. C. P. Villiers. 'Formerly, medical men and the Poor Law Board itself believed that there was much less necessity for greater space, paid nurses and other appliances than is now thought requisite', Gathorne Hardy asserted. 'We can only act up to the lights we have'. He could not refrain, however, from expressing surprise that, as recently as 1864, the House of Commons Committee on Poor Relief had recorded its satisfaction with the medical treatment of the poor generally. Nevertheless, he applauded the Chairman of that Committee (Mr. Villiers) for recommending that the authority of the Poor Law Board should be confirmed and strengthened, and, in particular, that more powers should be given for the purpose of effecting a better classification in workhouses.[1]

Gathorne Hardy's measure provided for such additional powers and for a new basis of classification. With dramatic emphasis, he defined his new policy and the use to be made of the authority for which he asked:

> There is one thing [he declared] which we must peremptorily insist on—namely, the treatment of the sick in the infirmaries being conducted on an entirely separate system; because the evils complained of have mainly arisen from the workhouse management, which must to a great degree be of a deterrent character, having been applied to the sick, who are not proper objects of such a system. That is one thing which I should insist upon as an absolute condition. I propose, therefore, that power shall be given to combine such districts as the Poor Law Board may think proper—whether parishes and parishes, unions and unions, or unions and parishes—under a more complete system of inspection and control.[2]

His main object, he continued, was to classify the inmates of workhouses, as the Poor Law Inquiry Commissioners had apparently intended when they reported in 1834 that the Central Board

> ... should be empowered to cause any number of parishes to be incorporated for the purpose of workhouse management, and for providing new workhouses where necessary and to assign to those workhouses separate classes of the poor. ... Each class might thus receive appropriate treatment; the old might enjoy their indulgences without torment from the boisterous, the children be educated, and the able-bodied subjected to such courses of labour as will repel the indolent and vicious.[3]

'In carrying out their intention', Gathorne Hardy went on, 'they seem to have come to a different conclusion, for, so far as I can see, no step was taken in this direction.'[4]

The aged, the sick and the infirm, he explained, had become the main occupants of workhouses since the time when they were originally designed for the purpose of deterring the able-bodied. Of nearly 27,000 inmates in the London institutions, less than 900 men and about 2,000 women were classed as able-bodied. Except for some 3,000 children, the

---

[1] *Hansard*, 1867, vol. clxxxv (third series), 8 February, cols. 151–58.
[2] Ibid., col. 163.   [3] Ibid., col. 160.   [4] Ibid.

remainder—about 21,000—were all sick, old or disabled. Of these, about 2,000 were classed as imbeciles or lunatics.[1] Gathorne Hardy proposed to legislate in accordance with the recommendations of his expert advisers, who had urged the necessity for greater space in the workhouses. In order to obtain this, he proposed, first, to remove the lunatics and imbeciles and to place them in new, separate establishments. This category would comprise the inoffensive cases who required 'none of the restraints nor the luxuries and advantages which were available for the other and more dangerous class in county asylums'.[2] Secondly, he would provide separate accommodation for seven to eight hundred needy persons suffering from 'fever' and smallpox. Prophetically, Gathorne Hardy expressed the hope that

> the time will come when by proper attention to the use of those remedies which science has discovered—vaccination on the one hand, and good sanitary arrangements on the other—we may be able to dispense with these hospitals almost entirely. We cannot, however, do so at present [he continued] and it is a most material thing for the people themselves, and for others in the workhouse, that, to avoid risk of spreading the disease, they should be removed.[3]

Hitherto, some of these cases had been treated in the charity-supported institutions of London, but, Gathorne Hardy urged, it was a matter of real necessity to build some entirely under poor law management. In the proposed new hospitals, he hoped to ensure resident medical officers, independent matrons and paid nurses, as well as to provide for medical instruction.[4]

Further, as 'half the pauperism of the country originated in sickness', it was proposed to erect dispensaries in different parts of the metropolis in order to prevent so many people coming into the hospitals. District medical officers would attend the outdoor poor at specified hours and would be obliged to keep written records of the drugs dispensed. This requirement was aimed to remedy the loose system of prescribing which was known to exist in the poor law medical service.[5] Gathorne Hardy explained that, although this might be considered a cumbersome procedure, it was carried out effectively in Paris and in Ireland. The dispensary system would help to prevent the spread of disease by providing early treatment.

It was estimated that the new schemes would cost about £60,000 a year to operate, a sum which could be met by a metropolitan poor rate of one penny in the pound. Capital costs would be in the region of £400,000. This would include £100,000 for institutions for the insane; £50,000 to £70,000 for isolation hospitals; a similar sum for additional

---

[1] See Chapter 1, Table 2. [2] *Hansard*, op. cit., col. 776.
[3] Ibid., col. 162. [4] Ibid., cols. 164–65.
[5] Mr. Gathorne Hardy cited instances where poor law patients sent a relative, sometimes a child, to the district medical officer. Medicine was dispensed on the basis of the second-hand description of the symptoms, sometimes with fatal results. He also referred to the practice in some workhouses of providing what was called 'house medicine', which was dispensed by pauper nurses to whoever applied for it (*Hansard*, op. cit., col. 166).

school buildings; and £120,000 for other sick paupers. These estimates were based on a rate of £50 per head for children and lunatics and £60 per head for the acute sick. An additional metropolitan rate of two-thirds of a penny in the pound would cover loan charges for the capital outlay.[1]

As the author of the Bill unfolded his plans, the additional degree of central control involved in each innovation appeared reasonable and not unduly excessive. The total effect, nevertheless, represented an appreciable diminution in parochial autonomy. The Poor Law Board was to be empowered to combine existing parishes and unions into 'Asylum Districts'.[2] The institutions for these new areas would be administered by boards of management composed partly of elected guardians and partly of Poor Law Board nominees, but the number of appointed members would not exceed one-third the number of guardians.[3] The object, Gathorne Hardy explained, was 'to make some persons responsible who might be volunteers and who would be removed if they did not discharge the duty which they had undertaken'. It was not intended that they should 'come into collision with the elected members'.[4] In effect, the inclusion of nominated members would be little different from the presence of Justices of the Peace[5] as *ex officio* guardians on existing boards, Gathorne Hardy explained, as he sought to allay fears of central interference in the local management of the projected hospitals.

Further, the Poor Law Board was to have authority to make similar appointments to any board of guardians or any district school board, should it be deemed necessary.[6] 'As a less expensive and more speedy remedy than a mandamus', the Poor Law Board would also be empowered to recruit nurses and other officers, if local boards neglected to make the requisite appointments.[7] Such action would only be taken in the case of those authorities who were 'continually considering, putting off, hoping that something would turn up to save them the necessity of complying'.[8]

Next, Gathorne Hardy intended to abolish Local Acts. Hitherto, the majority of the large parishes in the metropolis had been able to defy the central authority because they were administered under Local Acts by independent governing bodies, which were responsible for the management of the poor, in addition to a variety of other functions.[9] One such parish was that of St. Giles, Bloomsbury, where the pauper, Gibson, had died from neglect. These Local Acts had been among the greatest impediments with which the Poor

---

[1] *Hansard*, op. cit., col. 173.   [2] 30 & 31 Vict. c. 6 s. 6.

[3] Ibid., ss. 8–11. Nominees of the PLB were originally to be chosen from citizens rated at not less than £100 p.a., but Mr. Gathorne Hardy made it clear that he would be more than gratified if this figure were deleted and the choice were left to the PLB. In the Act, as passed, the qualification was reduced to £40 p.a., the same as for elected guardians (30 & 31 Vict. c. 6 s. 11).

[4] *Hansard*, op. cit., cols. 162, 777 and 778.

[5] Before 1834, local administration of the poor law in the counties had been in the hands of the Justices of the Peace. There was then little, if any, control by a central administrative authority. Since the 1834 Act, Justices of the Peace had been *ex officio* members of all boards of guardians.

[6] 30 & 31 Vict. c. 6 ss. 49 & 79.

[7] Ibid., s. 80.   [8] *Hansard*, op. cit., col. 773.

[9] *Encyclopaedia Britannica* (9th edn.) vol. xix (1885), p. 472.

Law Board had had to contend. 'Everything went wrong in consequence of this double government', Gathorne Hardy explained. 'I am willing to be responsible for the condition of the workhouses', he declared emphatically, 'if I have—and only if I have—power to enforce obedience to any orders I may issue.'[1] With the Local Acts out of the way, the whole of the metropolis would be under the administrative control of the Poor Law Board,[2] as intended by the 1834 Act. The Board was, therefore, asking for authority to direct that any London workhouse should be used as an asylum for the sick[3] or for any other class of the poor.[4] By this means, it would be possible to extend the scheme of classification begun by the separation of the infectious and the insane. Thus, the central authority was to be empowered to intervene in the administration and management of every area of relief in the metropolis, either immediately or when deemed necessary. When the reactionary element in the House expressed concern at the apparent undermining of local responsibility, Gathorne Hardy calmed their fears of bureaucratic domination by declaring that 'there was nothing in the Bill to abolish self-government: indeed under its provisions, local government would have the fullest scope for its exertions.'[5]

The President of the Poor Law Board then outlined the financial concessions which he proposed to offer. The burden of poor relief was to be more evenly distributed among the parishes and unions of London by the creation of a Common Poor Fund. Each locality would be obliged to contribute on a proportional basis, and each would be eligible to claim repayment for certain items of relief expenditure. These would include the cost of drugs, and the salaries of all officers, both medical and lay, employed by boards of guardians, managers of poor law schools, the new asylum boards and dispensary committees. The fund would also bear the cost of maintaining infectious and insane patients in the new hospitals.[6] Gathorne Hardy said little concerning the operation of the fund and nothing about its possible use as an instrument of coercion. The Bill, however, made it plain that it was to be under the control of the Poor Law Board, which would appoint a Receiver to administer it, and assess, on the basis of rateable value, each locality's contribution to the revenue of the fund. Claims were also to be subject to Poor Law Board orders.[7] The threat of central authority intervention in cases of non-compliance could be inferred from references to compensation payable from the fund to poor law officers whose contracts might be varied through the operation of the Act.[8]

The principle of collective responsibility for the support of the needy had been applied in the past within relatively limited areas. As early as the mid-sixteenth century, statutory collections had been made from the inhabitants of the more affluent neighbourhoods of

---

[1] *Hansard*, op. cit., cols. 774–75.

[2] 30 & 31 Vict. c. 6 ss. 73–78.

[3] Ibid., s. 18.   [4] Ibid., s. 50.

[5] *Hansard*, op. cit., col. 1864.

[6] Ibid., cols. 168–72 and 775. For details of the Metropolitan Common Poor Fund, see Appendix IV.

[7] 30 & 31 Vict. c. 6 ss. 60–72. To the office of Receiver of the Fund, the PLB appointed John Lambert, who had assisted Gathorne Hardy in drafting the 1867 Bill. His emoluments for the office were £400 p.a.

[8] 30 & 31 Vict. c. 6 ss. 59 and 69 (5).

cities and corporate towns for the purpose of relieving destitution in the poorer districts.[1] During the nineteenth century, the unit of relief was extended beyond the parish of Elizabethan legislation. The Poor Law Amendment Act of 1834 empowered parishes to combine into unions for the provision of workhouses; the Poor Law Amendment Act of 1844 permitted poor law localities in London and other large towns to combine into districts for the relief of the itinerant poor, and for the care of destitute children; while, under Mr. Villiers' Metropolitan Houseless Poor Act of 1864, all London parishes and unions were obliged to contribute to a common fund for the upkeep of casual wards for vagrants.[2] This system was to be extended for the purpose of financing Mr. Gathorne Hardy's medical reforms. Both Dr. Hart of the *Lancet* Commission and Miss Nightingale had advocated a general poor rate for maintaining the destitute sick of the metropolis.[3] This had been one of the salient features of the scheme which she had submitted to Gathorne Hardy and which he had declined to discuss with her.

The author of the Bill might escape Miss Nightingale in person, but her 'A B C' pursued him into the House. She campaigned furiously between the first and second readings of the Bill, particularly for the inclusion of provisions which would ensure improved nursing for the poor. In the course of an eloquent, if defensive, speech, Charles Villiers recited Miss Nightingale's hospital creed, and emphasized, in particular, the need 'for properly trained nurses to attend upon the sick', since this was 'almost more important than the attendance of doctors or the administration of medicine'.[4] He urged that the proposed hospitals should be superintended 'by persons whose education and interests qualified them for the post', since experience had shown 'the inappropriateness of the guardians superintending establishments for the sick'. Public hostility, he explained, had hitherto made it impossible for the Poor Law Board to obtain the necessary powers to act. Only now, when events had shown that the paupers required central protection from their local oppressors, was the moment opportune for such powers to be sought.[5]

---

[1] In 1555, it was decreed (2 & 3 P & M c. 5) that in cities and corporate towns not co-terminous with a single parish, the mayors and other head officers were to 'consider the estate and ability of every parish', and if they found that the parishioners of any one parish were 'of such wealth and haviour that they have no poverty amongst them, or be able sufficiently to relieve the poverty of the parish where they inhabit and dwell and also to help and succour poverty elsewhere further', they might then 'with the assent of two of the most honest and substantial inhabitants of every such wealthy parish' consider the needs of all the inhabitants of the town and 'move, induce or persuade the parishioners of the wealthy parish charitably to contribute somewhat according to their ability towards the weekly relief of the poor in the other parishes. When provision for the poor in this semi-voluntary manner proved inadequate, compulsion by magistrates was introduced by an Act of 1563 (5 Eliz. c. 3). Edwin Cannan, *The History of Local Rates in England in Relation to the Proper Distribution of the Burden of Taxation* (1927), p. 61.

[2] Under the Metropolitan Houseless Poor Act of 1864 (27 & 28 Vict. c. 116) the metropolitan unions contributed uniformly at the rate of one-eighth of a penny in the pound. The fund was administered by the Metropolitan Board of Works.

[3] Ernest Hart, 'The Condition of our State Hospitals', *Fortnightly Review*, iii (Dec. 1865), pp. 218–20; and Miss Nightingale's 'ABC' of Workhouse Reform, submitted to the President of the Poor Law Board (Mr. C. P. Villiers) in December 1865.

[4] *Hansard*, op. cit., Appendix, p. 4.   [5] Ibid., p. 6.

It had been anticipated that Villiers would display considerable hostility towards Gathorne Hardy and his Bill. During the latter's early days at the Poor Law Board, he had made his predecessor 'frantically angry' by asserting in the House of Commons that fresh poor law legislation was quite unnecessary, provided the existing Acts were properly understood and applied. Villiers had confided to Florence Nightingale that 'he was not going to sit down under this kind of thing' and that 'something more was needed to solve the poor law administration problem than a touch of Gathorne Hardy's magic wand'.[1] When the Bill was introduced, he had described it privately as 'a seven months child born in the Whitehall Workhouse'. (Gathorne Hardy had been at the Poor Law Board seven months, while Villiers had served there for as many years.)[2] But, so skilful and conciliatory was Gathorne Hardy's presentation of the Bill that Villiers declared his full support for the new policy, and criticized it only on the ground that it did not go far enough. 'The charge for the poor is as much a national charge as the interest on the National Debt', he declared, 'and it is only fair, when we can safely do so, to place it on the whole property of the country.'[3]

Miss Nightingale had mobilized another willing mouthpiece in the House, her devoted brother-in-law, Sir Harry Verney, Liberal Member for Buckinghamshire.[4] He advocated '*one* board for the uniform management of the sick poor of London . . . just as the general drainage of London was placed under the Metropolitan Board of Works.' His object was 'the cure of *all* the sick poor of the metropolis' who, he urged, 'should be placed under the care of trained nurses in a sufficient number of duly regulated hospitals'. The proposed Common Fund should be applied, he suggested, not only to the maintenance of the hospitals, but also to the cost of instructing the nurses.[5] One of the few amendments made to the Bill in committee was Miss Nightingale's recommendation, as presented by Sir Harry Verney, that the new hospitals should be used for the training of nurses as well as for medical instruction.[6]

To his radical critics, Gathorne Hardy explained that, as it was not possible in principle to distinguish between the outdoor sick and the indoor sick, he had thought it advisable to take only those classes of disease which could clearly be separated from the rest and which affected the health of the whole metropolis—fever and smallpox. 'These are not things, the relief of which can be traded in', he explained. 'Nobody will go into a smallpox or fever hospital who has not one of those diseases. Patients such as these endanger the health of the whole population. . . .'[7] As for the lunatics, it could not be contended that they belonged more to one part of the metropolis than to another. 'It is one of those items which cannot be jobbed: you cannot make lunatics for the purpose.'[8] To justify further the limitation of his scheme to certain classes of the sick, Gathorne Hardy explained that a sufficient

---

[1] C. Woodham-Smith, op. cit., p. 354.   [2] Ibid., p. 355.

[3] *Hansard*, op. cit., Appendix, p. 5.

[4] Sir Harry Verney, having failed to induce Florence Nightingale to become the second Lady Verney, married her elder sister, Parthenope Nightingale.

[5] *Hansard*, op. cit., col. 753.   [6] 30 & 31 Vict. c. 6 s. 29.

[7] *Hansard*, op. cit., cols. 171 and 775.   [8] Ibid., col. 170.

number of new hospitals for *all* the sick poor of London would be extremely costly and render useless existing workhouses. Moreover, the vast institutions required would be susceptible to 'hospital diseases'. 'In the smaller establishments, with all their defects, gangrene, erysipelas and puerperal fever did not intrude.'[1] In this way, Gathorne Hardy sought to suggest that immediate reforms of a more revolutionary nature were inadvisable. His real and concealed reasons were, doubtless, associated with the vast number of the sick poor in the London institutions, relative to the number of the able-bodied.[2] To remove 21,000 sick and infirm from the workhouses and place them in hospitals would leave the guardians with only about 11 per cent of their total indoor pauper population. If the 3,000 children were also removed, as Gathorne Hardy contemplated, and the thirty-nine boards of guardians were left with only 3,000 able-bodied inmates scattered in forty-three large institutions, the existing structure of poor law administration in London would disintegrate completely. The principle of local self-government, being as deeply ingrained as it was, the Bill would have risked defeat at the prospect of the vast majority of the London poor being re-housed at great expense and removed from the jurisdiction of the elected guardians to that of indirectly elected and centrally nominated hospital managers. It seemed more expedient to Gathorne Hardy to manoeuvre for new powers in the first instance, and to use these for consolidating his experimental scheme as and when the temper of local susceptibilities permitted.

Gathorne Hardy was diverted from defending his policy by objections to terminology. In the Bill, the new establishments were referred to as 'asylums', but throughout the debate Gathorne Hardy had spoken of 'hospitals'. Both Charles Villiers and Sir Harry Verney, among others, urged him to use this term in the Bill. Exception was taken to the word 'asylum', not on account of its association with the county institutions for 'lunatics', but because, as one Tory member explained, 'there were asylums for the blind, the deaf and dumb, for indigent gentlemen and decayed merchants. If the word were applied to receptacles for paupers, it might bring discredit on the others'.[3] Gathorne Hardy remained unmoved and the term 'asylum' was retained in the Bill to denote the establishments for the sick as well as for the insane.

The district hospital scheme, as expounded by Gathorne Hardy, left the House wondering what size the districts were intended to be. On occasion, he had mentioned one central board, but the context of such references suggested that he had in mind, not so much the management of the hospitals, as the administration of the Common Fund. When directly asked to specify the number of different boards which would be created under the Bill, Gathorne Hardy admitted that 'this has been one of the difficulties that have dwelt in my own mind'.[4] Miss Nightingale's emissaries suspected that Gathorne Hardy's mind was not irrevocably made up on this point, and they continued to urge—as she herself had done in her 'A B C'—that 'the *entire* medical relief of London should be under *one* central management'. John Stuart Mill, Member for Westminster, who also had been briefed in similar

[1] *Hansard*, op. cit., col. 164.
[2] See Chapter 1, Table 2.
[3] *Hansard*, op. cit., cols. 1611–13.
[4] Ibid., col. 776.

vein, made a persuasive and logical plea for a unitary authority. 'Why', he asked, 'had the Bill . . . preserved so much of the fractional character of the old system?' Its principles of administration seemed to him 'true and just', but the Bill was far from carrying them out to the extent which, he was persuaded, the House and the country would come in time to think desirable.[1]

> . . . It was a sound rule [he continued] that the administration of the same kind of things ought to be . . . on a large scale and under the same management. A central board would be under the eye of the public who would know and think more about it than about local boards. It would act under a much greater sense of responsibility. It was probable that a considerable number of powers now reserved to the Poor Law Board might safely be exercised by such a central board, which would to that extent preserve the principle of administration of the local affairs of the people by their own representatives. With a view to future legislation, it would be well worth considering whether the administration of relief of the sick for the whole of London should not be placed under central, instead of local, management. . . . The value of a central board to superintend the application of the resources of the whole Metropolis to the immediate exigencies of the distressed districts is obvious.[2]

Defender of individual liberty, John Stuart Mill was fundamentally opposed to social reform by the enlargement of State powers, but he did not wish to weaken the authority of the Poor Law Board, since the destitute were not a local but a national concern. Addressing the critics who had feared the creation of an intermediate board as a step towards centralization, he said that 'the denial of it would be a far greater step towards centralization. The powers which such a body was best qualified to exercise had become indispensable, and, in the absence of a central board, they would necessarily be assumed by a purely government board—the Poor Law Board'.[3] Charles Villiers, supporting John Stuart Mill's advocacy of a single hospital board, said that he had failed to find any provision in the Bill calculated to have that effect.[4] Replying to John Stuart Mill, Gathorne Hardy declared that 'an experiment would be made by the Bill, which to a certain extent would effect the object which the honourable Member had in view. . . .'[5] Either he had been converted by the exponents of a central board, or he had discovered unexpected support for his concealed intentions. For the first time during the debate, Gathorne Hardy made it clear that 'it was not proposed to have a board of management for each separate hospital, but one for each district; so that, if the metropolis were made one district, a central board would be created. . . .'[6]

One of the most difficult clauses which Gathorne Hardy had to defend was that which decreed that 'any order of the Poor Law Board under this Act shall not be deemed a General Order . . .'[7] 'General Orders' within the operation of the Poor Law Acts required the signatures of at least three Cabinet Ministers, members of the Poor Law Board, whereas

[1] Ibid., col. 1608.   [2] Ibid., col. 1609.   [3] Ibid., col. 1862.   [4] Ibid., col. 1611.
[5] Ibid., col. 1610.   [6] Ibid.   [7] 30 & 31 Vict. c. 6 s. 4.

'Common Orders', which also had the force of law, were signed only by the President and countersigned by the Permanent Secretary.[1] The system of 'Orders' was the principal means by which the central poor law department exercised its authority over local boards of guardians. The new measure would confer very great powers on the Poor Law Board—to take over buildings, buy land, sell property, grant compensation, alter poor law boundaries, administer a common fund, nominate hospital governors, and, if considered necessary, intervene in institutional management. Many such acts were to be executed by simple orders signed by the President of the Board. These would be statutory instruments, although they would lack the safeguards of Parliamentary sanction or shared responsibility: by this time the Poor Law Board had ceased to meet as a body. Gathorne Hardy confidently rode out the storm, and closed the discussion by declaring that 'it did not carry the matter further if the papers were sent round in a box for the signature of the President's colleagues. As soon as they saw his signature there, they added theirs as a matter of course, and there was an end of the matter.' He, as President of the Poor Law Board, was 'responsible for everything done'.[2] Assessed in their entirety, Gathorne Hardy's demands of Parliament appeared audaciously ambitious. In effect, he was seeking to extend the operations of the 'administrative State', introduced by the 1834 Act, and to endow the head of a central department with wide discretionary powers to devise the detailed means for implementing policies broadly defined in legislation. But, so sagacious was his judgment and conciliatory his manner, that he dispelled with relative ease the fears of despotic centralization which threatened to obstruct the passage of his Bill.

Gathorne Hardy had been persuaded that a pilot scheme for London was the logical approach to poor law medical reform. The capital, home of one-quarter of the total urban population of England and Wales,[3] was provided with the barest minimum of isolation accommodation. About one-sixth of the rate-aided poor of the country[4] was the responsibility of the metropolitan poor law authorities, and the ten largest of these had displayed an intractable degree of defiance to central direction on account of Local Acts. Further, by reason of the varying states of affluence and poverty of its constituent localities, London was particularly suited to a collective system of responsibility for its poor. A national scheme, as Villiers had intimated, was not yet feasible. Describing his Bill as 'a sketch which may hereafter be filled up',[5] Gathorne Hardy doubtless envisaged the completion of his reforms by subsequent legislation applicable to the provinces after the new measures had been adopted successfully in the capital.[6]

---

[1] *Hansard*, op. cit., col. 1674. 'General Orders' issued by the central poor law authority under the 1834 Poor Law Amendment Act were required to be communicated to the Home Secretary and formally laid before both Houses of Parliament.

[2] Ibid., cols. 1674 and 1686. [3] *Encyclopaedia Britannica* (9th edn.), vol. viii (1879), p. 221.

[4] Ibid., vol. xiv (1882), p. 832. [5] *Hansard*, op. cit., col. 1865.

[6] The Poor Law Amendment Act of 1868 (31 & 32 Vict. c. 122 s. 8) empowered provincial poor law authorities to provide separate infirmaries, but it was a whole generation before even a dozen unions in the larger towns got their separate infirmaries and dispensaries. They had no financial stimulus such as the Common Poor Fund. S. and B. Webb. *English Poor Law History*, op. cit., p. 321.

The legend of nineteenth-century *laissez-faire* was losing ground.[1] While *Hansard* records the animated and constructive debates on the Bill, Gathorne Hardy's personal diary best defines the climate in which the founding of England's first State hospitals was sanctioned.

> *February 9:* My Bill came on yesterday. . . . I got a most attentive hearing, and so far as talking went, universal approval . . .
> *February 24:* On Thursday night . . . my Poor Law Bill came on for second reading. . . . It was duly puffed by every speaker, and even Villiers had but small criticisms to make.
> *March 10:* On Friday evening, after long waiting, I at last got my Bill on, and the Committee carried me through 30 clauses with steady and earnest support. Indeed, I never saw anything like it.
> *March 12:* Last night I got through Committee with my Bill almost unchanged and ended amid loud cheers. Resistance to it was hopeless.[2]

On 14 March 1867, the Metropolitan Poor Bill was passed amid further enthusiasm and acclaim. Disraeli wrote exuberantly to the Queen describing 'the extraordinarily favourable impression made by Mr. Gathorne Hardy and his new poor law legislation'.[3] For the author of the Bill, it was a political triumph; for the reformers, the new measure was a victory, even if it fell short of all they had hoped. Miss Nightingale was angry, nevertheless, because Gathorne Hardy had not consulted her about the new hospitals and had failed to make direct provision for the improvement of workhouse nursing.[4] Giving vent to her disappointment, she scribbled on a draft copy of the Bill: 'Humbug!', 'No principles', 'Beastly!'. In calmer mood, she was able, later, to appreciate the advances which would be assured by the operation of the Act. 'This is a beginning. We shall get more in time', she wrote confidently to a friend.[5]

On 29 March 1867, the Bill received the Royal Assent. Six weeks later, Gathorne Hardy decreed that *all* the unions and parishes of the metropolis should be combined for the

---

[1] The intervention of the State in the field of medical care, under the 1867 Metropolitan Poor Act, adds support to Professor Brebner's denial of the commonly accepted view that 'laissez-faire' dominated British nineteenth-century politics. J. Bartlet Brebner, 'Laissez-faire and State Intervention in Nineteenth-Century Britain', *J. Econ. Hist.*, Supplement VIII, 1848, pp. 59–73. See also Ruth G. Hodgkinson's *The Origins of the National Health Service: The Medical Services of the New Poor Law, 1834–71*, passim.

[2] *Gathorne-Hardy, First Earl of Cranbrook, a Memoir*, ed. A. E. Gathorne-Hardy (1910), pp. 194–95. Gathorne Hardy kept a diary from the age of 23 until a few months before his death at the age of 92 (1906). In 1882, he began to summarize the contents of past diaries, but some entries, including the above, were left unedited.

[3] *Gathorne-Hardy . . . a Memoir*, op. cit., p. 194.

[4] Miss Nightingale's biographer, Mrs. Woodham-Smith, suggests that Miss Nightingale was, herself, to blame for this. She had written a letter to Gathorne Hardy reporting the victory of the Liverpool workhouse nursing scheme in which she gave a dramatic account of the difficulties encountered. He was either genuinely alarmed, or he was glad to find an excuse for postponing nursing reform; in any case he gave her letter as a reason for shelving the question. (C. Woodham-Smith, op. cit., p. 355).

[5] Letter written by Florence Nightingale in March 1867 to the Rev. Mother Bermondsey, cited by C. Woodham-Smith, op. cit., p. 355.

reception and relief of the London rate-aided poor suffering from smallpox, fever or insanity, and that, for this new hospital region—to be known as the Metropolitan Asylum District—a Board of Management should be constituted.[1] The Metropolitan Asylums Board was thus given statutory existence. Without disrupting the structure of London's poor law administration, Gathorne Hardy had instituted a central hospital system which would confer preventive benefits upon all constituent localities, and a Common Poor Fund which would equalize their relief burdens. Immediately after signing the birth certificate of England's first regional hospital board, the President left the Poor Law Board to take up his new appointment as Home Secretary.

During the following year, the implementation of the Metropolitan Poor Act was carried a stage further. Six 'Sick Asylum Districts' were formed. Each comprised four or five unions, which were ordered to erect a joint 'asylum' for the general sick poor.[2] Owing to the high cost of building, only two survived.[3] The constituent unions of the disbanded 'sick asylum districts' were re-grouped with a view to one of the existing workhouses in each of the new areas being allocated exclusively to the sick.[4] The remaining localities were instructed to 'provide infirmaries on sites detached from the workhouses'.[5] As a result, some twenty separate poor law infirmaries, with 10,000 beds, were established in London during the next decade.[6] For the outdoor sick, the guardians were urged to set up dispensaries under the Act; and during the same period all but three of the metropolitan unions and parishes successfully adopted this form of medical relief.[7]

State hospital services for the London poor were thus inaugurated. 'Gathorne Hardy's Act'—as it came to be known—proved to be the most important poor law measure for London between 1834 and 1929 and a significant step towards the socialization of medical care in this country.

[1] PLB (Metropolitan Asylum District) Order, 15 May 1867, to all metropolitan boards of guardians. R. G. Glen's *Poor Law Orders* (1898 edn.), p. 691. This was the only Order under the Metropolitan Poor Act of 1867 to be issued by Mr. Gathorne Hardy.

[2] *PLB Twentieth Annual Report*, 1867–68, pp. 17–18 (Cmd. 4039, HMSO, 1868).

[3] Central London and Poplar and Stepney Sick Asylum Districts, the formation of which was officially declared in PLB Orders dated 23 April and 2 May 1868.

[4] *PLB Twenty-first Annual Report*, 1868–69, pp. 16–18 (Cmd. 23650, HMSO, 1869) and *PLB Twenty-second Annual Report*, 1869–70, pp. xxxvi–xxxvii (Cmd. 123, HMSO, 1870).

[5] *PLB Twentieth Annual Report*, 1867–68, p. 18.

[6] See Chapter 5, Table 2.

[7] *Encyclopaedia Britannica* (9th edn.) vol. xiv (1882), p. 832. By 1880, twenty-seven of the thirty metropolitan unions had established forty-seven dispensaries. Some of them were set up only because the guardians feared the PLB would use its power over the Common Poor Fund under the 1867 Act (*PLB Twenty-second Annual Report*, op. cit., p. xliv).

PART ONE

The MAB—1867 to 1900: Three Decades of Nineteenth-Century Pioneering

'The Poor Law history of the last hundred years is, on the face of it, a record of mistaken beliefs fanatically adhered to, and of great evils tardily recognised and more tardily remedied. If we could look below the surface we would find, beyond a doubt, much Bumbledom, much cruelty and not a little corruption; but we would also find much more honest and conscientious service from both voluntary and paid workers, and not a little heroic devotion.'

Gilbert Slater, 'The Relief of the Poor', *A Century of Municipal Progress, 1835–1935*, (1935).

CHAPTER 3

England's First State Hospitals for Infectious Diseases

THE Metropolitan Asylums Board[1] embarked on its pioneering venture on 22 June 1867, when its sixty members met at the headquarters of the Metropolitan Board of Works in Spring Gardens, near Admiralty Arch. These premises—'cavernous and tavernous', as Lord Rosebery later described them[2]—were lent during weekends to the Asylums Board until it was able to find accommodation of its own. In accordance with the 1867 Act, fifteen members of the new hospital authority had been nominated by the Poor Law Board and the remaining forty-five had been elected by the metropolitan guardians, on the instructions of the Poor Law Board, to represent the thirty-nine unions and parishes[3] 'included in the Metropolis, as defined by the Metropolis Management Act, 1855'.[4] This new 'Asylum District', covering about 118 square miles and embracing a population of some three millions, was identical with the area within the jurisdiction of the Metropolitan Board of Works, and subsequently of the London County Council.

At this first meeting, a chairman was elected and five standing committees were set up.[5] A close contest resulted in the office of chairman being conferred on Dr. William Henry Brewer, JP, MD, MRCS, a coroner and one of the two representatives of the union of

---

[1] 'Metropolitan Asylums Board' will be abbreviated in the following text to M A B.

[2] A. G. Gardiner, *Sir John Benn and the Progressive Movement* (1925), p. 91.

[3] In 1867, there were thirty-nine metropolitan poor law districts. The six largest were allowed to have two representatives on the M A B, while the remainder each had one. By 1871, these districts had been reduced to thirty as a result of re-grouping following the dissolution of most of the 'sick asylum districts' referred to in Chapter 2. See Map I, following Appendix IV.

[4] 30 & 31 Vict. c. 6 s. 3. 'The Metropolis', as defined by the Metropolitan Management Act, 1855, was 'the Registrar-General's district' (*Hansard*, 1866, vol. 137, col. 701). This comprised the thirty-six registration districts used for the census of 1851. The Registrar-General's district had its origin in the Bills of Mortality which, since the sixteenth century, had been kept for parishes in the City and neighbouring populous areas, largely so that the Court and others might be warned of the coming of the plague and seek a safer retreat. As London grew, the Bills had been extended to more and more parishes, and when the Registrar-General was appointed, he continued the practice, using the area covered by the Bills as the basis of his metropolitan district. (Sir I. G. Gibbon and R. W. Bell, *History of the London County Council, 1889–1939*, p. 23).

[5] For details of the committee structure of the M A B, see Chapter 11 and Appendix I, Document IV. Of the five standing committees first appointed three were for the management of the three classes of patients —those suffering from 'fever', smallpox, and insanity—and the other two were general purposes and finance committees.

St. George's, Hanover Square, in John Stuart Mill's parliamentary constituency of Westminster. For the next fourteen years, the most crucial in the Board's history, its fortunes were to depend in large measure on the dynamic leadership of its first chairman.

For some months, the Board deliberated from Spring Gardens before moving into No. 6, Westminster Gardens, SW1, where it had acquired four rooms at a rent of £250 a year. The Poor Law Board, when notified, curtly reminded the M A B that such an arrangement was irregular without prior sanction. This early repression of the Board's aspirations towards a measure of autonomy presaged the relationship which was to develop during the next few years between the Asylums Board and the central authority. The M A B was recruited from an élite accustomed to arbitrary leadership, free competition of ideas and opinions, and intolerance of all but a minimum of State interference in the social and economic life of the country. Now, for the first time, a central department was entering the field of civilian hospital management, hitherto the monopoly of voluntary effort. Despite its extended powers for the purpose, the Poor Law Board was ill-equipped for its new role, since public health was entirely outside its province.

At the outset, the M A B was endowed with neither charter nor terms of reference beyond the provisions of the 1867 Act and the brief Poor Law Board order constituting the Metropolitan Asylum District.[1] The members of the new hospital authority assumed that they would be serving as governors of the projected establishments and that they would be granted ample latitude to govern, but the tone of the central authority's communications, in which they were referred to as 'Managers', left no doubt that their role was intended to be of a purely executive nature and subject to detailed control from Whitehall.

Undaunted, the pioneers began to study the fundamental problems of siting and designing the new institutions. For the fever and smallpox hospitals, they aimed to select localities which would be easily accessible to patients from every part of the capital, but without compulsory powers of purchase this was not easy. Concentrating on the neighbourhoods of Regent's Park, Victoria Park and Clapham Common, the Board eventually found three sites of about eight acres each in Hampstead in the north-west, Homerton in the north-east, and Stockwell in the south-west, at prices ranging from £12,000 to £15,000.[2] It was decided to build a 200-bed fever hospital and a 100-bed smallpox hospital on each site, with a view to providing for an estimated annual intake of from 4,200 to 4,500 'fever' cases and from 2,600 to 3,200 smallpox cases. On submission to the Poor Law Board, however, these projects were severely pruned, and it became necessary to limit the building at Hampstead—on the property known as 'Old Bartrams' off Haverstock Hill—to one fever hospital for one hundred patients. For mental cases, the Board decided to build two large institutions outside London, one north and one south of the Thames. A site of seventy-two acres was found at Caterham, Surrey, for £6,000, and one of eighty acres at Leavesden, Hertfordshire, for £8,600.

This was a beginning, but obstacles soon intervened. Not least of these resulted from

[1] PLB order to metropolitan boards of guardians, 15 May 1867.
[2] Capital expenditure of the M A B is discussed in Chapter 13.

local opposition at Hampstead, where the Board became involved in a dispute with Sir Rowland Hill of postage fame, who owned the property adjoining the M A B hospital site. The true agents of infection were not yet commonly understood and the 3,000-year-old miasmic theory still persisted. Sir Rowland Hill, with other local residents, fearful of fever-stricken paupers in their midst, sued the Board. The costly and protracted litigation which followed had far-reaching effects, not only for the fortunes of the M A B, but also for the development of public isolation hospitals in the country generally.

Further frustrations followed the submission of hospital plans to the Poor Law Board. These had been selected from designs invited from experienced architects. After retaining the plans for months, the central authority would return them with reduced dimensions and ill-advised criticisms.[1] The Managers became restive. Nearly two years had elapsed since the legislature had sanctioned the strengthening of London's inadequate defences against pestilence by the erection of infectious disease hospitals for the London poor. To the Managers' consternation, a communication was received from the Poor Law Board advising them that 'instead of erecting the whole of the three hospitals immediately, the more expedient course would be to erect only two of them in the first instance'. The Homerton and Stockwell institutions were considered sufficient. Only 'if further permanent accommodation should be found necessary' was the Hampstead hospital to be built.[2] Supported by medical opinion, the Managers voiced their concern at the unwisdom of this proposal and at the Poor Law Board's persistent quibbling on points of detail in connexion with the plans for the Homerton and Stockwell hospitals. Time-consuming correspondence continued until October 1869, when panic seized the Poor Law Board. The Lords of Her Majesty's Council had discovered 'threatenings of a serious epidemic of so-called relapsing fever[3] in London'. The Privy Council impressed upon the Poor Law Board that 'this evil can scarcely fail to attain very large proportions unless . . . steps are taken for ensuring that sufficient hospital accommodation may be provided for poor persons attacked with the disease'.[4] With the M A B hospitals still in embryo, the Poor Law

[1] On one occasion, the PLB, when commenting on an M A B hospital plan, complained that 'the staircase, 18 feet by 18 feet, to the residence of the assistant medical officers, considering that it is for their sole use, seems larger than necessary'. It was urged that a staircase half the size would be large enough for AMOs. (PLB letter to the M A B dated 15 April 1868). The Asylums Managers were obliged to explain that the 'staircase' on the plan was in fact a committee room!

[2] PLB letter to the M A B, 13 February 1869.

[3] Dr. Charles Murchison, writing in 1862 (*A Treatise on the Continued Fevers of Great Britain*, Chapter III), described relapsing fever, or famine fever, as a contagious disease chiefly met with in the form of epidemics during seasons of scarcity and famine. It was propagated by over-crowding, and prevailed in the most crowded localities of large cities, and, in the seventeenth and eighteenth centuries, was often confounded with typhus and enteric fever or incipient smallpox. It was characterized by an abrupt onset of feverish symptoms which disappeared about the fifth day. After a complete apyretic interval, the patient relapsed about the fourteenth day, the sickness running a similar course. This might be repeated twice or even five times. Before 1826, relapsing fever and typhus were regarded as modifications of the same disease, but after that date a distinction was drawn between the two. Epidemics of both often occurred simultaneously, the proportion of relapsing cases being greatest at the beginning of the epidemic.

[4] Privy Council letter to the PLB, 29 October 1869.

Board appealed in desperation to the London Fever Hospital.[1] The Privy Council reminded the vestries and district boards of 'the proceedings to be taken by them under the Sanitary Acts'. The Poor Law Board reminded the M A B of its duties under the 1867 Metropolitan Poor Act, and urgently ordered that it should 'take the requisite steps for providing temporary accommodation to meet the present emergency . . .'[2]

The Asylums Board thereupon convened a special fever committee with full powers to act as considered expedient and necessary. Forthwith a plan was formulated, and on 10 November 1869 it was presented personally by the committee to the President of the Poor Law Board, Mr. (later Lord) Goschen.[3] The committee suggested, and he agreed, that the Asylums Managers should negotiate with the Governors of the London Fever Hospital, Islington, for the erection of a temporary structure in the hospital grounds, the Board to pay rent and the cost of erecting and equipping. The committee impressed upon the President the need for utilizing the Hampstead site in anticipation of a serious epidemic. It lost no time in calling for designs and estimates for a temporary 90-bed structure which could be extended to 180 beds, if required, and erected within one month. Provisional assurances were secured in advance from the Poor Law Board that the requisite orders for equipping and staffing the hospital would be issued as soon as necessary. The Poor Law Board was asked to keep the fever committee informed of the accommodation being provided by the metropolitan poor law unions, while the Privy Council Office was requested to report regularly on the state of the epidemic. Both central departments readily deferred to the demands of the M A B fever committee, which had assumed complete control of the situation. Financial obstacles were removed and loans were made available by the Metropolitan Board of Works.

In December 1869, when it was apparent that the disease was gaining rapidly on the capital and that only two poor law unions had made any attempt to provide isolation accommodation, the M A B fever committee decided to erect the projected temporary hospital at Hampstead. By this time, the London Fever Hospital and the adjacent emergency structure were filled to capacity with over 400 cases, and many of the staff were stricken down. Building operations at Hampstead were speeded up and the fever committee set about staffing the temporary hospital within the month. Almost daily the Poor Law Board urged upon the Asylums Managers the necessity for hastening the completion of the structure. Christmas intervened, and the task of finding nurses and domestic staff at short notice became increasingly difficult. The chairman, Dr. Brewer, a devout churchman, tackled the problem personally. In Newport Market, Soho, in his poor law district, was a vagrants' refuge managed by nuns of the Anglican Society of St. Margaret. The mother house of the Sisterhood at East Grinstead had been founded in 1855 for the purpose of

---

[1] PLB letter to the Hon. Secretary, London Fever Hospital, 30 October 1869.
[2] PLB letter to the M A B, 30 October 1869.
[3] Mr. G. J. Goschen had taken office at the beginning of 1868, succeeding Lord Devon, who had filled the office of President during the intervening months since Mr. Gathorne Hardy's departure in May 1867.

nursing the poor, and the nuns had considerable experience of fever cases.[1] Dr. Brewer appealed to them for help and they readily responded. In order to maintain their essential community life, they stipulated that all the nursing and domestic staff of the hospital should be members of the Sisterhood. This was eminently satisfactory to the fever committee, and the nuns were engaged at the rates offered to temporary lay workers.[2] In one month, the 90-bed hospital had been erected, equipped and staffed. The cost of the temporary structures at Hampstead and Islington had totalled £12,000. On 25 January 1870, the Hampstead Hospital was opened for the reception of patients, the first of whom were Polish refugees from the East End of London. England's first State hospital was functioning.[3] The epidemic was under control.

Panic at the Poor Law Board now gave place to qualms concerning expenditure. The Asylums Managers were informed that 'the salaries at Hampstead appear to be very high. . . . In the London Fever Hospital the salaries for similar services are very much lower'.[4] This provoked the Asylums Managers to reply:

> . . . Although the salaries . . . are undoubtedly on a liberal scale, the Poor Law Board must remember that the engagements are entirely of a temporary character . . . and the employment is not without considerable personal risk to those engaged. The Managers would be glad to be informed if the Poor Law Board has ascertained whether the London Fever Hospital is able at a lower price to secure the services of servants who prove themselves in all respects efficient for the duties required of them. . . . The Managers believe it is true economy to provide their establishments with thoroughly efficient officers.[5]

[1] The East Grinstead Sisterhood, an Anglican religious community of the Society of St. Margaret, founded in 1855 by the Rev. John Mason Neale, was one of several such Orders established about this time for nursing the sick poor. In 1848, the St. John's Sisterhood, the first purely Nursing Order in the Church of England, was founded. This Order was the first to take over the entire nursing of a London hospital—King's College Hospital—while a sister Order, the All Saints Sisterhood, performed the same service at University College Hospital. At first Guy's, then the London and the Westminster Hospitals, were the sources of practical training. (J. Langdon-Davies, *Westminster Hospital—Two Centuries of Voluntary Service, 1719–1948* (1952), Chapter 5). Anglican nuns also nursed at the Chorlton poor law infirmary when it was established in the early 1860s. The practical experience of the nuns after training was gained in nursing the poor in their own homes. The great work, historically speaking, of these nursing Orders was the part they played in bridging the gap at the London hospitals between the ousting of the earlier uneducated, unreliable 'Sairey Gamp' type of nurse and the establishment of the new type of trained nurses drawn from the better-educated classes. (A. E. Pavey, *Story of the Growth of Nursing* (3rd edn. 1951)). For further information concerning nursing by religious communities, see: P. Anson, *The Call of the Cloister* (SPCK, 4th edn., 1964); R. E. Hutton, *St. Margaret's Convent, East Grinstead* (rev. edn., 1959); Eleanor A. Towle, *John Mason Neale, a Memoir,* (1906); *Memoirs of a Sister of St. Saviour's,* Mowbray's, (1903).

[2] The monthly rates of pay offered to the nursing nuns at Hampstead were: matron, £10; head nurse, £3; superintendent of night nurses, £4; ordinary nurses, £2 10s. Further details concerning remuneration of nurses in the service of the M A B are given in Chapter 12 and Appendix IV, Table K.

[3] Upon 'Old Bartrams', Hampstead, site of the first State hospital in this country, now stands the North-Western Branch of the Royal Free Hospital.

[4] PLB letter to the M A B, 2 February 1870.

[5] M A B letter to the PLB, 6 February 1870.

The medical press supported the Asylums Managers, and when the Poor Law Board objected to a wage of thirty shillings a month for a hospital kitchen maid, the *Lancet* recorded with relish the Managers' unanimous resolve to resign if their views were not respected, and commented:

> ... If the Poor Law Board wish to carry out their control to such details, they had better manage the whole affair. The fact is that the staff at Gwydyr House have been so accustomed to interfering with boards of guardians and have so frequently sanctioned contemptible expedients for saving money, that they have been tempted to try it on with gentlemen of intelligence and common sense, who know how wretchedly every sort of poor law officer is paid and how badly the public is served by them.[1]

No official regulations concerning hospital management existed at this stage and *ad hoc* orders were issued by the central authority when considered necessary. The M A B fever committee decided that the medical certificate and form of admission prescribed by the Poor Law Board 'were more detailed than was convenient', and drastically abbreviated them. When an infectious pauper arrived in a public cab, it reported the incident direct to the Home Secretary and reprimanded the guardians who sent him. The Poor Law Board did not intend the fever committee's emergency powers to continue indefinitely and impressed upon the Asylums Board that the legislature had intended the central authority to exert active, and not mere nominal, supervision over the new hospital services. The Managers, however, regarded Poor Law Board interference in organizational detail as obstructive and superfluous, and from now on took a firm stand.

In May 1870, the relapsing fever epidemic began to recede. Later in the year, the temporary structure at Hampstead was vacated and the London Fever Hospital resumed the reception of pauper cases, pending the opening of the new M A B isolation hospitals, which were still under construction.

[1] *Lancet*, 1870, vol. II, p. 225 (13 August).

CHAPTER 4

England's First State 'Imbecile Asylums'

I

WHEN introducing his Metropolitan Poor Bill in 1867, Gathorne Hardy had declared that he intended to initiate his workhouse classification scheme by building special establishments for poor law 'lunatics and imbeciles'.[1] At this time, the terms 'lunacy' and 'insanity' were loosely used for the whole of what is now termed 'mental disorder', whether of the nature of mental illness or of mental subnormality. Further, the terms 'imbecile' and 'defective' were used, equally loosely, for conditions associated with weakness of mind, and therefore applied to states of senile dementia and the end-results of mental illness, as well as to congenital defectiveness. Only the term 'idiot' was reserved definitively for the more severely subnormal.[2]

Before Gathorne Hardy's Act, the different methods of disposal of persons of unsound mind—in county asylums, poor law institutions, private licensed houses and voluntary hospitals—had resulted more from expediency than from statutory disposition. One of the main purposes of the 1867 Act had been to provide special hospitals for a particular group of the mentally afflicted—those 'idiotic, chronic and harmless patients' for whom the workhouses of London were the only available refuge.

The first attempt to regulate the institutional care of persons of unsound mind was the passing of an Act in 1774.[3] At that time, lunatics—to use the terminology of the period—were to be found in pitiable conditions in prisons, workhouses, public hospitals such as Bethlem, and private 'madhouses'. Nevertheless, the Act applied only to the private institutions. These were to be inspected and licensed by five Commissioners—all Fellows of the Royal College of Physicians—in the metropolitan area, and by Justices of the Peace in the provinces. The Act further required that admission should be on a medical certificate, and that notification of cases received, both in London and elsewhere, should be made to the Commissioners. Paupers, however, were excluded from the Act.

During the next four decades, standards of care in institutions for the mentally disordered failed to improve, and it became necessary for their regulation to be examined. A

---

[1] *Hansard*, 1867, vol. clxxxv (third series), 8 February, col. 161.
[2] For this elucidation of terminology, as well as of various other aspects of lunacy in the nineteenth century referred to in this chapter, the author is indebted to Dr. Alexander Walk.
[3] The Act for Regulating Private Madhouses, 1774.

Select Committee was accordingly set up in 1815, and re-appointed in 1816. By this time, thirty-four private licensed establishments functioned in London and upwards of forty in the counties. The Retreat at York, founded by the Quaker, William Tuke, had been opened in 1796; Guy's Hospital had a new lunatic ward; and a new Bethlem hospital had just been completed in Lambeth. In the provinces, there were a few other hospitals of ancient foundation, such as the York Asylum, where abuses had given rise to the enquiry. Twelve county asylums had been built under 'Wynn's Act' of 1808, but only one—that at Nottingham—was as yet fully in operation. The 1808 measure had empowered, but not compelled, Justices of the Peace in every county to provide establishments for the care of pauper lunatics, so that they might be removed from workhouses and prisons. Evidence received by the 1815–16 Committees revealed a generally noisome picture of the mentally disordered still suffering neglect in wretched conditions in workhouses, 'madhouses' and voluntary hospitals. Only in a few institutions were standards of care and treatment regarded as praiseworthy. These included the Nottingham Asylum (financed partly by the rates and partly by voluntary subscription), the York Retreat, and some of the licensed houses founded by medical men at the end of the eighteenth century. During the decade following the 1815–16 enquiry, however, most of the private institutions remained as bad as ever, despite the Committees' urgent demands for remedial measures.

Another Select Committee sat in 1827, largely as a result of agitation on the part of a new twenty-six-year old Member of Parliament, Lord Ashley (later Lord Shaftesbury) and Robert Gordon, a Dorsetshire magistrate. Their work on the Committee and subsequent publicity led to the passing of two Acts in 1828, one dealing with county asylums—their erection and management, and the care of pauper and criminal lunatics; and the other with private 'madhouses'. Under the Madhouse Act, a new Metropolitan Lunacy Commission was appointed consisting of fifteen members. Five were physicians paid at the rate of £1 an hour, and the remainder, including Ashley, Gordon and Wynn, were honorary. The Commissioners had greatly extended powers of inspection and licensing, and they made a significant improvement in the London area. Similar powers were bestowed on the Justices of the Peace, but progress in the provinces was less apparent. While private asylums were thus controlled, public institutions for the mentally disordered remained exempt, and single patients in care in the community continued to be unprotected.

When the 1834 Poor Law Amendment Act provided for the erection of large workhouses by the union of parishes, it was not intended that these institutions should become permanent refuges for pauper lunatics. Section XLV of the Act expressly prohibited the detention in a workhouse of 'any dangerous lunatic, insane person or idiot' for more than fourteen days. This wording, however, was taken by the guardians to imply that the detention of any who were not dangerous was allowable—an interpretation of doubtful legality. As the cost to the guardians of maintaining insane paupers in the workhouse was less than paying for their care elsewhere,[1] these patients were retained in the poor law

---

[1] In 1844, the average annual cost per head in a workhouse was £40; in a county asylum it varied from £100 to £350.

institutions, despite the absence of suitable accommodation and care, and in disregard of central recommendations, injunctions and statutory directives.

In 1838, a Select Committee of Enquiry into the operation of the poor law recommended the fusion of several unions for the purpose of maintaining a common lunatic asylum distinct from the county asylums. An attempt was made to implement this recommendation in a poor law Bill in 1839, but it was defeated by medical opposition on the ground that pauper patients would be deprived of what was regarded as superior treatment in the county asylums.

In 1842, the Poor Law Commissioners issued a directive to boards of guardians deprecating the improper retention in workhouses of any curable lunatics. It was urged that 'with lunatics the first object ought to be their cure by proper medical treatment, which can only be obtained in a well-regulated asylum'. But, at this time, not more than twenty county asylums had been established. In 1844, there were some 20,600 lunatics in all forms of care in England and Wales. Of this total, less than 3,800 were private patients, while over 16,800 were classed as paupers. These poor law patients were admitted without certification, and, once in care, were subject to no form of official inspection. For nearly twenty years, Ashley had been fighting to improve the lot of these patients in workhouses, while another champion of the rights of the mentally disordered, Dorothea Dix (1802–87), a former American schoolteacher, was agitating for improved conditions in asylums both in this country and the United States. Further light was brought to bear on the pressing need for reform by the results of a two-year survey carried out by the Metropolitan Lunacy Commissioners. Their report, published in 1844, showed that some 9,000 (about 75 per cent) of the total number of lunatics in the metropolitan area were still in workhouses, boarded out or in licensed houses, often in appalling conditions.

The following year saw the passing of 'Shaftesbury's Act', which became the basis for subsequent legislation. Under the 1845 Lunacy Act, a permanent Board of Lunacy Commissioners was created, and Justices everywhere—in counties and boroughs—were compelled to erect lunatic asylums to be financed by the local rates. Committees of Visitors were to regulate and superintend the asylums, which would be visited regularly by the Lunacy Commissioners in the London area and by the Justices elsewhere. The Commissioners were also obliged to visit all other establishments in which lunatics were in care. Safeguards governing admission and discharge were rigorously imposed. It was intended that all lunatic paupers should be transferred to the new asylums when built. Meantime, new procedures for the care of these patients in workhouses and licensed houses were to be observed. These included certification for admission, the keeping of records for the information of the Lunacy Commissioners, annual inspection by legal and medical Commissioners and the supervision of care and accommodation by special Visitors.

During the next decade, the system of licensing and methods of certification were tightened up; single patients were brought under supervision; and lunatics in workhouses and on outdoor relief were visited periodically and reported on by the union medical officer.[1]

[1] The Lunacy Act, 1853.

As the new county asylums gradually came into being, the guardians sent in, not only their mentally ill patients, but also their incurable defective cases, although the new institutions were intended to be places of treatment and cure. Delays in building the county asylums and the crowded state of those in operation rendered it necessary by the late 'fifties for the parochial authorities to take back their harmless chronic patients—by far the largest category of the mentally disordered. By 1859, there were some 36,000 lunatics in all forms of care in England and Wales—about 31,000 classed as paupers and 5,000 private patients. Over 17,000 of the paupers were in county asylums or on contract in licensed houses; about 7,000 were in workhouses; while a similar number were living 'with friends or elsewhere'. From the numbers recorded at this time, it is impossible to know how many patients were suffering from what we now call mental illness and how many from subnormality. When the Lunacy Commissioners made a study of mental patients in workhouses in 1847, they recognized three categories: 'the defectives from birth; the demented and fatuous; and the deranged or disordered'.[1] In the late 'fifties, many such patients were still being warded with sane inmates and attended by fellow paupers. Although forbidden by the Lunacy Commissioners, the use of mechanical restraints was tolerated because workhouse staffs could not manage without them.[2] A number of parochial boards, particularly in the metropolitan area, provided what they called 'insane wards', but these were generally ill-equipped and poorly staffed, and were created merely to avoid the extra expense of sending mental cases to other institutions. Later, however, in a few large provincial towns, including Liverpool, Manchester and Birmingham, special mental wards came to be developed in the poor law infirmaries with their own nurses and medical officer.[3]

In April 1859, while yet another Select Committee on lunacy was sitting, the Lunacy Commissioners published a special report on the insane in workhouses. They had decided that the time had come to publicize the problem and so pave the way to reform. In the course of this 80-page report, the Commissioners declared that any attempt to remedy the defects radically incident to the workhouse system would be impracticable so long as insane patients were detained in poor law institutions, whether mixed with other inmates or placed in distinct wards.[4] They recommended, as an alternative to extending the already overlarge county asylums,

> the erection of inexpensive buildings adapted for the residence of idiotic, chronic and harmless patients, in direct connexion with, or at a convenient distance from, the

[1] Lunacy Commissioners' Second Report, 1847.
[2] Lunacy Commissioners' Twelfth Report, 1859.
[3] Mental wards in *small* workhouses were not encouraged by the Lunacy Commissioners. They felt that to segregate the imbeciles from the other inmates deprived them of whatever cheerfulness, sense of protection or means of making themselves useful they might have in the body of the house (Twenty-first Report, 1868).
[4] Of the 655 workhouses in England and Wales in 1859, 10 per cent provided separate insane wards (Lunacy Commissioners' Twelfth Report, 1859).

existing institutions. These auxiliary asylums . . . would be intermediate between union workhouses and the principal curative asylums. . . .[1]

As with most of the Lunacy Commissioners' recommendations, this suggestion was left in abeyance.

Following the report of the 1859–60 Committee of Enquiry (July 1860), the Lunacy Act of 1862 was passed.[2] While empowering the Lunacy Commissioners to remove lunatics from workhouses to county asylums when considered necessary, the Act legalized the transfer of the harmless chronic insane from the overcrowded curative institutions to the workhouses. The Poor Law Board subsequently explained to guardians that it had not been contemplated that chronic patients should be generally received into workhouses, thereby constituting them all small lunatic asylums. Application to the Lunacy Commissioners for such transfers had to originate with the statutory Asylum Visitors, who would select only those poor law institutions which provided adequate accommodation, care and attendance. But of these there were relatively few.

In their early days, the Lunacy Commissioners had been hopeful of relying on the co-operation of the central destitution authority, but, as they found their recommendations constantly discarded and they had no power to enforce their suggested reforms, they came to voice their displeasure and alarm. Gathorne Hardy, during his first months at the Poor Law Board in 1866 was no less alarmed when he discovered that, as President of the Board, his authority was blunted by an absence of effective sanctions for compelling guardians to act upon such directives as were addressed to them. His powers thus limited, he was faced with the problem of remedying workhouse evils which stemmed from overcrowding, a situation which was aggravated by the presence of numerous inmates whose mental condition warranted their being in specialized care. The public asylums in the London area, as elsewhere, were also suffering from similar pressures. The number of county asylum beds was never sufficient to meet the demand. In addition to the 7,000 pauper lunatics which the metropolitan guardians maintained at this time in county asylums and licensed houses, there were in the London workhouses over fifty children and nearly 2,000 adults classed as 'insane'. These mentally afflicted adults formed part of the group designated 'Old and Infirm', which totalled upward of 14,000 and undoubtedly included, in addition, numerous senile dements and other weak-minded persons.[3]

When presenting his case for removing the insane from the London workhouses to new establishments, Gathorne Hardy approvingly endorsed the Lunacy Commissioners' recommendation for 'auxiliary asylums'.[4] The new institutions which he was proposing

[1] Supplement to Lunacy Commissioners' Twelfth Report, 1859.
[2] The 1862 Act is particularly noteworthy as pioneering, in a limited way, voluntary admission. It empowered any person who had been a patient in any type of mental hospital during the previous five years to enter a licensed house as a voluntary boarder, provided that he wrote personally for permission to two of the Lunacy Commissioners. This was soon afterwards extended to the registered hospitals.
[3] See Table 2 following Chapter 1.
[4] *Hansard*, 1867, vol. clxxxv (third series) 8 February, cols. 161–70.

were to accommodate the same broad category of 'harmless chronics', but they would not be administered by the same authorities as the existing curative institutions, but by a new body. As we have seen, this was to be the M A B.

To carry out its duties under the 1867 Act, the Asylums Board erected two large establishments at Leavesden and Caterham on sites which had been chosen for cheapness well out in the country. Originally designed for some 1,500 patients each, they were as nearly as possible identical in construction and consisted of three-storied blocks, each floor forming one enormous ward. These were opened in October 1870.

Poor Law Board regulations for the M A B imbecile asylums—as they were called at this time—had stipulated that admission required a medical certificate to the effect that 'the pauper is a chronic and harmless lunatic, idiot or imbecile . . .'.[1] But, despite this rule, Leavesden and Caterham were soon filled with patients of all ages suffering from every type of mental disorder, acute and chronic.[2] A large number of chronic insane were sent in from Hanwell and Colney Hatch, the county asylums of Middlesex. Heavy and sudden demands had been made upon nearly all the mental institutions near London following the 1867 Act. The Metropolitan Common Poor Fund, established under the Act, provided for the maintenance, not only of the 'insane poor' in the M A B asylums, but also of London rate-aided 'lunatics in asylums, registered hospitals and licensed houses'.[3] Guardians who were keeping patients in special insane wards in the workhouse were at a disadvantage, since they were paying for them out of the local poor rate, while those who had no segregation transferred to other institutions all cases for whom they could get medical certification, and claimed for their maintenance from the new common poor fund.[4] The indiscriminate demands made by the guardians on the imbecile asylums at Caterham and Leavesden continued for some years, notwithstanding the protests of the Lunacy Commissioners and the Asylums Board.

Lord Shaftesbury, who had been chairman of the Lunacy Commissioners since 1853, had foreseen some of the problems likely to arise in the running of the M A B asylums. While the Metropolitan Poor Bill was passing through committee in the House of Lords, he urged that the type of patient should be specifically defined and, further, that the same protection against the detention of sane persons in the new buildings should be provided as was the case in the county asylums.[5] When the regulations governing all M A B establishments were revised in 1875, the Local Government Board (which had absorbed the Poor Law Board) attempted to make the imbecile asylums' admission rules more explicit by adding the directive: 'No dangerous or curable person such as would . . . require to be sent to a lunatic asylum shall be admitted'. The amended regulations also

---

[1] PLB regulations, issued in October 1870, laid down that admission to an M A B imbecile asylum required an order signed by a relieving officer or a workhouse master and a certificate by a district or workhouse MO. Signed authorization on behalf of the guardians of the patient's home parish was also required.

[2] See classification of M A B patients according to mental disorder in Appendix III, Tables G (a) and (b).

[3] 30 & 31 Vict. c. 6 s. 69 (1).

[4] See note on the Metropolitan Common Poor Fund, Appendix IV.

[5] Lunacy Commissioners' Twenty-first Report, 1868, p. 74.

stipulated that no pauper should be prevented from quitting the asylum, either by himself or in charge of a relative or friend, unless the medical superintendent certified that he was 'not in a proper state to leave the asylum without danger to himself or others', a proviso which appeared to be at variance with the rule excluding dangerous cases.[1]

So great was the demand for beds at Leavesden and Caterham during their first five years that extensions had to be carried out. By 1876 about £172,000 had been spent on Leavesden (1,995 beds) and £183,000 on Caterham (2,052 beds)[2]—a much lower cost per bed than that of any contemporary county asylum.

Outside London, the institutional care of the vast majority of the mentally disordered continued to be divided between the county asylums and the workhouses. By the beginning of 1870, the number of poor law mental cases—acute and chronic—in England and Wales had risen in a decade by about 36 per cent to over 46,500. Of this number, approximately 25,500 were in county asylums, 1,500 in registered establishments, and 11,500 in workhouses. The remainder were boarded out or resided with relatives. The opening of the M A B asylums in the autumn of 1870 reduced the total number of insane patients in workhouses by about one-third, but it soon began to rise again and maintained a steady upward trend in step with the general increase in the number of mental patients in other institutions.[3] By 1876, there were nearly 65,000 mentally disordered persons in England and Wales. Pauper lunatics totalled 57,400: of these 15,000 were in workhouses and upwards of 4,500 in the M A B asylums.

For much of the remainder of the century, the reform of lunacy legislation was pursued on two fronts. On the one hand, were those who demanded increasing safeguards for the liberty of the subject, and were represented by the Lunacy Laws Amendment Association. On the other hand, were those who were convinced that the inspection system effectively removed the risk of improper incarceration, and were concerned primarily that complicated certification procedures should not deprive the patient of early diagnosis and treatment. The medical view, endorsed by Lord Shaftesbury, was voiced by Dr. Henry Maudsley before the Select Committee set up in 1877 to study anew the lunacy laws. Maudsley told the committee that mental ill health should be treated in the same terms as other illness without the stigma of certification and pauperism. But fears for personal liberty overshadowed the progressive approach.

Nevertheless, in the perspective of a century of effort, substantial advances had been achieved, largely as a result of Shaftesbury's personal endeavour and the patient work of his fellow Commissioners and associates. These gains were consolidated in the Lunacy Act

---

[1] LGB amended regulations governing the M A B imbecile asylums, dated 10 February 1875, superseded those originally issued by the PLB in 1870, which were not accepted by the M A B. See Chapter 5 following.

[2] For further details of the cost of the M A B imbecile asylums, see Appendix IV, Table B.

[3] The *actual* increase in 'insanity' may well have been slight. The rise in the numbers of the registered insane was due to a variety of reasons, including the diminishing death rate, the discouragement of outdoor relief, improved systems of registration, the growing disinclination of the community to tolerate irregularities of conduct, and the relegation of the victims to institutions for family convenience.

of 1890,[1] five years following the great reformer's death. The Act fell far short of Shaftesbury's hopes, since it perpetuated the close association between lunacy and the poor law and stressed the custodial as against the medical aspects. It survived in large measure, nevertheless, as the lunacy law of this country for another seven decades.[2]

II

We have seen that, notwithstanding the overall confusion attaching to the terms 'lunatic', 'insane' and 'imbecile' in the nineteenth century, it was recognized that 'idiots' (approximately the present 'severely subnormal' group) constituted a separate class, with its own problems and needs.[3]

Before the advent of the M A B, relatively little provision existed in this country for the care and training of idiots and imbeciles, as such. Attempts to improve severely defective children were first made in France, stimulated by the work of Dr. Jean-Marc Itard, who in 1798 initiated the practical study of the psychology of defect with a treatise on his attempts to educate the 'wild boy of Aveyron'.[4] By 1840, Dr. Séguin, a pupil of Dr. Itard, was directing a regular idiots' department at the Bicêtre in Paris. In 1844, the first German State institution for the training of idiots was set up in Saxony; while about this time other institutions for the same purpose were founded on a voluntary basis in Germany, Switzerland and elsewhere in Europe and the United States. In England, Samuel Gaskell, who as medical superintendent of the Lancaster Asylum had taken a special interest in the idiot children there, drew attention in 1847 to the work being done at the Bicêtre.[5] The Lunacy Commissioners in their second report, issued in the same year, also made a point of focusing interest on congenital mental defectives. They pointed out that 'though persons of this description are seldom fit objects for a curative asylum, they are in general capable of being greatly improved, both intellectually and morally, by a judicious system of train-

[1] A new feature of the 1890 Lunacy Act was the introduction of the 'reception order' by a magistrate or court at some stage in all cases, in addition to medical certification.

[2] In this section, an attempt has been made to place in its historical context the origin of England's first State institutions for harmless chronic demented and subnormal patients. Only the outstanding landmarks in the evolution of State intervention in the field of lunacy have been cited. Fuller accounts of the history of services for the mentally disordered are to be found in most public health histories, in particular, in C. Fraser Brockington, *A Short History of Public Health* (1956), Chapter XIII. The following studies of Kathleen Jones are devoted to the subject: *Lunacy, Law and Conscience, 1744–1845* (1955) and *Mental Health and Social Policy, 1845–1959* (1960). Detailed commentaries on certain aspects and philosophies of this process of reform include, in particular, Ruth G. Hodgkinson, 'Provision for Pauper Lunatics, 1834–71', *Med. Hist.*, vol. x, no. 2, pp. 138–54; and Alexander Walk, '"On the State of Lunacy", 1859–1959', *J. Ment. Sci.*, vol. 105, no. 441, October 1959, and 'Mental Hospitals' in F. N. L. Poynter (ed.), *The Evolution of Hospitals in Britain* (1964). The author is greatly indebted to these scholars for enabling her to draw on the results of their researches.

[3] The distinction between mental illness and subnormality was recognized in the fourteenth century when different legal provisions were made for the control and disposition of the property of a 'born fool', or idiot, and that of a 'lunatic', that is, a person 'who hath had understanding, but by disease, grief or other accident hath lost the use of his reason'.

[4] J.-M. Itard, *The Wild Boy of Aveyron*, trans. G. and M. Humphrey (1932).

[5] Samuel Gaskell, 'Education of Idiots at Bicêtre', *Chambers Edin. J.* (1847), pp. 20, 71, 105.

ing and instruction. . . .' That same year, the first 'asylum for idiots' in this country was established at Park House, Highgate, through the efforts of the Rev. Andrew Reed, the philanthropist, supported by Samuel Gaskell and by John Conolly, the former medical superintendent of Hanwell Asylum and champion of 'non-restraint'. Expansion was soon found necessary, and after a temporary stay at Essex Hall, Colchester, the patients were moved in 1855 to the purpose-built Earlswood Asylum, Surrey. Later, Essex Hall was reopened as the Eastern Counties' Asylum (1859); and other charitable institutions for the care and training of the severely subnormal were founded at Starcross, Devon (1864); at Knowle, Warwickshire (1868); and at Lancaster (1870). In 1886, these establishments were accorded a recognized status when the registration of all charitable and private hospitals for idiots became compulsory.[1]

Round about 1870, the county asylums of Hampshire, Warwickshire and Northamptonshire built separate 'idiot blocks', intended to provide training for subnormal children and young persons received under the Lunacy Acts. But, as we shall see in the next section, the M A B was the only public authority during the nineteenth century to establish a complete institution devoted exclusively to this class of patient.

III

At first, children as well as adults were admitted to the Caterham and Leavesden Asylums, where classification on a clinical basis was at best haphazard. After a year or two, however, the medical superintendents urged the Asylums Board to separate the children from the adults. This was agreed, and in 1873 the first children left Caterham and Leavesden for Hampstead, where they were housed in the Board's temporary fever hospital. Teachers were appointed, and the experiment of educating idiot children began. In 1878, after a temporary move to a disused orphanage at Clapton in north-east London,[2] the children were brought to Darenth, Kent, where the Board had established a new institution, complete with classrooms, to accommodate about 560 young patients. But when these children reached the age of 16, most of them were still unfit for discharge. In order to spare them from the detrimental effects of associating once more with the chronic adult patients, the Board erected a separate institution adjacent to the schools, with accommodation for 1,000. This was opened two years later, in 1880. The scheme was to receive into the schools children from 5 to 16 years; to subject them to a special course of education and manual instruction; to retain the 'improvable' after the age of 16 for training in the workshops set up in the adjacent institution; and to transfer the more severely handicapped older children—by far the larger group—to the remaining part of the new building.

This was the first attempt by a statutory body in this country to develop the potentialities of subnormal children: it owed much to the energy of the medical superintendent, Dr. Fletcher Beach. Sir Henry Burdett, the authority on hospitals, was so impressed with the scheme that he advocated the creation of such training establishments throughout the

[1] The Idiots' Act, 1886.   [2] Now the Salvation Army Congress Hall.

country as special county asylums under the existing laws.[1] Similar vision was, unfortunately, obscured in Whitehall by the accumulation in the metropolitan workhouses of large numbers of adult imbeciles. As Leavesden and Caterham were filled to capacity, the central authority in desperation ordered the M A B to admit these cases into the Darenth institution. The original purpose of the training experiment was suspended, while the schools and the new work centre were filled with helpless and hopeless cases.

IV

Meantime, a movement had been set afoot in this country to press the need for statutory provision for the mentally subnormal under the local authorities. In 1876, the Charity Organization Society initiated a study of the problem, and the attention of the Government was drawn to its findings by Lord Shaftesbury. However, the only action taken was the passing of the Idiots' Act in 1886. This provided a simple procedure for the admission of defective patients to the existing charitable institutions, and authorized local destitution authorities to place in these institutions idiots for whom they were responsible.

It was generally accepted at this time that the primary object of institutional care for the mentally subnormal was the prevention of their perpetuation by segregation. But the policy of the Asylums Board had a wider intention. It aimed to develop the potentialities of patients and to train them towards a measure of self-support. By stimulating their interest in activity, it was hoped to increase their satisfaction in living. Attempts were made to occupy adult patients, according to their capacity, in supervised tasks connected with the upkeep of the establishments, the gardens and farms. This progressive aim proved for the most part an unattainable ideal, mainly because only a minority of patients were able to participate. A large number were senile, paralytic, or too severely handicapped to co-operate. For eight years following the suspension in 1880 of the training and classification schemes, the Asylums Board attempted to resurrect these plans, but was thwarted by the ever-increasing flow of helpless chronic cases from the workhouses. By 1888, however, it had been possible to build ten pavilions at Darenth for five hundred children of school age and to acquire a site at Tooting Bec on which to erect an infirmary for sick and aged patients.

Results at the new Darenth establishment for children, though not spectacular, were more encouraging than the outcome of the occupational schemes for adults. All the children were unpromising subjects on entry; few had had previous experience of systematic instruction. Within two years of the opening of the school in 1888, only a small proportion of the five hundred were found to be totally ineducable. The majority made a

---

[1] H. C. Burdett, *Hospitals and Asylums of the World*, vol. 1 (1891), p. 154. Sir Henry Burdett (1847–1920), one-time secretary of the Queen's Hospital, Birmingham, and vice-president of the Committee of the Seamen's Hospital, was an active figure in hospital politics. He published the *Nursing Mirror*, *The Hospital*, and *Burdett's Hospital Annual*. He is probably best known for his international study of institutions for the care of the sick: *Hospitals and Asylums of the World* (1891–93) (4 vols.).

degree of progress; some even attained fair standards in the elementary subjects they were taught; while over sixty deaf and dumb children were instructed to read and speak on fingers.[1]

During the 1890s—twenty or so years after the first attempts of the M A B to educate mentally defective children[2]—a few local education authorities were beginning to provide for the instruction of children with physical and mental disabilities. In 1893, following the recommendations of the Royal Commission on the Blind, Deaf and Dumb, appointed in 1889,[3] the Elementary Education (Blind and Deaf Children) Act empowered school authorities to pay for the education and maintenance of blind and deaf children in residential schools. As a result of a study by the Education Department in 1898 of systems of instruction for mentally defective children,[4] the 1899 Elementary Education (Defective and Epileptic Children) Act empowered school authorities to organize special classes for feeble-minded children, and, where necessary, to board them out and provide transport. By the end of the nineteenth century, these two permissive measures, together with the Idiots' Act of 1886, were the extent of State intervention, outside the poor law,[5] on behalf of the mentally defective as a class.

V

By 1900, the M A B asylums at Caterham, Darenth and Leavesden were providing for nearly 6,000 patients. During the three-decade period since their inception, they had admitted nearly 24,000 cases. Of these, approximately 6,000 were discharged: about 1,400 of these were described as 'recovered', about 1,500 as 'relieved', and a similar number as 'not improved'. Most of the other discharges were transferred to county asylums.[6] All adult patients were certified under the Lunacy Laws, whether demented, chronic insane or subnormal.[7] Admission to the M A B asylums was through the metropolitan guardians,

---

[1] For the curriculum at the Darenth school for mentally subnormal children in 1890 and an analysis of their performance, see Appendix III, Table F.

[2] During the 1890s, the term 'mentally defective' was becoming the more usual one for the whole 'subnormal' group, while the higher grades were becoming the subject of increasing attention and study under the designation 'feeble-minded': see chapter 14 following.

[3] *Report of the Royal Commission on the Blind, Deaf and Dumb of the U.K.*, 1889; BPP, 1889, vols. xix and xx [Cmd. 5781].

[4] *Report of the Departmental Committee on Defective and Epileptic Children*, 1898; BPP, 1898, vol. xxvi, 1 [Cmd. 8746].

[5] The Poor Law Amendment Act of 1867, s. 21, authorized guardians to provide for the reception, maintenance and instruction of blind, deaf and dumb adult paupers in any institution established for such purposes. An Act of 1862 had made similar provision for handicapped children. The 1867 Metropolitan Poor Act provided for London's mentally defective paupers—adults and children—inasmuch as they formed part of the broad category of 'harmless chronics' eligible for the M A B imbecile asylums.

[6] See Appendix III, Table A, for statistics of the Leavesden, Caterham and Darenth institutions for the period 1870–1899.

[7] The M A B did not insist on certification for idiot children under 16, as they relied on a statement made by the Lunacy Commissioners in 1890 that they would not proceed against persons taking charge of such

who made application, not only for patients who were actual paupers, but also for former self-supporting citizens who required poor relief because of their mental incapacity. All were pauperized by admission, whatever their status or means on entry. Originally, the main object of the M A B imbecile asylums was that they should serve as 'receptacles for harmless chronic insane paupers'. It had not been envisaged that they would be anything more than custodial. The special treatment and systematic training provided at Darenth, and to a lesser extent in their other institutions, were due entirely to the independent and progressive approach of the Asylums Managers and their medical staff.

---

children without certification (M A B *Mins.* vol. xxiv, 1890, p. 363). When the children reached the age of 16, the M A B obtained dispensation from the necessity of obtaining a Justice's order for their retention as decreed by the Lunacy Act, 1890, s. 23 (3).

CHAPTER 5

The MAB Infectious Disease Hospitals: The First Phase—1870 to 1878

I

WHILE the mental health branch of the Board's work could not escape the repressive power of the poor law, the M A B services for the infectious sick encountered forces which resulted in State intervention in the field of medical care *outside* the poor law. These developments altered the traditional criterion of hospital admission from *lack of means* to *need of treatment*, and evolved in four progressive phases.

During the relapsing fever epidemic of 1869–70, the only M A B hospital in use was the hurriedly-erected structure at Hampstead. While the Asylums Managers were dealing with this unexpected visitation, building operations were being accelerated on the new smallpox and fever hospitals at Homerton and Stockwell. In July 1870, when the four units—two for 'fever' and two for smallpox—were approaching completion and plans for staffing them had been submitted to the central authority, the Asylums Board learned with frustrated amazement that the Poor Law Board considered it 'expedient that the Managers should open one fever and one smallpox hospital only, in the first instance, and defer appointing staff for the other two institutions until the number of patients renders it necessary that these should be made use of.'[1] Only eighteen months had elapsed since the ill-timed suspension of hospital building at Hampstead. The Board had already appointed, from among its own members, a management committee for each of the four hospitals. The committees straightway combined to study the situation. 'Compliance with the Poor Law Board's suggestion would not only stultify the exertions of the Asylums Board over the past three years', they affirmed, 'but it would be entirely contrary to the spirit of the intentions of the Legislature in passing the Act of 1867.' The committees' joint report recapitulated the rationale upon which the planning had been based, and emphasized the danger to which patients would be exposed if obliged to travel from one side of the metropolis to the other to reach the only available fever or smallpox hospital. Early in the autumn of 1870, this report was sent to the Poor Law Board, supported by the information that some 250 pauper cases of typhus and typhoid had been admitted recently to the London

[1] PLB letter to the M A B, 23 July 1870.

49

Fever Hospital; that smallpox was already threatening the East End of London; and that the voluntary smallpox hospital at Highgate was rapidly filling.[1]

As an anti-climax to this warning plea for effective action, the Asylums Board received two voluminous sets of Poor Law Board regulations governing the administration of the M A B isolation hospitals and mental institutions.[2] They were almost identically worded and were suggestive of the regimen of a penitentiary.[3] The functions of each officer were set out with minute precision. Of the fifteen articles specifying the duties of the medical superintendent, one prescribed that he was 'to govern and control all the officers, servants and other persons employed in the "asylum"'. (The central authority referred to all the M A B hospitals as 'asylums', while the M A B reserved this term only for its institutions for the chronic insane.) The 'house superintendent', whose functions were explained in twenty-three articles, was 'required to be over twenty-five years of age and qualified to keep accounts'. The matron, whose duties were those of a housekeeper, was to be responsible for female domestic staff on and off duty, and for nursing staff only off duty. Nurses, while on the wards, were to be directly responsible to the medical superintendent.[4]

While the Asylums Board was considering these regulations, the smallpox epidemic, which had been sweeping Europe, was gaining on the metropolis. Since early in 1868, extensive outbreaks had occurred in such widely separated places as Vienna, St. Petersburg, Hamburg and Dublin. Early in the autumn of 1870 Paris was invaded and by the beginning of November two hundred cases were reported in the East End of London. In the absence of hospital accommodation, these remained in workhouses and crowded dwellings.

When a major visitation appeared inescapable, the Poor Law Board sanctioned the opening of all four hospitals at Homerton and Stockwell, and the temporary building at Hampstead, and urged the Asylums Managers 'to act in this instance with the same promptitude as was shown with so satisfactory a result in the case of the outbreak of relapsing fever'.[5] The Managers thereupon made direct contact with Sir John Simon, Chief Medical Officer of the Privy Council; and his assessment of the situation confirmed their worst fears.

> ... The mortality from smallpox in London has been steadily increasing during the present year [wrote Sir John Simon]. Whether its further extension can be prevented depends to a large extent upon the special measures, vaccination and isolation, which shall now be taken, but, from the sanitary condition ... of some of the districts of

[1] Joint report of the M A B Homerton and Stockwell Hospital Management Committees, sent to the PLB, 8 October 1870 (M A B *Mins.*, vol. ix, pp. 181–83).
[2] PLB orders to the M A B, 6 October 1870, later superseded by LGB order, 10 February 1875.
[3] The 1870 PLB regulations (article 10) directed that every 'pauper' should be searched on admission for prohibited articles. This and similar rules were never enforced by the M A B (see Chapter 12).
[4] PLB regulations, op. cit., section on 'Duties of Principal Officers'.
[5] PLB letter to the M A B, 22 October 1870.

London where smallpox is most prevalent, there is a great reason to fear that the disease will increase, and that the epidemic will equal that of 1866–67.[1]

The MAB immediately appointed a management committee for the Hampstead Hospital—the only institution yet available—and authorized it to make all necessary arrangements. The Poor Law Board was asked 'to authorise the committee to proceed in the matter without adhering to the regulations prescribed in ordinary cases'. On 1 December 1870, the Hampstead Hospital was re-opened and very soon it was filled with small-pox cases from every part of London. The East Grinstead Sisterhood again came to the Board's assistance and supplied all the nursing and domestic staff. Initially, the outbreak was most prevalent among women and children. Wards were allocated accordingly, and the eighteenth-century practice of encouraging mothers to accompany and nurse their sick children[2] was revived. When further accommodation was required, the makeshift building behind the London Fever Hospital (formerly used for the relapsing fever out-break) was transferred to the Hampstead site, where the main structure was extended. By this means, a total of 450 beds was achieved at a cost of £13,000. For two months this was the only isolation accommodation available to the MAB. Irate boards of guardians descended upon the Managers and described the appalling conditions in their districts, where the stricken were crowded in workhouses, chapels and vestry houses. The Shore-ditch guardians upbraided the Board for the insufficiency of its isolation accommodation and demanded that it should receive immediately one hundred smallpox cases and two hundred imbeciles.

On 31 January 1871, the MAB smallpox hospital at Stockwell was opened, followed the next day by that at Homerton. Questioned in the House of Commons shortly after-wards, the President of the Poor Law Board (Mr. Goschen) was obliged to admit that there were then well over 1,200 known cases of smallpox in the metropolis and that only about half of these were isolated in the MAB hospitals.[3] Although the Homerton and Stockwell smallpox hospitals were officially open, they were unable to function adequately owing to the difficulty of recruiting staff at the rates of pay stipulated by the Poor Law Board; and it became necessary to revert to the scales originally recommended by the Asylums Board. These included 10s. 6d. a week for nurses,[4] a rate considered excessive by the central authority. By the beginning of March 1871, the Board was obliged to ask the London Fever Hospital to receive all its fever cases in order that the two fever hospitals at Homerton and Stockwell might be used for smallpox patients. The disease was of a particularly viru-lent type with a 17 per cent case fatality rate. With 1,200 smallpox beds, the Board now hoped to keep pace with the demand, but the epidemic raged unabated.

[1] Letter from Sir John Simon, Privy Council Office, to the MAB, 17 November 1870.
[2] G. F. Still, *The History of Paediatrics* (1931), p. 420.
[3] *Hansard*, vol. cciv (3rd series), 16 February 1871, col. 372.
[4] See Appendix IV, Table K, for nurses' rates of pay at various periods from 1870.

II

There were now signs of concern at the Poor Law Board. Dr. John Henry Bridges, FRCP, was sent to confer with the M A B hospital management committees. This was the beginning of an association which was to prove long and fruitful. Formerly a factory inspector, Dr. Bridges had been persuaded in 1869 by Mr. Goschen, friend of his school-days, to accept the post of medical inspector at the Board. An apostle of the philosophy of Comte and the religion of Humanity, he was integrated into the machine which controlled the lives of the helpless poor. To his duties he brought dedicated energy and reforming zeal. If such a class as 'hereditary paupers' really existed, he blamed the system. Among members of the Asylums Board he found men after his own heart; but his position at the Poor Law Board was not a happy one. He was hampered by 'the necessity of educating his official superiors, by the deadening futilities of red tape and by the undercurrent of opposition provoked by his religious views'.[1]

In accordance with Dr. Bridges' advice, the Asylums Managers set about finding additional sites for temporary isolation accommodation, and negotiated with the parochial authorities for the loan of some seven hundred supplementary beds. Meantime, the lay administrators of the Poor Law Board were invoking their powers under section 18 of the 1867 Act. Taking independent action, they ordered the appropriation of an old building belonging to the Islington guardians. Further, without consulting the Asylums Board or their medical inspector, they negotiated with the Commissioners of Works to make available a six-acre site at Battersea and arranged with the War Department to erect a hospital for four hundred smallpox patients. The Asylums Board was then assured that 'these arrangements have not been actuated by any wish to interfere in the general discharge by the Managers of their responsible duties but merely by the desire to render them every possible assistance in the present emergency'. 'One of the main objects', it was asserted, 'has been to save as much time as possible.' To this, the Managers replied that they were 'unable to enter into any engagement to take over a building, of which the plans—altogether unknown to them—might be unsuitable for the purpose and involve a very large charge upon London ratepayers for a very short period of time.'[2] After inspecting the site and the plans with representatives of the Poor Law Board and the War Depart-ment, the Managers declared that they wished to have nothing whatever to do with the project. The cost of erecting the building was estimated at £20,000. At the rate of £50 a bed, it was considered 'very inferior in all respects to the Hampstead Hospital which, despite its piecemeal construction, had cost no more than £45 per bed.' The catalogue of inadequacies concluded with a critical comment on 'one of the more peculiar features—the dead-house', which the War Department planners had designed as an appendage to the main building!'[3] A very angry reply was received, emphasizing that the Poor Law

[1] S. Liveing, *A Nineteenth-Century Teacher: John Henry Bridges, MB, FRCP* (1926), Chapters X and XIII, *passim.*   [2] PLB letter to the M A B, 4 March 1871 and M A B reply, 6 March 1871.
[3] M A B *Mins.*, vol. iv (1870–71), pp. 433–34.

Board had 'gone out of its way to facilitate the operation of the Managers and to save time, an object of such extreme importance.' The communication ended with a threat to take action under section 15 of the 1867 Act. This was tantamount to resorting to a mandamus and forcing the Asylums Board to proceed with the projected hospital at Battersea.[1] On taking legal advice concerning the powers of the central authority in this connexion, the Managers were 'fortified in the opinion at which they had themselves arrived'.

The M A B, although not convinced of the need for additional accommodation, offered to build a 200-bed hospital on an alternative site; but efforts to purchase land at Peckham and West Brompton belonging to two of the dissolved 'sick asylum districts'— Newington and Kensington—proved unsuccessful, and the Managers were obliged to charter from the Admiralty the hospital ship *Dreadnought*,[2] lying off Greenwich. Next, the Islington guardians refused the Managers access to the building which the Poor Law Board had ordered them to appropriate. Shortly afterwards, without prior notice, it was abandoned with some seventy unattended patients in it. Twenty-four hours later, the M A B had transformed it into a 300-bed convalescent annex to the Hampstead Hospital, which was now accommodating five hundred acute cases.

Despite their tireless efforts in the public interest, the Asylums Managers were incurring opprobrium and loss of prestige. A letter appeared in *The Times* charging the Hampstead management committee with maltreatment of patients and insufficient food supplies at the hospital. The writers were three assistant medical officers whom the committee had recently dismissed for irresponsibility. Not only had they kept unlicensed fighting dogs on the premises, but they had neglected their duties to frequent the George Inn at the hospital gates, after their daily issue of strong ale had been reduced by the committee from six to two pints. The central authority ordered an enquiry into the charges made against the management committee. On the completion of the evidence produced by the former AMOs, the hearing was suspended, as the young doctors' funds were insufficient to enable Counsel to continue with the cross-examination of the Board's numerous witnesses. In order that the enquiry might be completed, the central authority was obliged to sanction the cost from public funds. Most of the charges were proved to be grossly exaggerated and to derive from the exceptional circumstances of the epidemic. There were, for instance, only thirty-four ordinary nurses to look after some eight hundred patients. Eventually, the Board was absolved as a result of the investigation.

Meantime, Hampstead ratepayers continued to harry the M A B concerning the smallpox hospital in their midst. The Managers, however, were resolved to stand their ground, come what may. In an effort to reduce the incidence of infection in the locality, they attempted—possibly with memories of the Broad Street pump[3]—to organize the 'yielding'

---

[1] PLB letter to the M A B, 9 March 1871.

[2] The *Dreadnought* was formerly used as the Seamen's Hospital.

[3] In 1854, there was a disastrous outbreak of cholera in the parish of St. James's, Westminster, hitherto a healthy area. John Snow (1813–58), one of the earlier medical writers who considered the possibility of bacterial infection as the cause of 'fevers', traced the cholera cases of St. James's to one pump in Broad Street. Having persuaded the parish council to remove the pump handle, the outbreak ceased.

of communal pumps in Hampstead on Sunday mornings, only to be confronted with complaints from the poorer residents.

III

As the four hospitals at Homerton and Stockwell were now filled to capacity, with beds in the corridors, tents were hired from the War Department. With an admission rate of about five hundred a week, the number of cases under treatment at the height of the epidemic reached two thousand. By the middle of 1871, however, the outbreak appeared to be under control, and the fever hospitals at Homerton and Stockwell were returned to their original use; the Islington workhouse was restored to the guardians; and the *Dreadnought* was handed back to the Admiralty. Thereafter, the outbreak persisted spasmodically until January 1873. It was estimated that, for the period of the epidemic, the M A B hospitals had been able to admit only about one-third of London's smallpox victims and that twice as many had died from the disease at home as in hospital. The smallpox mortality rate in 1871—the worst year of the epidemic—was the highest ever recorded for the capital. Of every million of the metropolitan population, 2,421 died from the disease,[1] compared with a rate of 1,012 per million for the whole of England and Wales.[2] This loss of life was attributed mainly to neglect of vaccination and to excessive gin-drinking. Urban areas on the continent, however, were even more severely ravaged. In Vienna, the 1871 rate of death from smallpox was 5,369 per million, while that in Hamburg reached 10,750 per million.[3]

The 1870–73 epidemic had brought into relief the nineteenth-century trend of smallpox to concentrate on the capital while receding from the provinces. It had also emphasized the changing age-distribution of the disease. Formerly, children had been the chief victims of smallpox. During the latter half of the eighteenth century, between 80 and 90 per cent of smallpox deaths were of children under five. But from about the time when death registration was introduced (1837), the disease began to kill many more older people.[4] Free infant vaccination from 1840 and its statutory compulsion in 1853 and 1868 almost certainly reduced mortality from smallpox amongst infants. At first, the change was gradual, and then it became more rapid during the 1870–73 epidemic.[5] Of the 16,000 smallpox cases admitted to the M A B hospitals during this period, less than 1,000 (approximately 6 per cent) were under five years, while, of the 3,000 fatalities, less than 500 (about 16 per cent) were in this age group.[6]

[1] See Appendix II, Table A.
[2] Registrar-General's Annual Report for 1871.
[3] E. J. Edwards, 'The German Vaccination Commission', *Trans. Epid. Soc. Lond.*, 5, 27, 1885–86, cited by Professor Ronald Hare in *Pomp and Pestilence* (1954), p. 84.
[4] A. H. Gale, *Epidemic Diseases* (1959: Penguin Books), p. 63; and F. M. Burnet, *Viruses and Man* (1953: Penguin Books), p. 161.
[5] In the period 1851–60, smallpox deaths of children under five years in England and Wales were 62 per cent of the total; in 1861–70, 54 per cent; and in 1871–80, only 30 per cent (A. H. Gale, op. cit., p. 63).
[6] M A B *Mins.*, vol. ix, 1876, pp. 678–79.

IV

In July 1871, the Poor Law Board had been superseded by the Local Government Board. Merged into the new ministry were three scattered departments: the Public Health Division of the Privy Council; the Local Government Act Division of the Home Office; and the Poor Law Board itself. The office of Permanent Secretary had been given to John Lambert, formerly assistant to Gathorne Hardy. Lambert was meticulous and dogmatically 'poor law-minded'. To him, the new 'asylums' were not so much therapeutic institutions, as gambits in the poor law policy of deterrence. They would, he believed, facilitate the segregation of able-bodied paupers in disciplined deterrent workhouses.[1]

Although reduced to a division, the old Poor Law Board dominated the new Department, and relations with the M A B remained unchanged. Despite the efforts of the Asylums Managers to keep in check the worst epidemic of the century, no word of approbation was received from the central authority. When, towards the end of 1872, the outbreak began to subside, the Managers intimated that they 'would have been gratified if the Local Government Board had more specially recognized the manner in which hospital staffs had performed their duties under unprecedented difficulties during a long and severe strain upon their powers', and forthwith addressed a tribute to their personnel.

V

The management committees had worked strenuously throughout the epidemic period. One or more meetings were held each week at the hospitals, while individual members supervised day-to-day administration. This visitation of unprecedented severity had created problems which demanded immediate resolution and had rendered impracticable the precise application of the Poor Law Board hospital regulations. The management committees accorded the medical superintendent supremacy in all medical matters and freedom to pursue his clinical duties, while the house superintendent, whom they preferred to call the 'steward', was given responsibility, under their general direction, for all the non-medical aspects of the establishment. Although the matron came within the spheres of responsibility of both the medical superintendent and the steward, the Managers found it convenient to deal with her direct as if she were head of an independent department.

Following the epidemic, the Managers continued the system to which they had become accustomed. Not only were the central authority's regulations found to be unworkable in practice, but they involved two fundamental principles which were questioned by the Managers. The first concerned control. Was the Asylums Board to be a mere tool of the central authority? Or was it to be allowed to manage the hospitals with due latitude for discretion? The second concerned the sick for whom the hospitals had been created. Were

[1] For details concerning the policies and personnel of the Local Government Board created in 1871, see R. Lambert, *Sir John Simon (1816–1904) and English Social Administration* (1963), pp. 524–28, and *passim*; and B. Abel-Smith, *The Hospitals, 1800–1948* (1964), pp. 85–88.

they patients or paupers? A number of incongruities were pointed out to the Local Government Board, with the suggestion that it should 'make the regulations more applicable to hospitals of the nature of those under the charge of the Asylums Board'. Nine months elapsed. At the end of 1872, the Managers received, with some consternation, an extensive schedule of 'amended regulations', in which 'some additional provisions of an important character have been inserted'.[1] Resentment mounted when it was realized that, if adhered to, these regulations would completely undermine the system of management which had been built up since the opening of the hospitals. Based on the assumption of remote control by management committees, the re-issued regulations retained the principle of medical superintendence. Assistant medical officers were to work under the direction of the medical superintendent in the wards, and the steward likewise in the administrative offices. The tenor of the regulations suggested that the Local Government Board was intent on placing the M A B establishments on the same footing as workhouse infirmaries and of reducing the power of the hospital Managers.

After two years of acrimonious correspondence, the M A B requested the central authority 'so to frame its regulations that they would not be at variance with existing practice'. It was made clear that 'regulations applicable to workhouse infirmaries would not be found suitable for the hospitals of the Managers, as some differences must occur consequent on the varying circumstances of the several institutions', and it was suggested that the central authority's regulations might be replaced by one order empowering the management committees to prescribe their own rules, subject to the sanction of the Asylums Board. The M A B communication continued:

> ... The Board believes that in all the large London hospitals the duties of the medical men are strictly confined to those of a medical character and they are sure that such an arrangement is a wise one; ... in some other institutions where a contrary plan has been tried, it is well known that the medical superintendent has become to all practical purposes a medical steward, leaving the treatment of the patients to the assistant medical officers.[2]

The next move was the issue by the Local Government Board, on 10 February 1875, of an order embodying revised 'General Regulations'. This was accompanied by a note declaring the unacceptability of the Managers' views upon the relative positions of the medical superintendent and the 'house superintendent', but deferring to their wishes to the extent of referring to the latter as the 'steward'. Concerning the term 'pauper', the Local Government Board affirmed that 'as all the persons admitted into the asylums are persons maintained at the expense of the poor rates, the term "pauper" is the correct one, and there is not sufficient reason for substituting "patient"'. Thereafter, the Asylums Board always referred to the 'patients' and the Local Government Board persisted for the next twelve years in using the term 'paupers'.

[1] LGB letter to the M A B, 13 December 1872.
[2] M A B letter to the LGB, 22 December 1874.

In the exchanges which followed the 1875 order, the M A B declared that, if the Local Government Board 'insist on maintaining these regulations in their integrity, the Managers must definitely repudiate for themselves and throw upon the Local Government Board the responsibility for any failure that may occur in the management of the hospitals'.[1] Eventually, some of the regulations were modified by an admixture of ambiguity. For instance, in an attempt to clarify the duties of the chief executive officers, the Local Government Board decreed that, while authority was to be divided between the medical superintendent and the steward, the former was to assume overall responsibility 'for the good order of the asylum', although 'it was not necessary for the medical superintendent to interfere with the departments of other officers'.[2]

The voluminous correspondence which grew up around the 'amended' regulations resulted in the Managers' working 'bible' becoming a vast compendium of mandatory commands, prohibitions and advisory injunctions. The Board accordingly detailed its general purposes committee to compile a consolidated version of these fragmentary and sometimes conflicting 'regulations'. Meanwhile, the acceptance of personal responsibility by committee members became even more deeply entrenched in the administrative system, and each hospital continued to be governed by an oligarchy—the management committee—and operated by a triumvirate—the medical superintendent, the steward and the matron.

VI

In view of the potential need for additional accommodation, the M A B acquired reserve sites for emergency use in Fulham (West Brompton) and Deptford (Old Kent Road). By the middle of 1875, however, these were still unused. The existing hospitals had sufficed for the increased demand for scarlet fever beds during the outbreak of the previous autumn and for the relatively few smallpox cases since the 1870–73 epidemic. The makeshift building at Hampstead, which for a while had housed the Board's subnormal children, was being prepared for eventual use as a permanent smallpox and fever hospital. This aroused local opposition in renewed strength. Numerous memorials were addressed to the M A B and to the Local Government Board. Residents of Haverstock Hill, near the hospital, found an alternative site in Mill Lane, and tried to impress the Managers and the President with its superior merits. This led to hostilities between two opposing factions of Hampstead ratepayers. One or other, or both, descended periodically upon the President of the Local Government Board, Mr. Sclater-Booth, who remained unimpressed. Towards the end of 1874, *The Times* reported that one such deputation

> . . . was headed by six Members of Parliament and included representatives of residents and local bodies and the Provost of Eton, who was interested in property in the neighbourhood. After several hours, there were some who still desired to say 'a word or

[1] M A B letter to the LGB, 13 February 1875.
[2] LGB letter to the M A B, 18 February 1875.

two', but even the excited deputation had grown weary of the repetitions, and loud hushes met some who still attempted to intervene between the chief of the department and his visitors. After the President had made a statement, some others wanted to speak but the President said the subject was exhausted, and the deputation then retired much dissatisfied.[1]

These demonstrations culminated in the appointment in June 1875 of a House of Commons Select Committee, headed by Mr. Sclater-Booth, 'to report upon the action of the M A B with regard to the establishment of a fever and smallpox hospital at Hampstead'. Exhaustive evidence was received by the Committee from the Managers and the inhabitants of Hampstead. In its report, the Committee affirmed that the action of the Asylums Managers had been 'strictly in accordance with their duties, powers and responsibilities, as derived from the 1867 Act and from the sanction and control of the Local Government Board, so far as it was incumbent on them to be guided by that department'. Furthermore, the Committee saw no reason 'why Hampstead should claim the interference of Parliament for the removal from it of an inconvenience to which it had become subject by reason of the due execution of the provisions of a wise and beneficent law'.[2] The Committee, which warmly commended the Managers for the great services they had rendered to the metropolis, submitted, for the consideration of the House, whether compulsory powers of purchase, with corresponding powers of compensation, should not be conferred upon the Board. All the London Members of Parliament voted against the report.

VII

As the Select Committee had suggested that administrative offices should be erected on the two unused sites owned by the Board, 'so that there should be no ground for complaint that Hampstead was unduly made use of for the cure of paupers coming from the south and west of London', the sites in Fulham and Deptford were accordingly prepared for the erection of hospitals when required. The demand was manifested sooner than was expected. By the autumn of 1876, about 150 cases of smallpox were admitted to the Homerton and Stockwell hospitals. At Hampstead, the conversion of the temporary structure into a permanent building had been started. The Local Government Board, nevertheless, ordered that it should be opened forthwith for the reception of smallpox cases. For the third time, the East Grinstead Sisterhood took over the nursing and domestic work of the hospital. No sooner had the central authority's instructions been acted upon, than legal proceedings were taken against the Asylums Board by Sir Rowland Hill, and other Hampstead residents, to recover damages 'for a nuisance arising from the use of the hospital at Hampstead for smallpox and other infectious diseases, and for causing the

---

[1] *The Times*, 11 December 1874.
[2] *Report of the House of Commons Select Committee on the M A B Hospital at Hampstead, 1875*: BPP, 1875, vol. x (363), 643.

assemblage in the neighbourhood . . . of large numbers of persons suffering from such diseases. . . .' As the epidemic spread, it became necessary once more to use the fever hospitals for smallpox patients and to erect huts in the grounds of the Homerton and Stockwell establishments. In Dod Street, Limehouse, a private factory was taken over to accommodate severe cases occurring in the locality. This and other thoroughfares were marked off with plague flags as infected areas.

In August 1876, as the demands upon the Board's accommodation were mounting in a menacing manner and problem after problem presented itself, the Local Government Board sent a lay inspector to visit the hospitals. He discovered the 'consolidated' version of the central authority regulations, which had been issued to recently appointed staff. The verbal exchanges which ensued between the inspector and members of the management committees were followed by an official reprimand.

> The [Local Government] Board learn from their inspector [it read] that the officers of the asylums . . . have been supplied with certain rules printed by the Managers . . . purporting to be a consolidation of the regulations in force, but differing in many important respects from those issued by the [Local Government] Board. . . . The remarks of the committee to the effect that 'they can hardly believe that the Board will treat their Managers with such scant courtesy and so little confidence as to upset the system of management which they are desirous of perpetuating' appear to the Board to have no real foundation when regard is had to the concessions which were made in deference to the wishes of the Managers. . . .[1]

The Asylums Board retorted that the Local Government Board, in issuing its recent regulations, had acted unwisely for the public interests and that 'unless the policy which has dictated this line of treatment is altered, it will be impossible for the Managers to act with the Local Government Board in the same spirit of harmony as they have hitherto done'. The communication concluded by pointing out that, if the central authority

> . . . initiated what was to be done, the Managers merely giving effect to its directions, the result will probably be that this Board, hampered by the misguided regulations laid down by the Local Government Board, will be far less efficient for the good service of the inhabitants of the metropolis, and the public will learn how impossible really good work is when it is subject to the centralizing influence which the Local Government Board, through its officials, is so constantly exerting.[2]

In November 1876, a reply, signed by Sir John Lambert, reminded the Managers that

> . . . the Legislature has imposed on the Local Government Board the duty and responsibility of issuing such general regulations as they may deem proper for the good government of the Metropolitan District asylums, as well as of other Poor Law

[1] LGB letter to the M A B, 8 August 1876.
[2] M A B memorandum to the LGB, 20 October 1876.

establishments; acting under a sense of this responsibility, the President regrets that he cannot sanction the perpetuation by formal orders of a dual system of government, but must maintain the principle of unity of authority and the general supremacy of one superintendent.[1]

The Asylums Managers replied that they

... certainly do not wish for a dual system of government in their institutions. They have hitherto had unity of management, but that unity has consisted in the Managers themselves, by their several committees, being the real governing power. ... For a series of years this system has worked in all respects well and it must be a source of regret that the Local Government Board should now insist on its alteration.[2]

Sir John Lambert reiterated that

... the [Local Government] Board are distinctly of opinion that they would not be justified in sanctioning ... the principle of co-ordinate officers acting under the direction of the committee of management as it is obvious that gentlemen who may at any time seek to withdraw from their voluntary work cannot be held responsible for the order and discipline of the asylums in the same manner and degree as paid officers.[3]

By this time, Sir John Lambert had subjugated the medical element at the Local Government Board and was wielding undisputed power.[4] 'The office blunders on in the same dull, groping way', wrote Dr. J. H. Bridges in a personal letter in 1876,[5] while remaining a frustrated outsider in this controversy. Dr. William Brewer, who had earlier denounced the central poor law authority in the House of Commons as 'practically irresponsible' and its policy as 'notoriously fitful',[6] refused to be coerced by Sir John Lambert. And the system of personal supervision by committee members and day-to-day administration by the executive trio persisted unchanged in the M A B hospitals for many years to come.

Meantime, the Board had been planning the erection of hospitals on the two new sites in Fulham and Deptford to keep pace with the increasing demand for smallpox beds. Once again, after official approval of plans had been tardily granted and construction was in progress, the Local Government Board decided to limit the building programme to one hospital. The end of 1876 found the M A B hospitals with some five hundred smallpox cases and no sign of the outbreak receding. The Managers accordingly decided to proceed with building on both sites and to press meantime for permission to complete the two

---

[1] LGB letter to the M A B, 2 November 1876.
[2] M A B letter to the LGB, 16 November 1876.
[3] LGB letter to the M A B, 9 March 1877.
[4] Sir John Lambert had been instrumental in the eclipse of Sir John Simon, Chief Medical Officer of the LGB, and of his plans for the advancement of State medicine. (R. Lambert, *Sir John Simon* ... op. cit., pp. 573–75).
[5] S. Liveing, op. cit., p. 210.   [6] *Hansard*, vol. cc (3rd series), 25 April 1870, col. 1771.

units. The central authority eventually relented, and in March 1877 the Deptford and Fulham hospitals were opened, the former with thirteen, and the latter with ten, thirty-bed pavilions.

London was now at the height of the second smallpox visitation of the 'seventies. Characterized by an unprecedented proportion of haemorrhagic cases, it was regarded as the strongest analogy to the Black Death of the fourteenth century which had been witnessed since that time. During the epidemic period—from the second half of 1876 until the end of 1878—the M A B hospitals treated some 13,000 smallpox patients with a case fatality rate of about 19 per cent.[1] Outside the hospitals, the metropolitan rate of mortality from smallpox during 1877, the worst year of the outbreak, was 709 per million, compared with 2,421 per million for the record year of 1871.[2] The fact that about half of the deaths occurred in hospital, compared with about one-third during the previous outbreak, suggested that the traditional fear of hospitals was giving place to an appreciation of institutional medical care, despite the pauper stigma and disenfranchisement which entry to an Asylums Board institution entailed.

When founded, the M A B 'asylums' had been intended solely for the destitute sick. But during periods of pestilence, the wage-earning poor, as well as patients of other social classes, applied direct to the hospitals for admission. On medical and public health grounds, it was obviously inadvisable to turn them away. Many were dying and all were potential centres of infection. The medical superintendents admitted them. The Managers, appreciating the practical difficulties and futility of discriminating between the destitute and other patients, supported their medical staff, and then sought legal sanction for their action. Their representations eventually resulted in a modification of the official regulations, and medical superintendents were empowered to admit any patient who arrived without the required documents 'in such a condition that a refusal to admit him . . . might be attended with dangerous results'.[3] No poor law requirement could override the wisdom of defending both patient and public from the dangerous consequences of non-admission. Every case of fever or smallpox applying to the hospitals direct, instead of through the poor law authorities, was therefore regarded as an 'emergency' under the modified regulations. When it became apparent that a large proportion of patients were not of the class habitually relieved from the rates, the question of statutory provision to cover non-pauper maintenance charges had to be considered. An ingenious form of words was, therefore, inserted into the Divided Parishes and Poor Law Amendment Act of 1876 which made it possible, by implication, for such charges to be waived. In the case of a non-pauper being admitted into an M A B hospital 'under stress of urgency', the Board was authorized to exercise 'in respect of the recovery of all reasonable charges incurred', the 'like powers . . . as are conferred by the Poor Law Acts upon guardians over a pauper for the recovery of relief

---

[1] See Appendix II, Table B.   [2] Ibid., Table A.

[3] LGB regulations dated 10 February 1875, section ii, article 4. For admission to an M A B isolation hospital, a patient required an order signed by a poor law relieving officer and a certificate signed by a district or workhouse medical officer.

given ... by way of loan...'.[1] For the first time, non-paupers were provided for under the poor law. The initial statutory step was thus taken towards the provision of free isolation accommodation for all in need of treatment.

The proportion of non-pauper patients treated in the M A B hospitals during the 1876–78 smallpox outbreak was even higher than it had been during the earlier epidemic. In the hospitals' first eighteen months—up to mid-1872—of 16,459 admissions, only 4,792 had been in receipt of poor relief when sickness had overtaken them. Some 71 per cent therefore, were not paupers on admission. Of these, it was known that at least 235 had been admitted without the necessary relieving officers' orders; and the cost of maintenance—one shilling and threepence a day—had been recovered from 191.[2] When the 1871 census was taken, it was found that 82 per cent of the 223 male patients in the Hampstead Hospital were in regular gainful employment when admitted. Of these self-supporting patients, more than one-half were skilled artisans and well over one-fifth were 'white-collar' workers.[3] During the second smallpox epidemic, all M A B patients were asked (15 February 1877) whether they had ever before received poor relief. Only 10 per cent admitted that they had.[4] It appeared, therefore, that the vast majority were paupers in legal theory only.

VIII

The illusion persisted at the Local Government Board, nevertheless, that the practice of admitting non-pauper patients to the M A B hospitals was 'altogether exceptional'.[5] The sanitary authorities were circularized at the beginning of 1877 concerning their re-

---

[1] 39 & 40 Vict. c. 61 s. 42.   [2] See Table 1 at end of chapter.
[3] Report of Dr. Robert Grieve, Medical Superintendent of Hampstead Hospital, 15 April 1871 (M A B Mins., vol. v, pp. 39–41). The occupations of male patients were classified as follows:

Non-Paupers:		Paupers:	
Professional	6	Labourers	35
Master Tradesmen	2	Costermongers	3
Railway and Post Office		No occupation	2
Officials, etc.	8		
Shopmen and Clerks	24		
Domestic Servants	3		
Barmen, Waiters, etc.	9		
Skilled Artisans	94		
Omnibus Drivers,			
Carmen, Stablemen	26		
Porters	9		
Seamen	2		
	183		40

[4] Report of M A B general purposes committee, 22 February 1877 (M A B Mins., vol. x, p. 825).
[5] LGB Sixth Annual Report, 1876–77 (Cmd. 1865), HMSO, 1877, p. xxxiii.

sponsibility for non-destitute patients, and it was emphasized that the M A B hospitals were exclusively for paupers.[1] Replies from the local authorities showed that they could not, or would not, provide isolation accommodation for paying patients, which they were empowered to do under the 1866 Sanitary Act. The difficulty of obtaining sites, and fear of local opposition, were among their practical problems. Some of them appealed direct to the M A B, pointing out that, as the Board dealt with infectious disease among one class of the community and was supported out of the rates, an extension of its powers to enable it to deal with all classes would be more favourable to the sanitary and financial interests of London than would any separate action taken by the local authorities themselves.

A decade had passed since the creation of the M A B, and it now commanded some 2,000 isolation beds in five relatively equidistant units encircling the metropolis,[2] but in an epidemic these would be quite inadequate for London's 3·6 millions. Other hospital accommodation in the capital was still deficient, although it had increased to some extent during the past ten years. While the number of special beds of one kind and another remained about 3,000,[3] the bed complement of the general (voluntary) hospitals had risen to about 5,000,[4] and the workhouse infirmaries were providing more than twice that number.[5]

The M A B realized that the local authorities were trying to divest themselves of their statutory responsibilities. Nevertheless, their suggestions were considered with more than objective interest. The Board appreciated the folly of restricting fever hospitals to one section of the community and hoped to be empowered to provide isolation accommodation for the whole of the metropolis. Within the M A B system existed the means for merging poor law and public health requirements, but impediments to such integration persisted at the Local Government Board.[6] During the last phase of the old Poor Law Board, however, a flicker of hope had been kindled in this direction by Mr. Goschen's lip service to the wisdom of making medical services available to 'the poorer classes generally as distinguished from actual paupers'. He expressed the view that 'perfect accessibility to medical advice and free medicine at all times under thorough organization ought to be considered so important in themselves as to render it necessary to weigh with the greatest care all the reasons which might be adduced in their favour.'[7] These words were written

---

[1] Ibid. LGB circular to metropolitan vestries and district boards, 2 January 1877.
[2] See Map I, following Appendix IV (location of M A B hospitals in 1877).
[3] *Trans. NAPSS*, 1882, pp. 433–36; and *Lancet*, II, 16 July 1881, pp. 78–82.
[4] Ibid. See also Table I, Chapter I.   [5] See Table 2 at end of chapter.
[6] The civil servants of the P.L. Division of the LGB assumed that control of the poor law was the most important of all the civil functions of the government. They even continued to file all documents on whatever matter—sanitation or poor relief—according to poor law districts, a practice which subsisted until the advent in 1919 of the Ministry of Health (S. and B. Webb, *English Poor Law History*, op. cit., Vol. I, Chapter III).
[7] *PLB Twenty-Second Annual Report*, 1870, pp. xliv–xlv. At this time, there were estimated to be some 173,000 poor law patients in the country, of whom 54,000 were actually under medical treatment in poor law institutions (see H/C Returns 4 of 1867–68; 445 of 1868; and H/L 216 of 1866). This number was estimated by the Webbs (op. cit., p. 322) to be about one-fourth of *all* persons in England and Wales simultaneously under medical treatment, either at their own expense or paid for by charity or the poor rate.

into the Poor Law Board's annual report for 1870, compiled while London was suffering near-paralysis from the greatest smallpox epidemic it had ever known—a situation which could have been mitigated, if not averted, by the operation of such a free health service. The 1876–78 epidemic provided yet further evidence of the need for more comprehensive health services to protect the public from ill-controlled pestilence. In Ireland since 1851, all 'poor persons' who were sick had a right to free advice and medicine and it was not deemed poor relief.[1] But in England it was held that 'people must not be encouraged to be ill by the knowledge that they could be treated free at the expense of the State.'

The Asylums Board was determined to represent the need for encouraging all classes of the community to seek isolation when stricken with infectious disease. The reports of its management committees and medical superintendents urged that the central authority should be pressed to meet this need by providing a central hospital service for paying and non-paying patients alike, linked with a system of compensation for those who suffered financially by submitting to isolation for the benefit of the community. Typical of these reports, which were communicated to the Local Government Board with relentless regularity, was one from the management committee of the M A B Homerton Hospital in 1878, describing the impact of smallpox on the capital:

> . . . Smallpox has very seriously disturbed the health and comfort of the dwellers of London twice during the past seven years; it has not only destroyed a large number of lives which might have been saved, but has put the ratepayers to an immense expense for the maintenance of patients in the hospitals. Notwithstanding these deplorable results, and the lessons they teach, the same state of things is allowed to continue, year after year; no measures of a comprehensive character suited to the wants of this vast metropolis are being taken to arrest the ravages of the disease, beyond the mere sending of 50 or 60 per cent of the cases to the hospitals for paupers, while the remaining cases are permitted to stay in their own homes spreading the infection in every direction, and thus keeping the epidemic alive.[2]

The medical superintendent of the M A B Fulham Hospital emphasized

> . . . the need for encouraging the enormous class above the very poor to seek hospital treatment when suffering from disease, as well as the class of minor tradesmen who are focal centres of infection. Are the existing hospitals [he asked] to be utilised for all classes? Are the parishes to multiply infectious disease hospitals ad infinitum? Or are things to remain as they are, incompletely constituted?[3]

---

[1] Under the Medical Relief Charities Act of Ireland, 1851, any 'poor person' had the right to free advice and medicine. Each poor law union was divided into Dispensary Districts under the board of guardians, and the dispensary medical officers acted *ex officio* as medical officers of health under the sanitary authorities.

[2] Report of the Management Committee of the M A B Homerton Hospital, February 1878 (M A B *Mins.*, vol. xii, pp. 86–91).

[3] Report of Dr. Thomas C. Fox, Medical Superintendent, M A B Fulham Smallpox Hospital, 1 November 1877 (M A B *Mins.*, vol. xi, pp. 553–62).

The medical superintendent of the Board's Hampstead Hospital wrote:

> ... I hope the time will come when admission to these hospitals shall be freely asked and as easily obtained and when the burden of pecuniary loss borne for the safety of others can be distributed among those who enjoy safety. . . . That coming generations will look upon smallpox as a matter of tradition is perhaps too much to expect. . . .[1]

Lest it should escape the notice of the Local Government Board that the M A B lacked neither the willingness nor the vision to assume the role of London's central hospital authority for infectious diseases, it detailed its general purposes committee to formulate specific recommendations in the light of the local boards' attitudes concerning isolation hospital provision. It appeared that five of the thirty vestries and district boards had made some attempt to use their statutory powers to provide hospital accommodation; seven said they possessed no facilities; six advocated the creation of a central board for all infectious disease hospitals; and the remainder assumed, erroneously, that it was the duty of the Asylums Board to make provision for all cases.

As it was obvious that adequate provision for the isolation and treatment of epidemic disease in the metropolis did not exist, the M A B general purposes committee submitted the following recommendations:

(a) That such provision could be best made in a comprehensive manner by one central authority acting for the whole metropolis, not only for pauper patients but for other classes desirous of hospital accommodation;

(b) That such central authority should not be merely a department of poor law administration, but should have the powers of the Sanitary Acts conferred upon it;

(c) That either the M A B should be merged into such central authority or should itself be that authority, in which case its constitution should be altered and adapted to its enlarged duties and responsibilities.[2]

The central department was requested to give these suggestions urgent consideration, and local boards were invited to submit their views. It was clear from their replies that most of them were generally in favour of a central hospital authority, though some were averse to having 'the powers of the Sanitary Acts conferred upon it'.

Evidence of response—albeit ineffectual—on the part of the central authority appeared in two clauses inserted into the Public Health (Metropolis) Bill,[3] introduced into Parliament late in the 1876–77 session. These empowered, but did not compel, local authorities, either to combine for hospital purposes, or to contract with the Asylums Board for the reception of their non-pauper cases. The Bill was dropped; but in any case it would have done little to solve the problems of the M A B. While free from disease, the sanitary districts, as

---

[1] Report of Dr. Samuel Bingham, Medical Superintendent, M A B Hampstead Smallpox Hospital, for 1876–78 (M A B *Mins.*, vol. xiii, pp. 256–86).
[2] Report of the M A B general purposes committee, 22 February 1877 (M A B *Mins.*, vol. x, pp. 824–25).
[3] Public Health (Metropolis) Bill (No. 187), session 1876–77, clauses 56 and 64.

hitherto, would have done nothing to provide for their paying patients. In an epidemic, the measure would have imposed on the Board the moral responsibility of providing for all classes, whilst, in the absence of prior knowledge of probable requirements, it would have been unable to make adequate arrangements. Meantime, the local authorities, only too willing to take advantage of medical ethics and legal loopholes, went on sending their infectious cases to the M A B hospitals.

The Board continued to plan for the role of metropolitan public health authority with special responsibility for isolation accommodation, but, as the second smallpox epidemic of the 'seventies was subsiding, its aspirations suffered a temporary eclipse. On 29 November 1878, judgment against the M A B was given by Mr. Baron Pollock in the Hampstead Hospital law suit. After a trial lasting eleven days, the jury decided that the hospital, as hitherto used, was a legal nuisance, both in its incidence and in itself; and an injunction was issued for its closure.[1] With characteristic resilience, the Managers straightway proceeded to negotiate for a new trial.

This initial phase in the development of the M A B hospitals illustrated conclusively that the application of poor law principles and practice to infectious disease was a practical failure, even if it persisted as a legal fiction. Nevertheless, an initial—but as yet ineffective—step had been taken towards uniting in the hospital ward the 'two nations' which poor law policy perpetuated in English society.

[1] 4 QBD 433 (Hill *versus* Metropolitan Asylum District).

TABLE 1

**Cases received into the M A B Infectious Disease Hospitals from the date of opening
(between December 1870 and March 1871) up to 24 June 1872**

Hospital	Date of Opening	Total Number of cases received	Number of cases on the MOs' list, or otherwise in receipt of relief immediately before orders for their admission were given	Number of cases admitted without an order from the Relieving Officer
Hampstead	1 Dec. 1870 (for smallpox)	7,276		78
Homerton Smallpox	1 Feb. 1871	2,684		not known[1]
Homerton Fever	15 Feb. 1871	1,706		37
Stockwell Smallpox	31 Jan. 1871	2,641	4,792	120
Stockwell Fever	6 March 1871	1,858		not known[2]
	27 Dec. 1871) (after reopening for smallpox)	294		
Totals:		16,459	4,792	235[3]

[1] It was stated that relieving officers' orders were received *following* the reception of patients at the Homerton Smallpox Hospital.

[2] Number of cases admitted without orders prior to 27 December 1871 (when it was reopened for smallpox) not known but of 294 patients received after that date, 11 at least were granted *after* the admission of the patients.

[3] In 191 of these cases the cost of maintenance was repaid, amounting to £258 16s. 0d.

Source: House of Commons Return of M A B Fever and Smallpox Hospitals, 9 August 1872: BPP, vol. xlix, 1872 (424) 581.

TABLE 2

Metropolitan Workhouse Infirmary Accommodation in the late 1870s

Parish in which the Infirmary was situated	Parish to which the Infirmary belonged	Number of patients for whom accommodation was provided
Battersea	Wandsworth and Clapham	380
Bromley (Middlesex)	Poplar and Stepney	586
Camberwell	Camberwell	232
Chelsea	Chelsea	272
Chelsea	St. George's	776
St. George in-the-East	St. George in-the-East	307
Greenwich	Greenwich	247
Hackney	Hackney	322
Islington	Holborn	617
Islington	Islington	540
Kensington	Kensington	438
Kensington	St. Marylebone	744
Lambeth	Lambeth	622
St. Leonard, Bromley, and Mile End Old Town	London, City of	645
Newington	St. Saviour	1,010
Plumstead	Woolwich	213
Rotherhithe	St. Olave	180
Shoreditch	Shoreditch	470
St. Pancras	Strand and Westminster	523
St. Pancras	St. Giles and St. George (Bloomsbury), and St. Pancras	281
Whitechapel	Whitechapel	689
		Total: 10,094

Sources: Transactions: National Association for the Promotion of Social Science, 1882, p. 437; and the *Lancet,* 16 July, 1881, p. 80.

CHAPTER 6

The M A B Infectious Disease Hospitals: The Second Phase—1879 to 1886

I

THE next eight years saw radical changes in the epidemiological work of the M A B. These stemmed mainly from the revelation of deficiencies in the 1867 Metropolitan Poor Act which left the Board unprotected from the exigencies of common law; and from the investigations which ensued concerning the local impact of the M A B hospitals, their limitations and the demands made upon them. From these emerged improved measures of smallpox control and the prospect of escape from the grip of the poor law.

Despite the recession in the recent epidemic, the Board's isolation hospitals received some 3,600 smallpox patients during the years 1879 and 1880. During this period the number of London deaths from the disease reached nearly one thousand.[1] This level of mortality was attributed in the main to three factors: the lax administration of the metropolitan public health authorities; legislative anomalies which limited the class of patient legally admissible to the M A B hospitals; and the apparent disinclination of the government to remedy these defects.

The local authorities were constantly asking the M A B to accept their infectious non-pauper patients, and when informed by the Board that it was not legally empowered to do this, they suggested that the M A B should set up a separate department for the reception of such cases. On soliciting the views of the metropolitan vestries and district boards, the M A B learned that all but four were in favour of such an arrangement. A summary of these replies was sent to the Local Government Board, with the suggestion that an investigation should be made into the causes and conditions which had protracted the recent smallpox epidemic. No reply was received, but the Poor Law Amendment Bill, introduced into Parliament in the summer of 1879, included the provision—inserted three years before into the aborted Public Health (Metropolis) Bill—for empowering metropolitan sanitary authorities to contract with the M A B for the reception of their non-destitute patients. The Asylums Managers, who had not been consulted beforehand, represented to the Local Government Board, as they had done repeatedly in the past, that a more precise and

[1] See Appendix II, Tables A and B.

obligatory directive to the local authorities was required in order to ensure that adequate provision could be made for their patients. Beyond an acknowledgment, no further notice was taken of the Managers' protest, and the permissive provision passed into law.[1]

Responsibility for the destitute was clearly laid down in numerous statutory instruments under the poor law, but there was some ambiguity concerning the legal obligations of local authorities towards their independent poor when sick. Infectious non-pauper patients were not admissible into the sick wards of a workhouse except upon a Justice's Order under the 1875 Public Health Act.[2] However, if an infectious patient, though not utterly destitute, was without the means of obtaining medical attendance and nursing, it devolved upon the poor law authorities to supply 'the requisite relief'. If the patient had the necessary means and required to be removed to a hospital for isolation only, it devolved upon the sanitary authority, and not upon the guardians, to provide the accommodation. But, if the means of that patient became exhausted while he was isolated and the sanitary authority was unwilling to bear the cost of his maintenance in hospital, the 'non-pauper' patient's new state of destitution obliged the guardians to play their role under the poor law and to reimburse the sanitary authority from the poor rate.[3] This procedure—applicable to voluntary and local authority hospital admissions—varied slightly in the case of admittance to the M A B institutions, since no payment was exacted on entry, even if the patient was in a position to pay. The poor law guardians of the patient's locality were notified, and it was for them to use their legal machinery to investigate his means and to recover maintenance costs where possible.[4] In the stress of an epidemic, it was obviously impossible to discriminate between the non-destitute who could not afford medical necessities and those who could afford them and required isolation only. Practical difficulties thus impeded the satisfactory outcome of contractual or statutory provision for the care of the non-destitute suffering from infectious disease.

Having already estimated, by direct enquiry or by census returns, that between 70 and 90 per cent of their patients during the two earlier epidemics were not habitual paupers, the Asylums Managers made another attempt to assess the proportion of non-pauper admissions in 1880, when there was a recrudescence of smallpox. Local guardians were asked to report on the cases in which they had managed to recover all or part of the maintenance costs. On this basis, the proportion of 'non-paupers' was very low, ranging from 0·5 to 3·6 per cent, according to the locality of the hospital. Nevertheless, the proportion of patients who had not previously received public assistance was still substantial, varying from 78 to 93 per cent in the different institutions. In the existing state of the law, however,

[1] 42 & 43 Vict. c. 54 s. 15.
[2] 38 & 39 Vict. c. 55 s. 124.
[3] Glen's *Poor Law Orders* (11th edn., 1898), p. 274.
[4] The financial aspects of M A B hospital administration are described in Chapter 13.
It was not the duty of the M A B to distinguish between patients of the pauper class and others. Boards of guardians were the sole relief authorities to whom the legislature had delegated the responsibility and legal machinery for enquiring into the means of applicants for poor relief. (M A B letter to the City of London Guardians, 8 January 1883: M A B *Mins.*, vol. xvi, p. 798.)

once these self-supporting citizens entered the M A B hospitals for isolation and treatment, they were relegated to the pauper class and deprived of their civil rights. So far as the sanitary authorities were concerned, the law allowed them every means for evading their responsibilities. The only non-pauper cases which the M A B hospitals were legally empowered to accept, apart from the 'emergency' cases, were those for whom contracts were concluded at the voluntary instigation of the local authorities under the 1879 Poor Law Act. But, as the current irregular practices involved them in no financial commitments, the sanitary authorities made no contracts. The M A B hospitals, therefore, continued to treat, without statutory sanction and as a charge on the poor rate, a substantial number of patients who were legally the responsibility of the local authorities. Although the Board's position concerning this class of patient was slightly modified in legal theory, in practice it remained unchanged.

II

While the 1879 Poor Law Act was ineffective in extending the availability of the M A B hospitals to patients outside the pauper class, it nevertheless gave to the Board new powers to provide for patient transport. As early as 1818, a Select Committee had recommended a system for conveying infectious patients in the metropolis 'which would prevent the use of coaches or sedan chairs'.[1] Apart from the use of a hand litter by the 'House of Recovery' (as the London Fever Hospital was then called), no special means for removing the infectious sick existed in the metropolis, and the spread of infection remained unchecked. By 1867, nothing had been done to improve the situation. When the Metropolitan Poor Bill was being debated, it was proposed that provision should be made in the Bill for the allocation of a 'hospital carriage' to each of the projected 'asylums', but Gathorne Hardy expressed his belief that 'this most excellent suggestion' would be carried out under the clause providing for 'all necessary fixtures, furniture and conveniences'.[2] His successors, it seems, had not shared this assumption. Since the opening of the M A B hospitals, poor law patients had been moved in vehicles owned or hired by the parochial authorities. Old street cabs were frequently used and when not required these were often kept in mews alongside traders' carts. On occasion, the guardians arranged for discharged fever patients to be brought back from hospital in vehicles which had been used for smallpox admissions. Sometimes relatives accompanied the patient and made the return journey by public transport. For nearly a decade, the Asylums Managers protested to the guardians and to the central authority concerning these practices. Although the Board had refrained from suggesting that it should operate an ambulance service of its own, the Local Government Board made it clear that the M A B had no legal right to undertake the conveyance of the sick. In reply, the M A B described the unfortunate conditions which resulted from the

[1] *Report of the Select Committee appointed to examine the state of contagious fever in the metropolis*, 1818 (BPP, 1818, vol. vii, 332).

[2] *Hansard*, vol. clxxxv (third series), cols. 1697–98; 30 & 31 Vict. c. 6 s. 20.

lack of an organized system of patient transport during the current prolonged epidemic, and concluded:

> ... This is not the way to stamp out the epidemic. ... Unless more energy is displayed, the unspeakable miseries inflicted by it, not only on individuals but on whole families, will continue to be a scandal to the metropolis.[1]

A year later, the M A B was empowered under the 1879 Poor Law Act 'to provide and maintain carriages suitable for the conveyance of persons suffering from any infectious disorder'.[2]

III

Such hopes of improvement in the Board's status as the 1879 Act had raised were overshadowed at this juncture by anxiety concerning the outcome of the Hampstead Hospital law suit. In May 1879, however, after a three days' hearing, the Queen's Bench Division made an order dissolving the injunction to close the hospital and granted a new trial, with a direction that the costs of the first suit—in November 1878—should abide the result of the new trial.[3] By this time, Sir Rowland Hill was in failing health and in August 1879 he died.[4] His son, Pearson Hill, rallied the Hampstead plaintiffs, who appealed against the granting of a new trial. The Asylums Managers, on their part, appealed against the payment of costs. On 18 December 1879, the Court of Appeal set aside the ruling of the Queen's Bench Division and issued an order dismissing the Hampstead plaintiffs' appeal if, within a specified time, the Board paid the costs of the first trial. If that were not done, the plaintiffs' appeal was to be allowed. The following April, another writ of injunction was served on the Board, restraining the use of the Hampstead Hospital for the treatment of infectious diseases. The Asylums Managers then brought the order of the Court of Appeal to the House of Lords, where it was decided that the appeal should be heard on the question of the right of the Board, in point of law, to maintain the Hampstead Hospital in its existing state.[5]

The appeal was heard the following January, and judgment was given on 7 March 1881. On behalf of the Asylums Board, it was claimed that the smallpox hospital in Hampstead

---

[1] M A B letter to the LGB, 1 June 1878.

[2] 42 & 43 Vict. c. 54 s. 16.　　　　　　　　　　[3] 4 QBD 433.

[4] Sir Rowland Hill (1795–1879), one-time educationist, but better known as pioneer of the penny postage in 1839, came to Hampstead from Bayswater in 1848. After living at No. 2 Pond Street, he purchased Bartram House in 1854. On retirement, in 1864, from the post of Secretary of the Post Office, he received a parliamentary grant of £20,000 and retained his salary of £2,000 per annum as retiring pension.

[5] When the order of the Court of Appeal of 18 December 1879 concerning the granting of a new trial in the Hill *versus* M A B case was brought before the House of Lords, it received the designation of Appeal No. 1. In the first instance, it was argued on the question of competency, it being alleged by the plaintiffs (the Hampstead residents) to be in substance a mere appeal on costs. The House however, decided that it was not so to be considered (5 App. Cas. 582), but, before hearing the appeal on the facts, suggested that it would be advisable to hear the appeal on the question of the right of the appellants (the M A B), in point of law, to maintain the Hampstead Hospital for infectious diseases: this was designated Appeal No. 2.

had been erected near the properties of the respondents under statutory authority. The question raised was whether the appellants were not, in law, completely protected from liability. The 1867 Metropolitan Poor Act was invoked as evidence that the MAB had been constituted a public body by statute; that its duties were of a public nature; and that it was commanded by the Local Government Board to perform them.[1] Everything the Asylums Board had done had been done under statutory authority; every detail in the 1867 Act, it was asserted, showed that the legislature had contemplated the carrying into execution of a public work for the health and safety of the community. It was, therefore, impossible to apply to this case considerations of possible private inconvenience that might occur in the execution of that work. It was to be assumed that the legislature had anticipated such inconvenience and determined that it must be endured in consideration of the great public benefit that would result from it. Counsel for the respondents based their case on the fact that the 1867 Act conferred no compulsory powers on the Asylums Managers and contained no authority to act if action constituted a nuisance. The Lord Chancellor, Lord Selborne, re-affirmed that the Metropolitan Poor Act, so far as it related to an infectious hospital, contained nothing mandatory or imperative. He pointed out that the class of poor persons for which the hospital was to be provided was not specified in the Act. No *compulsory* power was given to acquire land for any asylum purposes. Included in the section of the Act specifying the objects chargeable to the Common Poor Fund was, he admitted, a reference to 'patients suffering from fever or smallpox', but, except for this and the fact that the general category of 'sick' necessarily included patients suffering from any kind of disease, there was *no* provision in the Act relating to infectious disorders. 'If express words, or necessary implication and intendment, must be shown in order to authorize the Poor Law Board or any managers of an asylum to create a nuisance in the exercise of the discretionary powers given to them, I can find none in this statute', declared the Lord Chancellor. The only sense in which the legislature could be properly said to have authorized the exercise of any of these powers, he argued, was that it had enabled the Poor Law Board to order certain things to be done, and the Asylums Managers to carry out their instructions 'if, and when, and where, they could obtain by free bargain and contract the means of doing so'. If the legislature had authorized some *compulsory* interference with private rights of property for the purpose of establishing the Hampstead Hospital for the treatment of infectious patients and had made provision for compensating those who might be injuriously affected by it, the case might have been judged otherwise. As the law stood, neither the Poor Law Board nor the MAB had any statutory authority to do anything which might be a nuisance to the plaintiffs without their consent. The Lord Chancellor, therefore, moved that the appeal should be dismissed with costs.[2]

In May 1882, the Law Lords heard the appeal concerning the rule for a new trial. This was unanimously granted.[3] About £40,000 of ratepayers' money had been spent on

---

[1] 30 & 31 Vict. c. 6 ss. 5, 6, 7, 15, 69.
[2] H/L 6 App. Cas. 193 (January and March 1881); *The Times*, 8 March 1881, p. 4, col. 1.
[3] H/L 7 App. Cas. 151 (May 1882).

litigation. Nothing had been achieved except a ruling that a new trial should take place. This was to be based, not on the statutory rights of the Board to create a nuisance, but on the question of fact—whether or not the treatment at the hospital of two to three hundred patients constituted a nuisance to neighbouring residents. By this time, these conditions no longer existed. The Hampstead Hospital had been closed since the end of 1878.

During the autumn of 1882, a serious outbreak of scarlet fever prompted the Asylums Managers to take legal advice concerning the possibility of using the Hampstead Hospital for fever cases. It was opened; and Mr. Pearson Hill immediately sued the Board for damages, once again. There were now two actions pending. £20,000 had originally been raised by the plaintiffs with the support of the Hampstead vestry, but by now the guarantee fund was £6,000 in debt and further appeals for public support were unproductive. As legal costs of both sides had fallen directly and indirectly on the residents of Hampstead, they finally threatened the Local Government Board with refusal to pay rates if litigation continued, and appealed to both parties to call a halt to legal proceedings. A settlement was effected out of court in 1883. The conditions included the purchase by the Board, from the executors of the late Sir Rowland Hill, of his residence, Bartram House,[1] and adjoining property for £13,000; the payment of £9,000 in full settlement of the two pending actions, and of £500 towards the cost of constructing an entrance at the opposite end of the hospital site and closing the approach from Haverstock Hill. There was also an undertaking to limit the number of smallpox cases under treatment in the hospital at any one time to forty.[2]

IV

While the Hampstead case was *sub judice*, the Managers decided to defer the acquisition of new hospital sites, although the appearance of numerous malignant smallpox cases early in 1880 had presaged another serious outbreak. The M A B strongly urged the Local Government Board to take statutory action to enable it to deal with a possible epidemic without being hampered by the deficiencies of the law. This plea was met with the suggestion that the Managers might erect huts or tents in the vicinity of their mental institutions in Kent. A canvas camp was accordingly established at Darenth. Such cases as could tolerate the journey were collected at the Board's Deptford Hospital and taken by road in hired four-in-hand horsed vehicles, which covered the distance of eighteen miles in three hours. This arrangement began in May 1881. Although third- and fourth-rate cities in America already had regulated ambulances in use, this was the first occasion on which a systematic transport service for hospital patients had ever been operated in London.

[1] Bartram House, when acquired by the M A B, was used as a nurses' home and also for committee meetings. Upon this site now stands the Hampstead General Hospital.

[2] The sparse references in existing M A B records to this out-of-court settlement have been supplemented by material in the archives of the Royal Free Hospital, which has been made available by the Administrator, Mr. R. G. Heppell, FCA, whose help is gratefully acknowledged.

The largest number of smallpox cases which could be treated at the Darenth camp was 640. There came a time when no more could be admitted. Sir Edmund Hay Currie, Vice-Chairman of the Board, had a brilliant idea. Two old wooden battleships were chartered from the Admiralty. A 90-gun ship, the *Atlas*, for acute cases, and a 50-gun frigate, the *Endymion*, for administrative purposes, were adapted at a cost of £11,000, and moored off Greenwich. The removal of patients to the ships direct from their homes and work-houses was then organized. A house in London Fields, East London, was rented to serve as an ambulance depot. A resident staff was installed; horse ambulances were provided; and the station was connected by telephone[1] direct with the Board's head office. Fierce local opposition followed. A writ was issued against the Board for recovery of possession. This was successful, but an arrangement was arrived at to enable the station to function until alternative accommodation could be found.

It was now mid-1881, and the epidemic, which had raged for nearly a year, had reached alarming proportions. The Board insisted on getting its legal position regularized. In view of the unfavourable House of Lords judgment in the Hampstead case in March 1881, the Managers renewed their representations to the Local Government Board and pressed for the immediate introduction of a Bill 'to define, and if requisite enlarge, the powers of the Asylums Board to enable it to perform in the present and any future epidemics, in a successful and satisfactory manner and without molestation, the duties which the Act of 1867 contemplated it should perform.'[2] In reply, the Managers were asked to suggest specific amendments to the law which, in their judgment, would be best calculated to resolve the difficulties in which they were placed.[3] The Managers suggested that 'an Act should be passed making it *compulsory* for the Asylums Board to provide hospital accommodation for all persons in the metropolis suffering from disease, infectious and other-wise. . .'. They also urged that legislation should be introduced to ensure that 'the same consequences should follow from the acts of the Asylums Board as if the hospitals now in existence, or to be erected in the future by the Board, *had been expressly sanctioned by Act of Parliament.*' Finally, the Asylums Managers emphasized the need for legislation which would make it obligatory for all cases of infectious disease to be notified to local authorities throughout the country.[4] The Local Government Board did not reply.

Meanwhile, encouraged by the decision in the Hampstead case, a number of Fulham residents took steps to prevent the Board's Fulham Hospital from being used for smallpox. An injunction was applied for in August 1881 but was refused. On appeal the following month, an interlocutory injunction was granted restricting the use of the hospital to small-pox admissions from a mile radius. The judgment was appealed against by the Board. But it was affirmed, despite evidence prepared by the medical superintendent to demonstrate

---

[1] Direct telephone lines between two users were in operation in large towns in the early 1880s, before the system of telephone 'exchanges' was adopted. (*Encyclopaedia Britannica*, vol. xxiii, 1888, p. 133.)

[2] Letter from the M A B to the LGB, 15 May 1881.

[3] LGB reply to the M A B, 18 May 1881.

[4] M A B letter to the LGB, 19 May 1881.

from over 150 histories of cases occurring within a mile of the hospital, that infection was derived from contact with non-isolated cases and not from the hospital by aerial convection. Shortly afterwards, the Board was pressed for fever accommodation and directed that scarlet fever cases should be admitted to the Fulham Hospital. Again the Board was sued for damages. The case was settled out of court for £6,000.

Concerned by now at the cost and inconvenience of public opposition, the Local Government Board instructed its inspector, Dr. W. H. Power, to make a detailed study of the incidence of smallpox in the vicinity of the Fulham Hospital. From his conclusions, it appeared that when smallpox cases were freely admitted into the hospital, the number of houses invaded in a special area within a mile radius of the hospital was four times greater than in other parts of the adjoining districts; and that, in the area itself, a regular and progressive increase of invasion existed as the centre of infection—the hospital—was approached. Such being the case in connexion with one hospital, it was assumed that it was the same for the others.[1] The hypothesis on which Dr. Power had worked was that infection had been conveyed through the air. As he dealt only with statistics of incidence and did not concentrate to any extent on human lines of communication, his conclusions did not prove one way or the other how the infection was conducted.

V

The Asylums Board had reached a critical stage in its development. Its hospitals at Hampstead and Fulham were severely restricted under legal injunctions, and similar proceedings were likely at Stockwell, Deptford and Homerton.[2] As the law now stood, the hospitals existed merely on the sufferance of the neighbourhoods in which they were located, and might be summarily closed at the height of an epidemic, leaving the disease to run its course uncontrolled. The health of the community was being endangered by an insufficiency of isolation accommodation which it was the statutory duty of the Board to provide. Yet the efforts of the Managers to carry out that duty were paralysed by the inadequacy of the powers conferred upon them by the legislature. Although thwarted by public opposition and official apathy, the Managers were in no doubt that their thankless task must continue.

At a plenary meeting of the M A B at the end of October 1881, Dr. Brewer rallied his colleagues to take the firmest possible line with the Local Government Board. Statutory action had to be taken, and taken without delay. Since the beginning of the year, 'the most horrible of all the ministers of death' had been stalking the streets of London uncontrolled,

---

[1] Supplement to the *Tenth Annual Report of the LGB*, 1881–82: BPP, 1882, vol. xxx, Part II, 1 [Cmd. 3290].

[2] The Hackney District Board was preparing a case against the M A B. Included among its objections were that the laundry at the Homerton Hospital was ventilated on to a main thoroughfare, and that the children clambered round the ambulances which waited at the entrance until the porter arrived. Meantime, the M A B was censuring the Hackney Board for not investigating more efficiently the slums of the locality.

and the number of the stricken was mounting day by day.[1] A letter from Dr. Brewer was addressed to the central authority insisting that

> . . . the time has arrived when the general purposes committee of the Asylums Board should seek an interview with the President . . . and ascertain whether the Local Government Board is prepared to take steps and, if so, what steps to enable the Asylums Managers to carry out their duties according to the spirit and intention of the Metropolitan Poor Act under which they were constituted. . . .[2]

Sir John Lambert, who had played a substantial part in assisting Gathorne Hardy to draft the 1867 Act, was now in the difficult position of having to advise his President, J. G. Dodson (later Lord Monk Bretton), on how to remedy its defects. The only possible way out of the impasse appeared to be the appointment of a Royal Commission. A fortnight after receiving Dr. Brewer's letter, Sir John Lambert replied that

> . . . the Government, having in view the difficulties attending this subject, have advised the issue of a Royal Commission to enquire into the whole matter and advise as to what further legislation is required. . . .[3]

Dr. Brewer never learned of this significant development. He died suddenly on 3 November 1881, four days following the despatch of his letter. After leading the Board valiantly through fourteen years of vicissitudes, he was deprived of witnessing this turning of the tide.

The Commission, which included a number of eminent medical men, was appointed in December 1881.[4] The main items in its terms of reference were: the nature, extent and sufficiency of isolation hospital provision by the MAB and the local authorities; the relative advantages of centrally- or locally-provided isolation accommodation; the expediency of continuing the existing isolation hospitals; the protection of the community; the operation of relevant legislation; and the protection of hospital authorities from liability to legal proceedings. The Asylums Managers took a prominent part in the submission of evidence.

The report, a significant contribution to the literature of public health, was presented to Parliament in August 1882.[5] Reviewing the past, the Commission declared despairingly that for many years London had been 'grappling with an evil influence' which 'is fitfully

---

[1] The only local authority which had made any effective provision was the Lewisham District Board. The St. Pancras and Islington vestries had been obliged to erect hospital encampments; these had been placed next to their burial grounds!

[2] MAB letter to the LGB, 30 October 1881.

[3] LGB letter to the MAB, 17 November 1881.

[4] Members of the 1881–82 Royal Commission on Smallpox and Fever Hospitals included: Baron Blackford (chairman), Sir James Paget, Sir Rutherford Alcock, Mr. A. Wellesley Peel, Mr. E. Leigh Pemberton, Dr. John Burdon Sanderson, Dr. A. Carpenter, Dr. W. H. Broadbent and Mr. Jonathan Hutchinson.

[5] *Report of the Royal Commission on Smallpox and Fever Hospitals*, 1882: BPP, 1882, vol. xxix, 1 [Cmd. 3314].

and sensibly gaining ground. . . .' Its main concern was the alleged ability of the Fulham Hospital to spread infection in the neighbourhood, and the possibility that the Board's other smallpox hospitals shared this power. It was accordingly urged that smallpox should be treated in isolated positions on the banks of the Thames or in floating hospitals and not in populous areas. Between fifteen hundred and two thousand smallpox beds, it was estimated, would be required for treatment outside London. Severe cases, which could not be moved so far, should be accommodated in the Board's London fever hospitals in a few small, isolated wards of annular design, rigorously separated from the fever wards and the administration. In any case, no urban institution should treat more than forty smallpox patients at any one time. The hospitals hitherto used for smallpox cases could provide about fifteen hundred additional fever beds; while a similar number of beds for convalescent fever cases in the country was also recommended. Concerning the legal position of the Asylums Board, the Commission urged that the power of arresting the Managers' operations by injunction should be removed; and that powers of compulsory purchase should be conferred upon the Board. The Managers' perennial plea for general compulsory notification of all infectious cases was also affirmed by the Commission. All London isolation hospitals, it was suggested, should be under the control of a central hospital authority composed for the most part of the existing M A B and reinforced by representatives of the local authorities. This body should also maintain a central ambulance service. Although unwilling to accept definitely the conclusions of the Fulham Hospital enquiry, the Commissioners evidently based their recommendations upon them. However, despite further detailed studies, they reached no definite conclusions concerning the means of spread, and merely recapitulated the reasoning of those who believed in aerial convection and of those who inclined to the hypothesis of contact infection. Both means, they cautiously recommended, should be eliminated in a sound administration.

The Commission's most fundamental proposition was that the provision of hospital accommodation for infectious diseases should be entirely disconnected from the poor law and treated as part of the sanitary arrangements of London. Emphasizing the view that preventive practice and poor law principles were incompatible, the Commissioners affirmed that provision for the infectious sick was

> . . . not to be treated solely with reference to the periodic relief of the indigent sick but as a question also of public safety, with primary reference to the extirpation of epidemic infectious disease, subject to the obligation of doing all that humanity demands for the benefit of individual sufferers. . . .[1]

Particularly noteworthy was the Commission's recommendation that poor law patients and others should be treated alike. Separate wards might be made available for paying patients, but the Commissioners were doubtful whether, in cases of ordinary accommodation, payment should be claimed even from those who could afford to pay without

[1] *Report of the Royal Commission on Smallpox and Fever Hospitals*, 1882: BPP, 1882, vol. xxix, 1 [Cmd. 3314], p. vii.

difficulty. This was the first time that Parliament had been presented with a scheme of public hospital provision for the free use of all in need of treatment, irrespective of class or ability to pay.

VI

Immediately following the issue of the Royal Commission's report, the M A B took steps to carry into effect the internal reforms suggested. These included the construction of separate hospital entrances for patients and tradesmen; longer periods off duty for nurses; and stricter visiting and disinfection regulations. But the Board could do little else until the central authority initiated statutory action. Three months passed without any move on the part of the Local Government Board. Becoming restive, the Managers urgently enquired what steps it intended to take on the Commission's report.[1] In reply, the M A B was informed that 'the Government cannot at this time undertake to state what measures they may be able to bring forward during the next session of Parliament'.[2] The Asylums Board thereupon directed its general purposes committee to seek an interview with the Prime Minister, Mr. Gladstone, with a view to discussing the advisability and practicability of the M A B taking immediate steps to put into effect the Commission's recommendations concerning the provision of country hospitals and the organization of London ambulances.[3] A communication was despatched to the Prime Minister at the end of 1882 emphasizing the Board's difficulties—the impediments, the harassing conditions, the heavy costs to ratepayers, the absence of statutory protection, the lack of local authority hospital provision and, finally, 'the very unsatisfactory announcement' made by the Local Government Board. Voicing the Managers' sense of urgency, the M A B communication concluded:

> . . . It is impossible to conceive any question more pressing or requiring more immediate consideration, or one more likely to be fraught with serious and complicated consequences than that which the Asylums Board desires to have dealt with, seeing that it affects not only directly the health and lives of a large portion of the population of this vast metropolis, but also indirectly the health and lives of the community at large.[4]

In January 1883, a member of the Prime Minister's staff was directed to reply that:

> . . . Mr. Gladstone regrets that he is not able to receive a deputation on a matter which is beyond the province of his own department. Indeed, he could not undertake at the present time to receive any deputation whatever, having been enjoined to abstain from all business other than that which is absolutely necessary.[5]

[1] M A B letter to the LGB, 26 November 1882.
[2] LGB reply to the M A B, 29 November 1882.   [3] M A B *Mins.*, vol. xvi, p. 747.
[4] Letter from the Chairman of the M A B to Mr. Gladstone, Prime Minister, 22 December 1882.
[5] Letter from Mr. Gladstone to the Chairman of the M A B, 11 January 1883.

Mr. (later Sir) Edwin Galsworthy, who had succeeded Dr. Brewer as chairman of the M A B, insisted early in February 1883 on seeing the President and senior officials of the Local Government Board. At the close of the interview, he was under the impression that the Managers' problems had been understood and that legislation would be promoted forthwith to safeguard their position. He asked that the outcome of the discussion should be embodied in a confirmatory letter, but when he received this communication, it revealed an insufficient appreciation of the essence and magnitude of the difficulties discussed. Concerning legislation, the Local Government Board referred to a Bill 'promised during the current session for the extension of municipal government to the metropolitan area' and assured the chairman that 'it would not interfere with the action of the M A B in providing additional accommodation. . . .' The only question affecting the M A B which might arise in connexion with the Bill was 'whether the care and management of patients of the non-pauper class should not be clearly shown to devolve on the sanitary authorities rather than upon the Asylums Board'.[1] This was quite irrelevant to the recommendations of the Royal Commission, which had envisaged one central hospital authority in London for infectious patients of all social classes. In regard to additional accommodation, however, the Local Government Board agreed that floating hospitals might be established in the Thames some distance down river for the less acute smallpox cases. Buildings for convalescent cases, it suggested, could be erected 'on land at no great distance from the ships which could probably be secured without compulsory powers of purchase'. Concerning the conveyance of patients, the Local Government Board assented to Mr. Galsworthy's suggestion that the M A B should acquire paddle steamers and transform them into river ambulances. In the last resort, the central authority agreed to consider legislation for the compulsory purchase of riverside sites for wharves.

The Asylums Managers were not satisfied. The acquisition of a few hospital ships would not provide the 1,500 fever beds and 2,000 smallpox beds recommended by the Royal Commission. However, they began their extra-metropolitan system of smallpox treatment by purchasing from the Admiralty the *Atlas* and the *Endymion*, which had been on charter. In addition, they acquired the *Castalia*, a disused cross-Channel steamer, and equipped her as a hospital ship. The floating hospitals were moored in Long Reach, some seventeen miles below London Bridge. In addition to the 350 beds which the ships would provide, and the 200 beds for severe cases left in the five London hospitals, at least another 1,000 smallpox beds would be needed outside the metropolis to meet future epidemics. Additional land was therefore purchased at Darenth and prepared with roads, gas and water. It was planned to erect ten 100-bed blocks at a rate of £100 per bed. The cost of acquiring and equipping the hospital ships totalled some £96,000, a rate of nearly £275 per bed. Next, two paddle steamers were bought for £10,000 and fitted up as ambulance ships. A pier was constructed at Long Reach and wharves were established at Blackwall, Rotherhithe and Fulham at a cost of £42,000. Each wharf was equipped with an examination room, an isolation ward for patients found unfit to make the journey,

[1] LGB letter to the M A B, 16 February 1883.

and other wards for cases of doubtful diagnosis. Plans were also put in hand for extending the land ambulance service which had been inaugurated during the 1880–81 smallpox epidemic. Finally, a site was acquired at Winchmore Hill in north London on which to erect a 500-bed convalescent fever hospital. Like the Darenth project, this was designed for partial opening to meet the state of demand.

VII

In view of the difficulties which still beset the Board whenever it attempted to acquire land for a hospital, an ambulance station or a wharf, the Asylums Managers continued to press for compulsory powers of purchase. The Local Government Board was now perturbed, however, with the prospect of an outbreak of cholera. When the Managers were approached concerning the reception of cholera patients, they firmly declined to accept an undefined responsibility in view of their experience with other infectious diseases. They made it clear to the Local Government Board that they did not intend to relieve the sanitary authorities of their responsibilities in this connexion unless their own commitments were precisely laid down. It was finally agreed that the M A B should be responsible for finding accommodation for up to fifty patients in the early stages of an outbreak. Thereafter, each local authority was to be responsible for providing its own hospital accommodation. On this occasion the views of the Asylums Board were respected. A Bill was introduced setting out the arrangement agreed upon and decreeing that the M A B should be deemed 'a local authority under the Diseases Prevention Act of 1855' for the purpose of providing for cholera patients.

For the M A B, these provisions were, however, the least important of the innovations introduced by the new measure—the Diseases Prevention (Metropolis) Act of 1883.[1] The Board was at last endowed with compulsory powers of purchase.[2] Although these were limited to the acquisition of landing places for the ambulance ships and did not extend to hospital sites, their conferment represented a break-through in the legislative dilemma. Furthermore, the Act affirmed that no person should suffer disability or disqualification by reason of admission to an M A B institution for infectious diseases.[3] M A B hospitals, nevertheless, remained poor law establishments, administered by a poor law authority and maintained out of the poor rates, but the stigma of pauperism had been removed from patients. These two provisions represented the only statutory implementation to date of the numerous recommendations made in the Royal Commission's report. Nothing was included concerning compulsory notification of infectious disease. The Act was valid for one year only, but was renewed annually for another eight years.[4] It would seem that qualms existed at the Local Government Board lest the long-term acceptance of this measure might undermine the punitive principles of the poor law.

[1] 46 & 47 Vict. c. 35.   [2] Ibid., section 6.   [3] Ibid., section 7.
[4] The provisions of the Diseases Prevention (Metropolis) Act, 1883, were recapitulated in section 80 of the consolidating Public Health (London) Act, 1891 (see chapter 7).

VIII

Before the Asylums Board was able to complete its building programme, smallpox again invaded London—the fourth large-scale epidemic since the advent of the M A B. Now that treatment in the Board's hospitals was no longer considered to be parochial relief, there was an unprecedented demand for admission, despite the liability to maintenance charges which non-pauper patients still incurred. The new site at Darenth was made into a huge hospital encampment in the spring of 1884. Soon it was taxed to the utmost. It was decided that a 'lady superintendent' was needed. Dr. Bridges, of the Local Government Board, offered to find a suitable candidate. Miss Isabella Baker, possessed of Nightingalian qualities, had already been induced by him to stand as first woman guardian for Holborn. Again, she responded to his persuasion, and in the summer of 1884, she found herself under canvas at Darenth in the midst of 1,100 smallpox patients from all parts of London. Nothing was ready when she arrived. She described how the patients 'came pouring in from the ships across the river with their goods and chattels like the children of Israel passing through the Red Sea'. The average number of arrivals was one hundred a day. Everything had to be provided for them, and one of her proud achievements was 'obtaining a separate brush and comb for each patient, a luxury hitherto unknown'.[1]

During this epidemic, the Asylums Board was forced by the rapid influx of patients to dispense with all hampering restrictions. Non-pauper cases were accepted on the application of Medical Officers of Health. The only proviso was that a medical certificate should be handed to the ambulance nurse when the patient was collected. Pauper cases were received on the application of any poor law official and admission orders were sought later. In the past, the Asylums Managers had found it necessary to act in advance of legislation, and they were now confident that, as they were serving the best interests of the public, their action would eventually receive statutory sanction. In the earlier development of preventive medicine, growth had nearly always been stimulated by expansion in methods of administration and then followed by legislation in the fulness of time.

In the autumn of 1884, the Board again approached the central authority concerning the situation which had resulted from the permissive powers of the local authorities to contract with the M A B for the reception of infectious non-pauper patients under the 1879 Act.[2] Up to this time, no vestry or district board had entered into any such agreement with the Asylums Board. Patients above the pauper class were being admitted to the M A B hospitals on public health and humanitarian grounds. The Asylums Board strongly represented to the central authority that explicit legal sanction should now be given for the admission of all such patients. The practical effect of section 7 of the Diseases Prevention (Metropolis) Act of 1883, which abolished the pauper stigma, had been to remove the distinction between pauper and non-pauper cases. The Asylums Managers were informed in reply that no Local Government Board order was necessary to enable them

[1] S. Liveing, op. cit., p. 196.
[2] M A B letter to the LGB, 26 October 1884.

to contract with the local authorities, but that any arrangement entered into would require central authority sanction.[1] The Asylums Board thereupon submitted to the Local Government Board the draft of a circular which it proposed to address to the metropolitan vestries and district boards. This contained an offer to admit local authority patients into M A B isolation hospitals at a fixed fee of four guineas a case. This would be chargeable to the vestry or district board and recoverable from the patient, as the local authority saw fit. The Board made it clear that it could not undertake to make any class distinction in the treatment of patients in the isolation hospitals.[2] The Asylums Board was informed by the Local Government Board that it could not make an open offer in this way and that it would have to enter into a separate contract with each authority.[3] Thereupon, the M A B sent to each of the forty metropolitan vestries and district boards a form of contract, drawn up on the lines of its circular, and invited comments. Not one authority agreed unconditionally to enter into a written agreement. Fourteen agreed in principle, with modifications; fifteen disapproved; seven offered alternative schemes; and four did not reply. Most of them questioned the justice of exacting a fee and suggested that expenses should be a charge, either on the Metropolitan Common Poor Fund, or on a sanitary fund set up for the purpose. The Asylums Board sent a summary of these replies to the central authority, and declared that it could take no further action in the matter 'unless and until the Local Government Board shall see fit to obtain from Parliament such additional powers as will render compulsory, instead of optional, the conditions of section 15 of the Poor Law Act of 1879'.[4] No reply was received to this communication.

IX

So far the M A B had failed to move the central authority to secure its legal recognition as an isolation hospital authority for the whole of London. But it could look back from 1886 over two decades of substantial achievement. It now had 1,900 fever beds in its six London hospitals—the North-Western (Hampstead), the South-Western (Stockwell), the North-Eastern (Homerton), the Western (Fulham), the South-Eastern (Deptford) and the Northern (the new convalescent hospital at Winchmore Hill).[5] On the Darenth camp site and the nearby Gore Farm estate, plans were well advanced for the provision of one thousand smallpox beds in permanent buildings to supplement the accommodation of the hospital ships, now 'modernized' with electrical equipment. With its characteristic pioneering spirit, the Board had never hesitated to break new ground. The banishment of large numbers of smallpox patients from populous areas to hulks on the river was a revolutionary experiment. It was as yet too soon to judge whether it would result in a significant advance

[1] LGB letter to the M A B, 6 December 1884.
[2] M A B *Mins.*, vol. xviii, 1885, p. 1180.
[3] LGB letter to the M A B, 2 March 1885.
[4] M A B letter to the LGB, 7 October 1886; 42 & 43 Vict. c. 54 s. 15.
[5] In 1882, each M A B London hospital became known by its geographical location and no longer by its district name, at the suggestion of a Hampstead resident, Mr. B. Woodd Smith.

in pestilence control. Since the inauguration of its ambulance service in 1881, the Board had established three permanent stations adjoining the hospitals at Deptford (1883), Fulham (1884) and Homerton (1885), at a total cost of £25,000. These depots were served by resident staff and equipped with ambulance vehicles and horses.[1] Nurses for smallpox cases were quartered at the stations, but for fever cases they were drawn from the staff of the adjoining hospital in order to avoid cross-infection. The stations were maintained in readiness to transport patients at any time of the day or night from any part of London on receiving orders from the M A B head office in Norfolk Street, Strand, with which they were linked by direct telephone lines. The advent of the telephone in the early 1880s had materially increased the efficiency of the Board's isolation hospitals. It became possible to arrange more promptly than previously for the removal of patients; and in times of pressure, the M A B head office, which was also in telephonic communication with all its institutions, was able to direct the allocation of patients to the nearest hospital with vacant beds. The Board's centralized ambulance service was still the only organized system of patient transport in London, and its efficiency had already stimulated demands for a similar public service for the conveyance of accident and other cases in the capital.[2]

Since the M A B hospitals were first opened, they had treated upward of 57,000 small-pox patients and borne the brunt of four serious epidemics. Some 30,000 'fever' cases had also passed through the Board's hospitals. Of these, about 60 per cent were scarlet fever patients and the remainder were chiefly typhus and enteric cases.[3] By now, the M A B hospital system for infectious diseases had become accepted as an essential part of London's public health administration. But, at this very juncture of relative stability, forces were afoot to reform the municipal government of the metropolis.[4] For the M A B, the future was enigmatic, but the past had witnessed a definite, if limited, step forward in preventive medicine.

[1] For illustrations of M A B ambulance carriages at this period see figure 2.

[2] In 1882, a year after the inauguration of the M A B ambulance service for infectious cases, the Duke of Cambridge presided at a public meeting convened to consider the establishment of a similar service for non-infectious cases in London. Money was raised by private subscription, but the service came to an end when the ambulances wore out. (*Trans. NAPSS*, 1882, pp. 392–95.)

[3] See Appendix II, Tables B and D, showing statistics of M A B smallpox and fever hospitals during this period.

[4] Schemes of London government reform were debated during the Gladstone administration which fell in 1886 and Lord Salisbury's second administration which followed it, but it was not until 1888 that the Local Government Bill was introduced, incorporating the idea of a central body for 'such work as is essentially metropolitan in character'.

CHAPTER 7

The MAB Infectious Disease Hospitals: The Third Phase—1887 to 1891

I

THE major preoccupation of the Asylums Board during the next five years was to see the M A B services for infectious patients legally divorced from the poor law and made freely available to all citizens of London in need of isolation and treatment. The Board's infectious disease hospitals were now admitting all cases on the production of a certificate signed by a registered practitioner. The involvement of the relieving officer in admissions procedure had always been an unnecessary impediment from a medical point of view and was now nothing but an anachronism. In by-passing the relieving officer and accepting a medical certificate as the sole passport to entry, the Managers were serving the best interests of the community and the individual patient. Nevertheless, they were acting illegally, and therefore pressed the Local Government Board for permission to receive all patients solely on the application 'of any duly qualified practitioner'. But the central authority clung tenaciously to the tenets of the poor law. In 1887, an amended Local Government Board order regulating the admission of infectious patients stipulated that every 'poor person' was to be 'admitted upon an order . . . signed by a relieving officer or a master of a workhouse . . . and a certificate signed by either a poor law medical officer or by some other registered medical practitioner.'[1] When the Asylums Board suggested that the reference to the relieving officer should be deleted from the regulation on account of the inconvenience and delay which his intervention entailed, the Local Government Board declared that it was not empowered to issue such an order and that, in any case, M A B medical superintendents were already authorized to receive any person who was in such a condition that a refusal to admit him might have dangerous results.[2] This safeguarding concession, however, had been wrested from the Local Government Board in 1875,[3] before the M A B ambulances were in use and when advanced cases frequently arrived at the hospital gates without medical certificates or poor law admission orders. The need at that time, the Managers

---

[1] LGB order to the M A B, 7 July 1887, in substitution of article 3 of LGB order dated 10 February 1875.
[2] LGB letter to the M A B, 14 November 1887.
[3] See Chapter 5.

pointed out, had been to regularize the reception of these emergency cases. Now, it was 'absolutely necessary to obtain from Parliament, without further delay, powers to enable the M A B to admit to its hospitals *all* persons suffering from fever or smallpox, solely on the application of a duly qualified medical practitioner.' The Managers added that some 40 per cent of recent admissions had applied without orders from any poor law official.[1] In the absence of a prompt reply, a deputation of Asylums Managers called upon Mr. C. T. (later Lord) Ritchie, President of the Local Government Board, to press their demands. The interview was followed shortly by a communication intimating that the central authority 'would consider the question with a view to legislation'.[2]

II

At this time, the Local Government Board was already considering legislation on another issue which concerned the M A B. Diphtheria was now causing more than usual alarm in London. Although an important disease in France during the first half of the nineteenth century, diphtheria was almost unknown to British doctors until 1855. During the next few years, it became widespread in this country.[3] At first, it appeared to affect rural areas more than towns, but by the 1880s this tendency was negligible. Since 1859, when deaths from diphtheria were first entered separately in the Registrar-General's returns, the mortality rate for London had always been in excess of that for the whole of England and Wales. In 1886, the Society of Medical Officers of Health and boards of guardians, supported by London coroners, appealed to the Asylums Board to admit diphtheria cases into the fever hospitals. The diphtheria bacillus had been discovered and isolated during the past three years,[4] but the use of a resistant serum for treating the disease was as yet only a hypothesis in the minds of certain German research workers.[5] Tracheotomy was the only means of saving advanced cases and this demanded prompt hospital co-operation. The Asylums Managers felt it was their duty to admit diphtheria cases, particularly as the voluntary hospitals had become less inclined to accept infectious patients of any kind since the founding of the M A B institutions. Isolation accommodation was still considerably below the epidemic potential of the diseases already admissible, so the Local Government Board was consulted. The question as to whether diphtheria could be regarded as a 'fever' within the meaning of section 69 of the Metropolitan Poor Act of 1867 was deliberated for some weeks in Whitehall. Finally, the Royal College of Physicians was asked to advise. The President, Sir William Jenner, replied:

---

[1] M A B letter to the LGB, 23 November 1887.

[2] LGB letter to the M A B, 16 December 1887.

[3] *Second Report of the Medical Officer to the Privy Council* (Sir John Simon) for 1859. See also A. H. Gale, *Epidemic Diseases* (1959), pp. 93–94.

[4] The diphtheria bacillus was first discovered by Klebs in 1883 and was isolated by Löffler in 1884 (F. Löffler, *Mitt. Reichsgesundheilsamt*, 2 (1884), 421).

[5] Behring and Wernicke, *Dtsch. Med. Wschr.* 39 (1892), 873.

... If the words in the Act had been for persons suffering from 'fevers', I should most certainly have considered diphtheria to be included under the term 'fever', but the separation of smallpox from fevers seems to signify that the word 'fever' was intended to include only fever of a special type ... to which the word 'fever' is specially applied, as scarlet fever, typhus fever and typhoid fever.[1]

After further consideration, the Local Government Board decided that the 1867 Act did not cover diphtheria and that, therefore, special legislation was required to regularize the admission of diphtheria cases into the M A B hospitals. Meantime, mortality from the disease in London continued to increase. Another year passed and there was still no sign of legislation, either concerning the treatment of diphtheria cases in the Board's fever hospitals or on the wider question of abolishing the poor law channels for the admission of infectious patients generally. Despite fifteen years of preventive and curative work, the public health functions of the M A B infectious disease hospitals appeared to be still unrecognized by the central authority.

III

By the autumn of 1887, the Asylums Managers had a serious scarlet fever epidemic on their hands. The hospitals were treating some 3,000 cases—nearly four times the highest number under treatment on any previous occasion during the past decade. These, it was estimated, represented only one-third of all the scarlet fever cases in London at this time. Additional pavilions were, therefore, hurriedly erected at the Winchmore Hill Hospital, and £31,000 was spent on temporary accommodation. The 1887 influx was attributed at the time to the extended use of medical certificates by non-poor law doctors; to the growing desire of Londoners to enjoy the advantages of institutional treatment; and to the decreasing reluctance of parents to allow their children to enter hospital. These factors, doubtless, accounted in part for the accelerated demand for fever beds, but the 1887 outbreak was later assessed as exceptional in character. In any case, it marked the beginning of a decade of increasingly numerous scarlet fever admissions to the Board's hospitals.

Meantime, the Local Government Board continued to deliberate upon the demand of the Asylums Managers for compulsory powers to enable them to acquire land for hospital extensions; and the Asylums Managers, without waiting for statutory authorization, proceeded to plan for future demands. A brick-hut hospital for six hundred smallpox beds was designed, at an estimated cost of £66,000, for the Gore Farm estate adjoining the Darenth hospital camp. For the first time in the Board's history, speed in providing smallpox accommodation was not of paramount importance. Since smallpox had been treated on the hospital ships, London had enjoyed unprecedented immunity from the disease,[2] although its incidence had reached epidemic dimensions in other large towns, including Sheffield, Manchester and Bristol, as well as Paris.

[1] Letter from the President of the Royal College of Physicians to the LGB, 18 July 1886.
[2] See Appendix II, Table A.

IV

In February 1888, the Asylums Managers renewed their pressure on the Local Government Board concerning outstanding issues requiring legislation. In reply, the President intimated his intention of introducing a Bill which would provide for the admission of diphtheria cases to the Board's fever hospitals. Meantime, 'if the M A B were determined to admit diphtheria', the Local Government Board would 'sanction the expenditure incurred with a view to removing any difficulty with the Auditor'.[1] Immediately, the M A B hospitals began to receive all diphtheria patients seeking admission, irrespective of class. From 23 October 1888 until the end of the year, 96 cases were treated.

By the time the overdue permission to receive diphtheria patients was received, an epidemic of measles of exceptional severity had broken out in London, as in other parts of the country. In the Metropolitan Asylum District, deaths from measles averaged 133 weekly during the winter of 1888–89. This level was far in excess of mortality from small-pox for any comparable period in the Board's history, except during the memorable epidemic of 1870–72, which only slightly exceeded it. Emergencies in the past had been used by the Board to lever the central authority into action. Again, it represented to the Local Government Board London's need for a central isolation hospital authority which would provide for patients of all classes suffering from acute infectious disease in any form. The Asylums Managers felt that the moment was opportune to press their case, not only on public health grounds, but also because changes in the Board's status, either for better or worse, seemed imminent. The recent Local Government Act of 1888 had dealt with the area of the metropolis—the Metropolitan Asylum District—as if it were a separate county, both for administrative and for non-administrative purposes. This was surely the juncture which would determine the future of the M A B as a sanitary authority with special responsibility for infectious diseases. Reasoning on these lines, the Asylums Board declared to the Local Government Board that:

> . . . the paramount duty of a sanitary authority being the prevention of death from preventible cause, it would seem to follow that, whether deaths are occasioned by fever, smallpox, diphtheria or measles, equal precautions should be adopted. . . . The isolation of measles, which has increased in extent and virulence during the past few years, cannot much longer be delayed . . . and will doubtless be dealt with by such central sanitary authority as may ultimately be charged with the supervision of the health requirements of the metropolis. . . . In present circumstances, with insufficient accommodation for its basic needs and still without sanction to acquire sites for hospital extensions, the Asylums Board is powerless to help in the current measles epidemic. . . .[2]

No reply was received to this communication.

Apart from political considerations, the Asylums Managers were genuinely distressed

[1] LGB letter to the M A B, 17 October 1888.
[2] M A B letter to the LGB, 14 February 1889.

at the extent of sickness and death from measles, especially among children, and at their powerlessness to remedy the situation on account of official inertia and public apathy. 'If the mortality which characterized last autumn's epidemic of measles had affected the adult population instead of children', observed the Board's chairman in 1889, 'public opinion would probably have insisted upon provision being made for the proper isolation and treatment of patients afflicted with this disease'.[1] Such was the general attitude towards the welfare of the rising generation at this time that nearly a quarter of a century was to elapse before public hospital provision was made for London children suffering from measles.[2]

V

Meantime, the Asylums Managers continued to press the Local Government Board for explicit legal sanction to admit fever and smallpox patients above the pauper class to their infectious disease hospitals, and also to convey them in M A B ambulances, since non-destitute patients who wished to get to an M A B hospital, or any other destination in London, were obliged to use public transport. The Managers also persisted in their demands for compulsory powers concerning the purchase of hospital sites, and at the same time reiterated the need for obligatory notification of infectious disease. In these representations they were supported by the Sanitary Institute, the Association of Medical Officers of Health, and the National Association for the Promotion of Social Science.[3]

These determined efforts eventually met with a substantial measure of success in the Poor Law Act of 1889,[4] which conferred upon the M A B some of the public health functions for which it had been pressing. Subject to Local Government Board regulations, the Asylums Board was empowered to admit into its hospitals *any* person who was not a pauper and who was reasonably believed to be suffering from fever, smallpox or diphtheria. A relieving officer's order was still required in the case of paupers but this might be obtained after admission instead of before.[5] Where the non-pauper patient could afford to pay, the guardians of the parish in which he lived were empowered to recover maintenance charges.[6] In default of this recoupment, the Act permitted the guardians to charge these expenses to the Metropolitan Common Poor Fund.[7] With the scope of admissions legally extended, it followed logically that patients of all classes should be carried in M A B ambulances, and the Board was authorized under the Act to convey all persons suffering from any infectious disorder, not only to and from hospital, but anywhere else when required.[8] The new measure also provided that M A B isolation hospitals should be used as medical schools.[9] One of the Board's constant hazards had been a widespread

---

[1] *M A B Annual Report* for 1888–89, p. 120. [2] See Chapter 15.

[3] At all its conferences during this period, the NAPSS (Health Section) discussed the reforms for which the M A B was pressing, e.g. *Trans. of the NAPSS*, 1882: T. Gilbart-Smith, 'What reforms are desirable in the administration of hospitals?', pp. 390–448; also: W. H. Michael, 'Notification of infectious diseases', *ibid.*, pp. 448 et seq.; also ibid., 1881, p. 532; 1880, p. 608; 1876, p. 478.

[4] 52 & 53 Vict. c. 56. [5] *Idem*, section 3 (1). [6] *Idem*, section 3 (2).

[7] *Idem*, section 3 (3). [8] *Idem*, section 6. [9] *Idem*, section 4.

deficiency in diagnostic skill in the field of zymotic disease and this had been deplored repeatedly in the reports of M A B medical superintendents. Clinical instruction in London's 'sick asylums' had been authorized in the 1867 Metropolitan Poor Act,[1] but this provision had been rescinded before the first M A B hospital had been erected.[2] So far as powers of compulsory purchase were concerned, the 'nuisance' element inherent in siting new hospitals caused the legislature to limit the powers conferred upon the Board to land adjoining its existing institutions.[3] Statutory authorization to extend the scope of admissions was therefore of restricted value without legal sanction to acquire new hospital sites compulsorily in other parts of the capital. Despite its limitations, however, the 1889 Poor Law Act represented a significant advance for the M A B isolation hospitals system. For the first time in poor law history, institutions for the destitute sick had been made legally available to patients of all social classes.[4]

VI

The year 1889 saw yet a further step forward on the public health front and a response to another of the Board's perennial demands. In October, the Infectious Disease (Notification) Act[5] was passed. This applied to eleven diseases,[6] including cholera, smallpox and the fevers treated in the M A B hospitals. The Act made it obligatory in London for details of all cases of these diseases to be communicated promptly by general practitioners to local Medical Officers of Health, who were required to furnish the M A B with copies of the relevant medical certificates within twelve hours of notification.[7] The local sanitary authority paid a fee to the doctor reporting the case—two shillings and sixpence for private

[1] 30 & 31 Vict. c. 6 s. 29.   [2] 32 & 33 Vict. c. 63 s. 20; see Chapter 17.

[3] 52 & 53 Vict. c. 56 s. 5. The newly-acquired powers of compulsory purchase were severely limited in the case of the M A B Fulham hospital. Under the London and North-Western Railway Act, introduced as a private bill shortly after the 1889 Poor Law Bill, the Railway acquired the Lillie Bridge Grounds adjoining the M A B hospital for sidings. Despite steps taken to oppose the bill, the only relief obtained by the M A B was a decision by the House of Lords for the bill to include a provision for the banning of shunting from 10 p.m. to 6 a.m.

[4] In 1889, after non-paupers were legally admitted into the M A B hospitals, the LGB authorized medical officers of poor law infirmaries to admit urgent cases without a relieving officer's order (e.g. Special Order to Mile End Old Town, dated 10 October 1889). In 1876, LGB inspectors had been instructed to induce the provincial boards of guardians to unite in establishing out of the poor rates hospitals for infectious diseases which should admit non-paupers on payment (MS. minutes, Manchester Board of Guardians, 17 February 1876), but outside London, boards of guardians failed everywhere to respond to the LGB recommendation. (S. and B. Webb, *English Local Government*, vol. i, pp. 326–333.)

[5] 52 & 53 Vict. c. 72.

[6] The 1889 Infectious Disease (Notification) Act applied at first to only eleven diseases: smallpox, cholera, diphtheria and membranous croup, erysipelas, scarlatina, typhus, typhoid, enteric, 'relapsing', 'continued' and puerperal fevers. A clause permitted the LGB to add further diseases. By the Public Health (Amendment) Act of 1890 (adoptive), the sanitary authorities were endowed with further powers of supervision and coercion.

[7] At first, the response of district Medical Officers of Health to the demands of the 1889 Infectious Disease (Notification) Act was incomplete and erratic, so that the M A B weekly returns were consequently not as comprehensive as they might have been during the first year or two of the operation of the Act.

patients and one shilling for others—and was reimbursed by the M A B from the Metropolitan Common Poor Fund. Outside London, the Act was only permissive.[1] Cholera, however, was compulsorily notifiable under the 1875 Public Health Act; and fifty provincial towns, with an aggregate population of nearly four millions, were already empowered by Local Acts to enforce notification of infectious disease. Following the 1889 Act, nearly one thousand sanitary authorities, with an aggregate population of upwards of sixteen millions, voluntarily adopted its provisions. Including London's four and a quarter millions, the obligatory notification of infectious disease therefore applied to some twenty-four of the twenty-nine million inhabitants of the whole country at this time.[2]

Now that this measure of pestilence control had reached the Statute Book, the Asylums Board was far from satisfied with its provisions so far as they applied to London. The Act contained nothing mandatory concerning the ultimate use to be made of the data received from the local authorities, apart from a directive that the M A B should communicate to the recently created LCC such returns of infectious disease as that authority 'should from time to time require'.[3] The Local Government Act of 1888, under which the LCC had been created, lacked precision concerning the public health functions of the local authorities which the Council was intended to supervise, and the M A B doubted whether good use would be made of the returns once the Council received them. In the past, the Board had taken the initiative in supplying local sanitary authorities with details of M A B hospital admissions, classified according to districts of origin. This had had useful results. Now that the M A B was to serve as a receiving centre under the Act for all metropolitan notifications, it decided to establish a systematic clearing house for all available information concerning infectious disease in London. These data were collated and processed under the direction of the Board's statistical committee, and comprehensive tabular statements were published and circulated weekly to all metropolitan medical officers of health. This procedure was of twofold importance. First, as every metropolitan local authority was furnished regularly with up-to-date information concerning the spread of infection, both in its own and contiguous districts, it was enabled to take prompt measures of control. Secondly, the M A B was able to obtain, for the first time, an authentic and relatively comprehensive picture of the state of disease in the metropolis as a whole, thus making it possible to regulate existing accommodation and assess future requirements with greater precision and economy.

During the first year of operation of the 1889 Notification Act, the M A B statistical committee made a study of its effectiveness and concluded that certain amendments were urgently required. The exemption under the Act of cases occurring in other London hospitals considerably diminished its value. Likewise, the clause exempting from notification establishments belonging to the Crown provided an appreciable factor of uncertainty.

[1] Notification of infectious disease was made compulsory throughout the country by the Notification of Infectious Disease Extension Act, 1899.

[2] Sir H. Burdett, *Hospitals and Asylums of the World*, vol. iii (1893), p. 109.

[3] 52 & 53 Vict. c. 72 s. 10.

There were in London some 130 hospitals in which infectious cases might possibly be under treatment. Although a number of these were voluntarily notified by the medical officers of these institutions, many remained unreported. As the M A B statistical committee also regarded as inadequate the medical certificate which had been designed for use under the Act, it was suggested to the Local Government Board that, in addition to the name and address of the patient and the name of the disease, the certificate should indicate the patient's sex and age, as well as the address of the certifying medical practitioner, and a statement as to whether he attended the patient privately or as medical officer of a public body or institution. The limited information required by the Local Government Board might be adequate in provincial towns, the Asylums Board pointed out, but in London, with its large population and numerous independent local authorities, it was insufficient.[1] The Local Government Board replied that 'the amendments suggested were not required for the purposes for which the system of notification was rendered compulsory'.[2] With their habitual pertinacity, the Asylums Managers persisted in their efforts to bring about the required improvements. When, two years later, a public health code was conferred upon London, infectious cases in hospitals were included in the notifications system,[3] although it continued for a quarter of a century to exclude the infectious occupants of palaces, barracks, police stations and prisons.[4]

VII

In 1891, twenty-nine earlier enactments were revised and codified in the Public Health (London) Law Consolidation Bill. Of these, the Diseases Prevention (Metropolis) Act of 1883[5] and the Poor Law Act of 1889[6] most closely affected the administration of the M A B isolation hospitals system. In addition to confirming the powers which the M A B had derived from these enactments, the 1891 Bill renewed the existing, but unused, powers of the metropolitan sanitary authorities to provide hospitals and ambulances for paying patients as well as temporary medical assistance for 'the poorer inhabitants' of their districts. An important innovation under the new legislation was the power it conferred upon magistrates to order the detention in hospital of infectious patients who lacked suitable alternative accommodation.[7]

During the Committee stage of the Bill, discussion was focused on the general prin-

---

[1] M A B letter to the LGB, 6 November 1889.
[2] LGB letter to the M A B, 4 December 1889.
[3] Public Health (London) Act, 1891 (54 & 55 Vict. c. 76 s. 55).
[4] Local Government (Emergency Provisions) Act, 1916, section 5 (b), provided, as a temporary measure, for the notification of infectious disease contracted by members of H.M. Forces and employees of the Admiralty, Army Council and Ministry of Munitions. This provision was extended from time to time under the Expiring Laws Acts.
[5] 46 & 47 Vict. c. 35 s. 7, which abolished poor law disqualifications of M A B infectious patients.
[6] 52 & 53 Vict. c. 56 ss. 3 (1), 3 (2) and 6 (see section V of this chapter).
[7] 54 & 55 Vict. c. 76 s. 82.

ciple of payment for treatment in sanitary authority hospitals. At the instigation of Mr. Pickersgill, Member for Bethnal Green, the clause providing for payment by patients in these hospitals was eventually deleted. During the Second Reading, a strong body of opinion urged the re-insertion of the payment clause on the ground that, if gratuitous treatment were given in these hospitals, 'there would be nothing to prevent the establishment of free dispensaries all over London'. Those who upheld the principle of free treatment sought to strengthen their case by emphasizing the public health aspect of isolating infectious patients. All this discussion was purely hypothetical, since no metropolitan sanitary authority had availed itself of its powers under earlier legislation to provide a hospital of any kind. Mr. C. R. (later Lord) Ritchie, President of the Local Government Board, drew the attention of the House to this fact, and explained that the only hospitals in question in the Bill were, therefore, the M A B fever and smallpox institutions. He would, he said, consider whether any amendment was required in the body of the Bill itself in order to make it clear that the waiving of hospital charges applied 'only to hospitals for infectious diseases'. He conceded that it was 'all a matter of inducement'; and, 'considering that the amount that would be received would be infinitesimal', he thought the arguments in favour of payment 'ought not to be allowed to weigh against the general good, which was that persons suffering from infectious disease should go into some place where they could be properly treated. . .'.[1]

The Act eventually made it explicit that expenses incurred by a non-destitute patient who was not suffering from infectious disease should be a simple contract debt due to the authority from the patient.[2] While no local authority in the metropolis provided a hospital, this provision remained a dead letter. So far as concerned expenses incurred by infectious patients in the M A B hospitals, the Act incorporated the section of the 1889 Act which authorized the admission of non-pauper patients into the Board's hospitals,[3] but it omitted the reference to the power of the parochial authorities to recover maintenance costs from such patients.[4] Thus amended, the relevant section of the 1889 Act, when embodied in the 1891 Act, was reduced to: 'The said expenses shall be repaid to the board of guardians out of the Metropolitan Common Poor Fund.'[5] The 1889 Act had empowered boards of guardians to charge the maintenance costs of non-pauper patients against the Common Poor Fund only in cases where they had failed to collect all or part of the amount owing.[6] The destitution authorities, which were liable to the M A B for the hospital expenses of patients in their respective districts, had taken the line of least resistance and recovered from the Fund the whole of the charges of both their pauper and non-pauper cases.[7] All patients in the M A B isolation hospitals—destitute, wage-earning and affluent alike—had

[1] *Hansard*, 1891, vol. cccliv (third series), cols. 1589–1601.
[2] 54 & 55 Vict. c. 76 s. 76.   [3] 52 & 53 Vict. c. 56 s. 3 (1).
[4] 52 & 53 Vict. c. 56 s. 3 (2).   [5] 54 & 55 Vict. c. 76 s. 80 (3).
[6] 52 & 53 Vict. c. 56 s. 3 (3).
[7] The Webbs could find no evidence between 1889 and 1891 of any attempt by any metropolitan board of guardians to recover costs from non-destitute infectious patients. (S. and B. Webb, *English Local Government*, vol. i, p. 326, n. 3.)

thus been maintained at public expense since 1889, and probably for many years before. The 1891 legislation, by waiving all M A B hospital charges, accorded statutory sanction to what was already an arbitrary practice. The new public health measure also endorsed the complete dissociation of the M A B isolation hospitals from the poor law, and confirmed the removal from the infectious sick of those disqualifications by which the poor law punished the misfortune of poverty.[1]

The 1891 Act thus implemented the long-ignored recommendations submitted by investigating bodies during the previous three-quarters of a century. In 1818 the Select Committee appointed to study contagious fever in the metropolis had urged the establishment in London of free isolation hospitals.[2] In 1854, another Select Committee of Enquiry had put forward the revolutionary notion that medical relief should not pauperize the recipients as did other forms of relief.[3] The 1881–82 Royal Commission on Fever and Smallpox Hospitals had suggested the abolition of hospital charges, even where these could be paid without hardship, and had emphasized the desirability of dissociating from the poor law all treatment of infectious disease.[4]

Nothing in the 1891 Public Health (London) Act altered the poor law status of the Asylums Board, but it transformed the M A B fever and smallpox hospitals from pauper institutions into England's first free State hospitals. On and after 1 January 1892, every citizen of London suffering from infectious disease was legally entitled to admission into an M A B hospital for gratuitous treatment, irrespective of ability to pay, and subject only to the production of a medical certificate. A new and important principle of social administration had been inaugurated. Members of a dependent class—the infectious sick—were to be treated by the community, not in respect of their economic circumstances, but by reference to their medical needs. Unobtrusively, the State had penetrated a sphere hitherto the monopoly of charity.

[1] 54 & 55 Vict. c. 76 s. 80 (4). The Diseases Prevention (Metropolis) Act of 1883 (46 & 47 Vict. c. 33 s. 7) abolished the denial of the vote to M A B patients, except in parish elections. The complete removal of electoral disqualifications for all sick paupers was effected by the Medical Relief Disqualification Act of 1885 (48 & 49 Vict. c. 46 s. 2).

[2] *Report of the Select Committee of 1818 appointed to examine into the state of contagious fever in the metropolis:* BPP, 1818, vol. vii (Cmd. 332), p. 6 [178].

[3] *Report of the Select Committee of 1854 appointed to enquire into the mode in which medical relief is administered in the unions of England and Wales:* BPP, 1854 (348), vol. xii, 431 (recommendation no. 5).

[4] See Chapter 6.

CHAPTER 8

The *MAB Infectious Disease Hospitals:*
The Fourth Phase—1892 to 1900

I

THE omission of a few words in the 1891 Public Health (London) Act had created for the Asylums Board a new universe comprising four and a quarter million Londoners of all classes. At the time of its inception twenty-four years earlier, the Board's responsibilities had been limited to the infectious and insane members of the pauper population of 163,000.[1] From 1892, when the 1891 Act came into operation, until the end of the century, the Asylums Board was concerned both to meet the immediate expansion in demand, which the new legislation imposed on its isolation accommmodation, and to plan for long-range changes in the modes of man and microbe.

New hospitals were needed. The Board aimed to provide one fever bed for every one thousand inhabitants of London and sufficient accommodation to meet effectively any future outbreak of smallpox. By this time, the Board commanded some 2,350 fever beds in seven hospitals, a ratio of one bed to approximately eighteen hundred of the metropolitan population. Nearly 1,500 smallpox beds were already available, although many were in temporary structures on the riverside encampment at Darenth. A decade earlier, the 1881–82 Royal Commission had recommended the provision of an additional 1,500 fever beds, making a total of 3,000, and of 2,000 smallpox beds. But at that time, the population of London was smaller; non-paupers were ineligible for treatment; compulsory notification was not in force; the Board's ambulance systems had not been established; diphtheria was not an admissible disease; and smallpox hospitals were still located in populous London districts. To meet the changes of the past few years and to provide for future contingencies, the Board planned to build five new fever hospitals—all, except one, south of the Thames—to accommodate 2,000 acute, and 800 convalescent, cases.

Suitable sites were becoming scarce by this time. Apprehensive of local opposition, the central authority held a public enquiry into each proposed purchase. Objectors were invited to appeal and often succeeded in their appeals. The Asylums Board had never been granted

---

[1] The total number of paupers relieved in London at the end of 1867 was 163,179 (38,173 indoor and 125,006 outdoor) (*PLB Twenty-first Annual Report*, 1868–69, pp. 272 and 280).

compulsory powers for the purchase of new hospital sites. Although charged by Parliament to provide isolation accommodation for the whole of London, the Board was more hampered than any irresponsible private individual and was obliged to pay considerably higher prices for land. Two years was the usual interval between the selection of a site and the Local Government Board's decision regarding purchase. A fever hospital for 500 patients could not be erected, equipped and staffed in less than a further two years.

In 1890, the Board had already anticipated the expansion programme and selected a site of 28 acres at Tottenham for a new hospital for North London. The price was £12,000. After two years' deliberation, the Local Government Board decided against its acquisition. The Asylums Managers thereupon found alternative building land at Tooting. This was submitted to the same inquisition, with identical results. Meantime, a violent outbreak of scarlet fever had beset the capital. Admissions to the Board's fever hospitals during 1892 exceeded 13,000—more than twice the annual average for the previous five years. On occasion, over 4,000 patients were under treatment. As the demand for fever beds increased, the Managers pressed the Local Government Board to reconsider the purchase of the Tottenham and Tooting sites. In the absence of a prompt response, the M A B conferred emergency powers upon its general purposes committee. In two weeks, the committee had arranged for the erection around the existing hospitals of temporary huts to accommodate one thousand cases. When these were full, eight hundred more beds were hurriedly secured. But even these were insufficient to keep pace with the epidemic. For the first time in their history, the M A B fever hospitals were obliged to refuse admissions. Vacancies left by deaths and discharges were given to applicants housed in the worst conditions, while arrangements were made for some of the London general hospitals to admit enteric cases. This situation prompted the Local Government Board to sanction the appropriation of the Tottenham site. Within seven weeks, a temporary structure—the North-Eastern Hospital[1]—was designed, equipped and staffed. In October 1892, it opened with 500 beds. The Board now had upwards of 4,700 fever beds—twice the number available five months before.

II

Providing for patients suffering from 'fever', diphtheria and smallpox was not the extent of the Asylums Board's public health functions. Under the 1891 Public Health (London) Act, it was liable to be endowed with 'the powers and duties of a sanitary authority. . . .'[2] The Asylums Managers had assumed that this provision had been inserted by Mr. Ritchie, President of the Local Government Board when the Act was passed, by way of implementing their recommendation that a central board—ideally the M A B—should be appointed in London to co-ordinate and supervise the functions of the local sanitary

[1] A model of the M A B North-Eastern Hospital at Tottenham, now known as St. Ann's General Hospital, is shown in figure 1. Architectural notes will be found at the beginning of Appendix II.

[2] 54 & 55 Vict. c. 76 s. 85.

authorities with a view to improving public health administration. Instead, Mr. Ritchie's successor, Mr. H. H. Fowler (later Viscount Wolverhampton), imposed upon the Asylums Board *ad hoc* emergency duties when the country was threatened with pestilential invasion from the continent. In 1892, for example, at the height of the scarlet fever epidemic, the Asylums Board was ordered at short notice to make arrangements to guard against the introduction into England of Asiatic cholera.[1] The disease had swept across Europe and eventually decimated Hamburg. Despite its other preoccupations, the M A B convened a special cholera committee, which included a specialist in the disease, Dr. Arthur Shadwell, and the LCC Medical Officer of Health, Dr. Shirley Murphy. Two thousand beds were made available by arrangement with the general hospitals and workhouse infirmaries, and thirty cholera receiving stations were set up throughout London. These precautions were maintained for the next two years. During this period, only one bed was required in London, although four isolated cases at Gravesend, Cardiff, Grimsby and Hull caused some alarm.[2]

Meantime, metropolitan Medical Officers of Health were appealing to the Local Government Board to sanction the allocation of M A B ambulances for the use of influenza cases. 'Russian influenza',[3] as it was known, had reached Western Europe, and it was feared that it would spread to London. The question of M A B ambulances being used in such a contingency was pondered for so long in Whitehall that the danger passed before a decision was reached. Consequently, influenza was never included among the diseases for which treatment and transport could be legally provided by the M A B hospital services.

III

The threats of cholera and influenza were accompanied in 1893 by a recrudescence of scarlet fever and an outbreak of smallpox. The need for additional accommodation was becoming acute. Again, the M A B demanded powers for acquiring building land, and permission to appropriate the Tooting site was eventually obtained. Again, a makeshift hospital was erected. 'The Fountain'—as it was called—provided four hundred more fever beds, at a cost of £117,000. Patients received into the Board's fever hospitals during 1893 totalled 14,500, but it had been necessary to turn away some 6,000 applicants for whom no beds were available. The continued high incidence of scarlet fever in London and the insufficiency of beds in the M A B hospitals created acute public concern. A battery of parliamentary questions between June and September 1895, however, resulted in building sites being made available to the Board. Within a few months, three new hospitals were in course of construction—the 'Park' at Lewisham, the 'Grove' at Tooting, and the

---

[1] Before 1892, Asiatic cholera had not appeared in England since 1866. (A. H. Gale, op. cit., Chapter 5.)

[2] Dr. Arthur Shadwell's report on the 1892–93 cholera epidemic in Europe and the arrangements made for the sick in London is appended to M A B *Mins.*, vol. xxvii, pp. 752–58.

[3] The 1889–92 pandemic of influenza was the beginning of a new chapter in the history of the disease, not only in this country but also in Europe and North America, and probably throughout the world. (A. H. Gale, op. cit., p. 47.)

'Brook' at Woolwich.[1] In 1896, authorization was also granted by the Local Government Board for the purchase of a 136-acre site at Carshalton, upon which to build an 800-bed convalescent hospital. This eventually became known as Queen Mary's Hospital for Children.[2]

Legislation did not dispel immediately the 'taint' of pauperism hitherto associated with the Board's hospitals, but by the mid-1890s they had begun to acquire the impress of social acceptability. In August 1897, the Prince of Wales (later King Edward VII) formally opened the new Park Fever Hospital at Lewisham—the most up-to-date of the Board's institutions according to contemporary standards—and declared it to be 'dedicated to the public'. Only then was the transition from pauper to public health status in effect complete.

IV

Rapid growth in the M A B hospital system during the terminal decade of the century was accompanied by changes in the prevalence and treatment of the 'crowd diseases'. Discoveries were reported almost annually. The diagnostic development of the Klebs-Löffler bacillus[3] and the newly-discovered antitoxin treatment for diphtheria[4] had both immediate and far-reaching significance for the M A B fever hospitals. Following the introduction in 1894 of the antitoxin treatment, diphtheria deaths in hospital steadily declined, while admissions rapidly increased.[5] In the long term, these advances led to the establishment by the Board of its own pathological and serum production laboratories.[6] The adoption of the new techniques opportunely coincided with the opening of the Board's hospitals to medical students for clinical instruction,[7] followed by attempts to improve nursing standards and organization.[8] With these innovations, began a new scientific approach to the study and treatment of infectious disease which was to alter the character of the M A B isolation hospitals in the coming century.

The incidence of disease, it has been said, expresses a conflict between two constantly-evolving, dynamic forces—man and the attacking microbe.[9] In this perpetual struggle, the agents of disease continue to change while man advances. William Farr wrote in his 1873 annual letter to the Registrar-General:

> ... the infectious diseases replace each other and when one is rooted out it is apt to be replaced by others which ravage the human race indifferently whenever the conditions of healthy life are wanting. They have this property in common with weeds and other forms of life—as one species recedes, another advances.[10]

---

[1] See Map II, following Appendix IV, for the location of M A B hospitals in 1900.
[2] See Chapter 18.   [3] F. Löffler, *Mitt. Reichsgesundheitsamt*, 2 (1884), 421.
[4] Behring and Wernicke, *Dtsch. Med. Wschr.* 39 (1892), 873.
[5] See Appendix II, Table D.   [6] See Chapter 17.   [7] Ibid.   [8] See Chapter 12.
[9] W. H. Bradley, 'Notifiable Infectious Diseases: A Re-Assessment', *R. Soc. Hlth. J.*, vol. 79, No. 4, July–August 1959, p. 484.
[10] Cited by W. H. Bradley, op. cit.

So it was with the diseases which the M A B hospitals had been treating for more than two decades. Planning programmes could not ignore their changing incidence and character.

Scarlet fever had been declining progressively.[1] Reporting in 1890, Dr. W. Gayton, medical superintendent of the Hampstead (North-Western) Hospital, pointed out that during the thirty-four years from 1840 to 1873, deaths from scarlet fever in London had exceeded 82,000, while during the next seventeen years (1874 to 1890) 'in spite of the still crowded dwellings of the working classes', they had numbered about 31,000, 'a state of things undreamed of in past years'.[2] The annual average of some 600 scarlet fever deaths during the last quinquennium of the century, in a more densely populated London, was likewise quite 'undreamed of' by Dr. Gayton when writing on the eve of London's 1891 Public Health Act. The death rate—and probably the incidence—of enteric fevers (typhoid and paratyphoid) had been declining since 1871. By 1890, a static point had been reached which was maintained until the end of the century.[3] This decline, which was attributed to purer water supplies, was more marked in the mortality of adults and of older children than in that of babies.[4] Typhus also had been declining rapidly during the latter half of the nineteenth century, although it remained a leading cause of death among the poor of industrial areas.[5] Diphtheria had become widespread and was increasing. From about 1880, it began to overtake scarlet fever as one of the most fatal of the infectious diseases of childhood, and in the quinquennium 1886–90 actually took the lead. Thereafter, it was overtaken by measles and whooping-cough but long remained one of the leading causes of death in children.[6] Disastrous as smallpox had been in London since the beginning of death registration (1838), it was a mere shadow of what it had been in the eighteenth century. Despite admitted inaccuracies in the bills of mortality, epidemiologists agree that deaths from smallpox, relative to those from other causes, diminished towards the end of the eighteenth century and that this trend was maintained broadly, with intermittent flaring-up, throughout the nineteenth century in London, as in the country generally.[7]

V

To what extent, if at all, London's vulnerability to smallpox would be influenced by the new measures of control—notification and treatment away from populous areas—it was, at this juncture, too early to foretell. Although the average annual rate of death from smallpox in London had fallen to two per million during the six years immediately following the removal of smallpox cases out of the capital, the disease had not yet been eradicated.

[1] A. H. Gale, op. cit., p. 91, fig. 11.   [2] *M A B Annual Report* for 1890, p. 35.
[3] See Appendix II, Table D.   [4] A. H. Gale, op. cit., p. 139.
[5] Ibid., pp. 74–75.
[6] Sir John Simon, *Second Report to the Privy Council for 1859*, section on diphtheria; and A. H. Gale, op. cit., pp. 93–94 and 139.
[7] C. Creighton, *A History of Epidemics in Britain*, II (1894), p. 612; L. H. Greenwood, *Epidemics and Crowd Diseases*, I (1935), p. 239; A. H. Gale, op. cit., pp. 55–63; W. H. Bradley, op. cit.

An epidemic between 1893 and 1895 brought some 4,500 cases to the river hospitals.[1] This represented over 90 per cent of all notified cases, a degree of control never before achieved. Contemplating the possibility of repeated outbreaks, the Asylums Managers decided to build a 900-bed smallpox hospital near Dartford, in Kent, and eventually to do away with the hospital ships, which were costly to administer and subject to numerous hazards.[2] They submitted plans to the Local Government Board and applied for sanction to purchase a site of 218 acres, the Joyce Green estate. While the central authority approved the purchase of the site, it contended that four hundred beds would be adequate. Aware of the insidiousness of the disease, the M A B senior medical staff insisted on the need for preparedness. After two years' deliberation, the Local Government Board conceded that, in the event of an outbreak which could not be met by existing buildings, consent would be given for the erection of temporary accommodation.[3] The Asylums Managers were not satisfied; their experience had shown that temporary building to meet emergencies was unnecessarily costly. Resolving that 'it would be imprudent to consume more valuable time at this juncture in negotiations with the Local Government Board', they decided on strategic action. While work was in progress on the pavilions for the four hundred beds approved by the central authority, representations concerning the need for a 900-bed structure would continue. Once the basic services were laid on, it would be pointed out that the whole project could be completed on a permanent basis far more economically if undertaken while the builders' plant was on the spot. When, during the last year of the century, there were signs of an impending outbreak of smallpox, the central authority found it difficult to resist the fact that a hospital, on which £222,000 had already been expended, could be completed and doubled in value for an additional £77,000. The 986-bed Joyce Green Hospital was thus secured for future generations.

VI

During this period of expansion and change, the Managers' battles with bureaucracy were not limited to hospital building. The rented premises which the M A B had occupied in Norfolk Street, Strand, for the past thirty years had become inadequate. The Board's total personnel now exceeded 5,000. Some 3,000 served in the fever hospitals; about 1,000 in the mental institutions; 550 in the smallpox hospitals; and some 300 in the ambulance services; while about 150 were required at the head office. Legislation decreed that the M A B should administer hospital, ambulance and statistical services; but when application was made for permission to build an office from which these activities could be directed, the M A B was informed by the Local Government Board that no statutory authority

---

[1] See Appendix II, Table B.

[2] The three M A B hospital ships, providing 300 smallpox beds, cost over £9,000 a year to administer during the last decade of the nineteenth century, apart from the cost of the river ambulance service, which averaged £8,000 a year.

[3] LGB letter to the M A B, 27 August 1896.

existed for the raising of money for this purpose.[1] The Managers thereupon urged the introduction of legislation to remedy this situation. Meantime, they negotiated with the Land Committee of the Corporation of the City of London for the acquisition of a site at the corner of Victoria Embankment and Carmelite Street. Purchase was made conditional on permission being received before the end of the current session of Parliament for raising a loan for the building. In August 1897, after three months of active negotiation, authorization was granted to the Asylums Board to purchase the site, at a price not exceeding £53,000, for the erection of a head office.[2] Within three years, the M A B central staff was installed in the new headquarters.

Despite the increased stature of the Asylums Board, its main functions were still limited to the institutional treatment and transport of patients suffering from certain acute infectious diseases and to the care of chronic insane paupers. The provision in the 1891 Act which empowered the Local Government Board to confer upon the M A B the status of a public health authority[3] was never implemented beyond the imposition of *ad hoc* emergency functions. The opportunity to establish—in collaboration with the LCC and the metropolitan local authorities—a comprehensive public health body for the whole of London was lost for a generation. The M A B remained nominally a poor law authority; and so long as the poor law survived it was to inhibit the development of public social service.[4] Only by a persistent, if imperceptible, undermining of the poor law had it been possible to open to the public the doors of the M A B 'pauper asylums' for infectious diseases; and this had demanded an exceptional alignment of blind fortuitous forces and purposive endeavour.

[1] LGB letters to the M A B, 4 December 1896 and 3 May 1897.
[2] LGB letter to the M A B, 31 August 1897.
[3] 54 & 55 Vict. c. 76 s. 85.
[4] During the nineteenth century, public social service was almost synonymous with the administration of the poor law. Even when a service was extended beyond the pauper class, it was usually entrusted, as a subsidiary function, to the poor law guardians. (T. S. Simey, *Principles of Social Administration* (1937), p. 35 *et seq.*)

9

CHAPTER 9

From Poor Law to Public Health Status: The Forces of Transition

BAGEHOT regarded progress in the history of mankind as rare and exceptional, depending on an uncommon combination of energy and balance of mind.[1] Implicit in Bagehot's philosophy—and indeed in most socio-philosophical theories of social change—is the thesis that voluntary acts of individuals or groups are an important factor in bringing about changes in the structure of societies. On analysis, such acts are shown invariably to be motivated by social maladjustments or 'tensions'. But the changes which eventually result are often found to stem, not so much from the original, predetermined acts, but rather from their unintended outcome. An effect designed to serve certain ends comes in the course of its development to serve others. New needs may arise; obstacles may be encountered. At a particular moment in time, there is a convergence of elements derived from different sources, the impact of which determines a new direction.[2] Of such a nature was the translation of the M A B isolation hospitals system from poor law to public health status.

The social malaise induced by the inhumanity of the Victorian poor law between the 1830s and 1860s led to a demand for separate provision for the care of the destitute sick and finally to the creation of special hospitals for these dependants of the State. This was the predetermined goal; but an outcome, unforeseen by the original reformers, was the convergence of independent forces which had been set in motion during this process. This had the effect of diverting developments into channels which led eventually to the establishment of this country's first free State hospital service for the general public.

One of the worst features of the nineteenth-century poor law was the absence of a specific policy governing the care of the destitute sick. Only when the fatal neglect of paupers in metropolitan workhouses was forced upon the attention of the public was an attempt made to rescue the sick from the punitive conditions designed to deter the able-bodied. The awakening of the public conscience and the mobilization of the legislature was due initially to individual and privately organized activity aimed at poor law medical reform. These purposive strivings culminated in 'Gathorne Hardy's Act' of 1867, the creation of the M A B in the same year, and the opening in London, three years later, of

---

[1] W. Bagehot, *Physics and Politics* (1872).
[2] Professor M. Ginsberg, 'Social Change', *British Journal of Sociology*, vol. ix, 3 (September 1958).

the first special hospitals for sick paupers. An immediate goal had been achieved, but the vicissitudes to which it became subject created further difficulties and fresh demands. During the next decade, these necessitated a reappraisal of the hospitals' functions in relation to public needs. The tangled skein of events during this period were linked by 'Acts of God', on the one hand, and Acts of Parliament, on the other. The reactions of individuals and groups to these phenomena and enactments mediated the connexion between the first State 'asylums' for the destitute sick and the public isolation hospitals of a later age.

Throughout history, pestilence has proved a powerful agent of social change, not only as a demographic factor, but also as an efficient cause through the reactions of those involved. In the early days of the M A B hospitals, infectious disease revealed the failure of the metropolitan sanitary authorities to provide hospitals for patients above the pauper class. As a result, visitations of smallpox to the capital caused the M A B institutions to be inundated with non-pauper patients for whom they were not legally intended. This situation set in motion three independent currents of activity which, nevertheless, contributed blindly to a common end.

First, the excessive demands made upon the M A B hospitals rendered it necessary to regularize the illegal, but expedient, admission of non-paupers suffering from infectious disease. Initially, the official regulations governing hospital management were modified to permit the reception of 'emergency' cases. Subsequently, the 1876 Poor Law Amendment Act gave statutory sanction to the waiving of maintenance charges in respect of these patients. Three years later, in the absence of institutions of their own, the metropolitan sanitary authorities were empowered—by the Poor Law Act of 1879—to contract with the Asylums Board for the admission of their non-destitute infectious patients into the M A B hospitals. Neither of these piecemeal attempts to patch up public health deficiencies proved effective in practice. The legalized 'emergency' admissions served merely to perpetuate the existing situation in which any non-pauper patient suffering from an acute infectious fever or smallpox, who applied direct to an M A B isolation hospital, was received and subsidized from the poor rates; while the sanitary authorities, finding this procedure financially advantageous, refrained from contracting with the M A B. These two measures, nevertheless, are noteworthy in that they represent the first poor law enactments to provide for the medical care of non-destitute patients in pauper institutions.[1] To this extent, they furthered the erosion of traditional poor law principles which was begun by the 1867 Metropolitan Poor Act.

Secondly, the unforeseen use of the M A B isolation hospitals by infectious patients outside the pauper class brought into relief ideological differences between the Asylums

---

[1] 39 & 40 Vict. c. 61 s. 42, and 42 & 43 Vict. c. 54 s. 15. There was no statutory authority before 1876 for admitting a non-pauper patient into the sick ward of a workhouse except upon a Justice's Order under the Public Health Act of 1875 (38 & 39 Vict. c. 55 s. 124) in the case of a person suffering from a dangerous or infectious disorder 'if such a ward could be considered a hospital within the meaning of the Act'. (Glen's *Poor Law Orders* (1898: 11th edn.), p. 274, n. 1.)

Managers and their masters in Whitehall concerning the character of the hospitals and the precise role of the M A B in their administration. Broadly, the central department viewed the new 'asylums' as part of a poor law classification system in which the separation of the sick facilitated the stricter application of deterrent measures to the able-bodied paupers. The M A B, on the other hand, was concerned mainly with public health considerations, and regarded the hospitals as the sanitary defences of London. During their first decade, the Asylums Managers sought to administer their institutions on voluntary hospital lines[1] and to promote their use by all needing isolation and treatment in the metropolitan area, irrespective of class or ability to pay. These objectives were discouraged by the central authority, which at this time was prone to an anti-medical bias and inflexible 'poor law thinking'.

Thirdly, the location of the M A B smallpox institutions in populous areas aroused fears among local residents, who engaged the Asylums Board in protracted and fruitless legal disputes. This litigation revealed the fact that any, or all, of the M A B isolation hospitals might be summarily immobilized if local residents claimed that a fever or smallpox hospital constituted a 'nuisance' in common law. This was possible because the 1867 Act, under which the M A B came into being, was declared by the Law Lords in 1881 to contain no mandatory provision whatever for the erection of isolation hospitals by the Asylums Board. The private right of individuals to freedom from nuisance arising from any action of the M A B was upheld.[2] In the existing state of the law, the Asylums Board could be divested of its power to perform its statutory functions and London deprived of a means of protection from infectious disease.

The irresponsibility of the sanitary authorities; the irreconcilable philosophies of the M A B and the central authority; and the near-paralysis of the Board's hospitals through drafting defects in legislation combined to create an *impasse*. This convergence of intractable elements became the preoccupation of the Royal Commission appointed in 1881 to investigate the isolation hospitals of London. Its recommendation that treatment for infectious disease should be completely divorced from the poor law was as revolutionary as Gathorne Hardy's declaration in 1867 that the care of the destitute sick should be conducted on a system entirely dissociated from the workhouse.[3] Also without precedent were the Commission's suggestions that all infectious patients—paupers and non-destitute alike—should be accommodated together in the general wards of the M A B hospitals, and that maintenance charges should be waived even where these could be paid without hardship.[4] As a result of these deliberations, a new direction was given to the fortunes of the hitherto ill-fated M A B isolation hospitals.

During the ensuing decade, most of the Commission's recommendations were em-

[1] Administration of the M A B hospitals is discussed in Chapter 12.
[2] H. L. 6 App. Cas. 193 (March 1881).
[3] *Hansard*, vol. clxxxv (third series), col. 163 (8 February 1867).
[4] *Report of the Royal Commission on Smallpox and Fever Hospitals*, 1882, BPP, 1882, vol. xxiv, 1 [Cmd. 3314].

bodied in legislation which nibbled unobtrusively into the poor law. The Diseases Prevention (Metropolis) Act of 1883 removed the pauperization and the civil disabilities hitherto inflicted upon patients admitted to the M A B hospitals.[1] Further advances resulted from the Poor Law Act of 1889, which empowered the Board's hospitals to receive *all* confirmed cases of fever, smallpox and diphtheria.[2] Under the Act, M A B ambulances— hitherto restricted by the 1879 Poor Law Act to the transport of pauper cases—were permitted to convey any infectious patient to any part of London.[3] The Infectious Disease Notification Act of 1889,[4] which created a new measure of pestilence control, revealed the true extent of the need for adequate isolation provision in London and resulted in greater demands on the M A B hospitals. In 1891, the consolidating Public Health (London) Act confirmed the open door of the M A B infectious disease hospitals, and decreed that maintenance costs of all patients, of whatever status, should be paid from the Metropolitan Common Fund, the collectivist system inaugurated by the 1867 Metropolitan Poor Act.[5] One of England's first social services of modern times was thus created out of a pauper hospital system.

The progress from poor law to public health status had not been influenced in any marked degree by advances in the scientific knowledge of disease—a powerful force in the movement towards specialization, and thence to socialization, in the general sector of hospital provision. It was not until the decade following the acquisition of public health status that the M A B isolation hospitals were affected by bacteriological discoveries.[6] Before these advances, however, the fear of disease, with but imprecise knowledge of its aetiology or mode of communication, was the most potent promoter of the primacy of public health needs over poor law principles. Following the Gladstonian Reform Acts of 1884 and 1885, the voice of fear could make itself even more clearly heard in the House of Commons, which, to a greater extent than ever before, had become effectively representative of public opinion and the centre of legislative power.

The first statutory stepping stones from the poor law of the nineteenth century to the social legislation of the twentieth were, in effect, the product of persistent reforming endeavour, motivated by social maladjustments and aided by maturing public opinion, pestilence and the force of fear.

[1] 46 & 47 Vict. c. 35 s. 7. [2] 52 & 53 Vict. c. 56 s. 3.
[3] *Idem*, s. 6. [4] 52 & 53 Vict. c. 72.
[5] 54 & 55 Vict. c. 76 s. 80 (3). The Metropolitan Common Poor Fund is described in Chapter 13 and in Appendix IV.
[6] See Chapter 17 concerning developments in the M A B hospitals following the introduction of the antitoxin treatment of diphtheria. Other bacteriological discoveries of the terminal decade of the nineteenth century included the plague bacillus (Kitasato and Yersin: 1894); trypanosoma, the cause of sleeping sickness (Bruce: 1894); the dysentery bacillus (Shiga: 1897); the transmission of malaria and yellow fever by mosquitoes (Ross: 1899).

CHAPTER 10

Infection and Prevention in the Metropolis—
1870 to 1900: An Evaluation

I

By the end of the century, the M A B infectious disease hospitals had been functioning for three decades. During the greater part of this period, London, in common with other rapidly expanding urban areas, had been fighting a losing battle against disease. Only during the last decade of the century was any significant advance apparent in London's war on pestilence. By this time, two new weapons were in use—free isolation accommodation and compulsory notification. It is obviously impossible to estimate to what extent, if at all, these influenced the course of disease and death in London, since they formed only part of a complexity of contributory factors, which included improved sanitation, education, housing and living standards generally. Nevertheless, a comparison of infectious disease mortality rates obtaining in London during the decennium before the advent of the M A B hospitals (1861–70) with those prevailing a generation after their creation (1891–1900) suggests that the hospitals—together with obligatory notification—may well have played some part in the diminution of death from infectious diseases. From Table 1 following[1], it will be seen that during the latter period, the average annual rate of death from smallpox in London was 266 per million less than during the earlier period; while mortality from scarlet fever and the group 'typhus, enteric and the simple continued fevers' was reduced by 945 and 757 per million respectively. On the other hand, there was an apparent annual increase of 321 diphtheria deaths per million during the last decade of the century. On balance, therefore, deaths from all the diseases treated in the M A B hospitals showed a net average annual reduction of 1,647 per million during the third decade of their operation. In London's population of over 4·5 million, this represented an average annual total of some 7,400 lives apparently saved during the years of free isolation provision and obligatory notification. Although numerous other factors would have been concerned in this apparent saving of life, these two measures were the only ones directly aimed at such a result.

While compulsory notification was in force in most parts of the country during the

[1] Tables referred to are set out at the end of this chapter unless otherwise indicated.

last decade of the century, London was unique in the extent to which it was provided with isolation hospitals and ambulances for the infectious sick.[1] The question naturally arises as to whether the lack of these amenities appreciably affected mortality rates outside the metropolis. If London rates of death from the M A B diseases are compared with those for the country as a whole during the pre-M A B decennium and the 1891–1900 decennium (see Table 1 following), it will be seen that the metropolitan decline in death rates during the intervening period was greater than that for the whole of England and Wales. During the 1861–70 decennium, the rates of death in London from smallpox and the infectious fevers were higher than for the country as a whole, although the rate for diphtheria was lower. During the 1891–1900 decennium, London's rate of death from smallpox at 10 per million was lower than the annual average of 13 for England and Wales. The London death rate for diphtheria, however, had worsened, being 500 per million compared with 262 per million for the country as a whole. While London's rate of mortality from scarlet fever had improved considerably, it was still higher than the rest of the country at the end of the century. But when mortality from all the M A B diseases is considered, London shows a higher rate of improvement than the country as a whole—a decline of 1,647 deaths per million a year, compared with a decline of 1,590 for the whole country. When deaths from diphtheria[2] are excluded, the advance in London's public health position is even more marked—an annual decline of 1,968 deaths per million a year, compared with the decline of 1,665 deaths per million for England and Wales. The Asylums Board may, therefore, have had just cause for claiming some credit for London's relatively superior rate of improvement so far as concerned deaths from the diseases treated in the M A B hospitals. The extent of the hospitals' contribution obviously cannot be disentangled from the total epidemiological situation, particularly as this would have been affected by the changing behaviour of the causal organisms of the diseases. In the case of scarlet fever, for instance, the significant difference in mortality between the 1860s and the 1890s was accounted for largely by the phenomenal severity of the disease during

[1] At the time of the Bristowe-Holmes Report on Hospitals in the UK (1863), op. cit., and for a generation after, Newcastle was the only town in the UK, apart from London, to have a special fever hospital. It is significant that rates of mortality from the acute infectious fevers in Newcastle were consistently lower than in other provincial towns, according to the Registrar-General's Summaries of Births, Deaths and Causes of Death in London and Other Great Towns.

[2] Compared with the rest of the country, London's diphtheria mortality rates were very much higher from about 1880 onwards:

Diphtheria mortality rates per million

Date	England and Wales	London
1861–1870	187	179
1871–1880	121	122
1881–1890	163	259
1891–1900	262	500

(Registrar-General's 63rd Annual Report (1900), pp. civ–cv.)

the earlier period. Historically, scarlet fever has exhibited alternately mild and severe phases, apparently associated with some biological change in the causal agent and not conspicuously with social change. One phase of severity began about 1830 and reached its peak in 1863, when more than 30,000 people died in this country from the disease. The high level of mortality from scarlet fever which occurred during the three to four decades of this phase was described by Creighton as 'one of the most remarkable things in our epidemiology'.[1] After 1863, it gradually became progressively milder throughout the country.

This cyclical diminution in the severity of scarlet fever renders even more complex an assessment of the contribution of other possible factors to this improvement during the last third of the century. Nevertheless, it is not without interest to observe the close association betweeen the decrease in metropolitan rates of death from scarlet fever—as well as from enteric fever[2]—and the increase in M A B admissions of patients suffering from these diseases—increases which were induced primarily by the steady relaxation of poor law restrictions in the course of the hospitals' phases of change between 1870 and 1900. During the first two of these three decades, the M A B was fighting for the legal right to treat all cases of infectious disease on the basis of medical rather than pecuniary need. From Table 2 below, it will be seen that scarlet fever admissions rose from a yearly average of some 550 during the first phase (1871–78), when only the destitute were legally admissible, to more than three times this figure during the second phase (1879–86), when admission regulations were slightly relaxed; to an annual average of over 5,000 during the third phase (1887–91), when regulations were further relaxed; and to over 13,000 during the fourth phase (1892–1900), when all restrictions were abolished. During these four periods, scarlet fever death rates in the metropolis fell steadily from some 560 per million, during the first phase, to about 190 per million during the fourth phase. Despite the long-term recession in the severity of the disease, this association between M A B admissions and metropolitan mortality suggests that deaths in London from scarlet fever were very probably influenced, at least to some extent, by the progressive relaxation of poor law admission regulations. In any case, a similar decline may be observed (Table 2) in the London death rate from enteric fever as admissions to the M A B hospitals increased.

Before indices of incidence were available, it could not be known to what extent the steady increase in demand for admission to the Board's hospitals was due to the gradual relaxation of admission regulations, to population growth, to a greater prevalence of the diseases treated, or to a new-found preference for hospital rather than domiciliary treatment. Only after 1889—when notification was enforced by statute—was it possible to make reasonable assumptions. When the number of cases admitted to the M A B hospitals is expressed as a percentage of the number of cases notified in London each year during the last decennium of the century (see Table 3 (ii) following), it will be found that, for each of the diseases treated, the proportion of notified cases entering the Board's fever hospitals

[1] C. A. Creighton, *A History of Epidemics in Britain* (1894), cited by A. H. Gale, op. cit., p. 91.
[2] See Appendix II, Table D.

progressively increased, with only slight fluctuations, throughout the period. For instance, the proportion of notified scarlet fever cases entering hospital rose from 43 per cent in 1890 to 75 per cent in 1900, while the proportion of notified diphtheria cases admitted increased from 18 per cent to 72 per cent during the same period. Motives are always complex, and domestic and financial factors may have been involved in this steady expansion in the use of the M A B fever hospitals. Nevertheless, the marked increase in the demand for beds following the abolition of deterrents to admission may be interpreted broadly as an index of the unsatisfied needs and desires suppressed by poor law impediments during the earlier phases, irrespective of the ebb and flow of epidemics.

The relaxation of admission restrictions would appear to have contributed to a decline in mortality, not only among the metropolitan community as a whole, but also among patients in hospital. Since the treatment, skills and amenities available in the M A B hospitals were more conducive to the successful outcome of infectious illness than conditions outside, the greater the number of cases admitted, the greater the chance of a larger number of recoveries. Scarlet fever cases comprised about two-thirds of the M A B fever hospital population. Hospital statistics of scarlet fever cases during four significant periods are, therefore, used here to illustrate the effect on M A B case fatality rates—or, conversely, recovery rates—of the factors influencing entry to hospital. From Tables 4 A–D following, it will be seen that, during the hospitals' first sixteen years, 1871–86 (4A), when all patients were 'pauperized' on entry, the total number of scarlet fever admissions averaged about 1,000 a year. During this sixteen-year period, the crude fatality rate among scarlet fever patients was nearly 12 per cent, while 23 per cent of children under five died in hospital from the disease. In 1887 (4B), patients were admitted to the M A B hospitals on the certification of *any* registered medical practitioner, whether in the poor law service or not. Within three years, 15,000 scarlet fever cases were treated—not far short of the total number admitted during the preceding sixteen years. With this extension in the scope of admissions, the crude case fatality rate fell to 9 per cent, while that for the 'under-fives' fell to 19 per cent. During 1890 and 1891 (4C), the first two years of compulsory notification in London, when more cases were brought to light, upward of 12,000 scarlet fever patients were admitted to the Board's hospitals. The crude fatality rate then fell to 7 per cent, while that for the 'under-fives' fell to 17 per cent. Following the total abolition of all restrictions under the 1891 Public Health (London) Act until the end of the century (4D), scarlet fever admissions averaged about 13,400 a year. The crude fatality rate then fell to below 5 per cent, while hospital deaths among the 'under-fives' dropped to 11 per cent. These were less than half the corresponding rates for the first sixteen-year period, 1871–86 (4A), while in some age-groups the fall was even greater.

A similar marked decline occurred in hospital deaths from diphtheria.[1] This improvement, however, was due mainly to the new antitoxin serum treatment, which was introduced in 1894 and practised experimentally until about 1897, when it came into regular

[1] See Appendix II, Tables H 2 (A) and (B), showing age and sex distribution of M A B diphtheria admissions and deaths before and after the introduction of the antitoxin treatment (1888–94 and 1895–99).

use.[1] From this time onwards greater numbers of diphtheria patients applied for admission to the M A B fever hospitals and the hospital case fatality rate progressively fell (see Appendix II, Table D).

Since compulsory notification brought to the hospitals a larger proportion of mild cases of all admissible diseases, the later years of the century might have been expected to witness a fall in case fatality rates, apart from the intervention of other factors. Nevertheless, the marked relationship between increasing admissions and rising recovery rates throughout the thirty years under review suggests that, allied to improved clinical practice and rising standards of living, the factors which encouraged entry to hospital—relaxation of admission restrictions, compulsory notification and improved hospital amenities and treatment—contributed in large measure to the fall in hospital fatality rates, as well as to the decline in metropolitan mortality from the acute infectious fevers.

The social and demographic interest attaching to the part played by the M A B fever hospitals in this saving of life is heightened by the fact that the vast majority of patients were children.[2] When the M A B fever hospital population is analysed according to age, patients under fifteen years are found to represent 84 per cent of the total number of admissions and over 86 per cent of all deaths (see Table 5 following). Only about 8 per cent of patients suffered from enteric fever or typhus—infections to which children are much less susceptible than they are to scarlet fever and diphtheria. When these 8 per cent are excluded from the calculation, children under fifteen are found to comprise 88 per cent of admissions and 96 per cent of deaths. Although it is known that scarlet fever and diphtheria were predominantly diseases of childhood, the role of the M A B fever hospitals becomes clearer when it is realized that they were mainly paediatric institutions. The Board's resistance to restricted entry thus represented, not only a defence of medical ethics and common humanity, but a fight for the lives of those in whom the future was vested. There is no yardstick for measuring the impact of health and welfare services in the sphere of human suffering, but in caring for these children, the M A B was also conferring social and economic benefits upon their families and the wider community. Parents in fever-stricken homes were relieved of the anxiety and fatigue inseparable from nursing sick children; working-class breadwinners were spared from loss of efficiency and earnings; while the young patients were saved from the hazards of inadequate home-nursing and the after-effects, sometimes permanent, which deprivation of specialized care and convalescence entailed. By the end of the century, these benefits had been bestowed by the M A B hospitals upon 170,000 London children, of whom 90 per cent had been restored to health. But for the inhuman rigidities of the poor law, hundreds more might have been saved.

Even when free entry had been obtained for all London victims of scarlet fever,

[1] The antitoxin serum treatment for diphtheria was initiated by the New York public health authorities in 1895, the year following its introduction in London by the M A B hospitals. In five years, the treatment had halved the rate of death from diphtheria among children under ten years. (Sir A. Newsholme, *The Last Thirty Years in Public Health* (1936), p. 320.)

[2] See Appendix II, Tables H 1 to H 4, for age and sex distribution of M A B scarlet fever, diphtheria, enteric fever and typhus admissions and deaths during the 30-year period to the end of the century.

diphtheria, enteric fever and typhus, there were still a number of infections which the Board's fever hospitals were not empowered to treat. During the last decade of the century, the principal acute infectious diseases accounted for some 12,000 metropolitan deaths a year—about 14 per cent of deaths from all causes (see Tables 6 (A and B) following). On average, about 2,000 of these fatalities resulted each year from measles, 2,000 from whooping-cough and over 4,000 from diarrhoea. As in the case of scarlet fever and diphtheria, most of these victims were young children. How many more risked death and disablement through unskilled nursing at home cannot be known. Cases of these diseases were neither notifiable nor admissible to the M A B hospitals during this period of the Board's history, despite the thousands of children dying from these conditions each year. The infections which the M A B isolation hospitals were authorized to treat accounted for only about one-third of the total number of deaths from the principal zymotic diseases in London.

II

While it may be assumed from statistical evidence that the M A B *fever* hospitals served in some measure, during their first thirty years, to control the prevalence and mortality of the diseases they were authorized to treat, it is more difficult to assess the impact of the Board's *smallpox* establishments upon the health of the capital during this period. London, as the emporium of the nation, seasonal resort of the wealthy, and centre of world trade and finance, was particularly susceptible to the importation of communicable disease. Of the 42,000 smallpox deaths in England and Wales during the 1871–73 nationwide epidemic, nearly a quarter occurred in the capital.

It is questionable whether the disease was controlled or encouraged as a result of the presence in London of the M A B smallpox hospitals between 1871 and 1884. During this period, some 58,000 cases were treated in institutions situated in populous metropolitan areas.[1] Although certain precautions were taken in the smallpox hospitals to counter contagion,[2] the invading virus was provided, nevertheless, with ample scope for propagation, by whatever media it travelled. The same entrances were used by patients, tradesmen, visitors and staff; and wards and laundries were ventilated on to the busy streets. While these conditions persisted, London experienced four large-scale visitations. The 1881 report of the official investigation into the incidence of smallpox in Fulham had suggested that

[1] Treatment in the M A B smallpox hospitals consisted mainly of salines with large quantities of chlorate of potash and gargles of the same agent. Stimulants were prescribed in extreme cases of exhaustion. Wards were darkened during the acute stages. To avoid pitting, the face was painted with a strong solution of nitrate of silver. The general consensus of medical opinion at this time (1870–1900) was that drugs were of little or no use in the treatment of smallpox in the early uncomplicated acute stages. But a host of complications and sequelae were always likely to arise and these each demanded special treatment and remedies.

[2] To prevent contagion in the smallpox hospitals, sheets saturated with a solution of chloralum were suspended from frames placed around the beds. Objects handled by patients were disinfected with carbolic acid. Letters were subjected to two hours' disinfection by iodine. Such visitors as were allowed were also subject to disinfection with iodine and carbolic acid before leaving.

the M A B hospital in that district was responsible for spreading the disease to a distance of at least a mile, independent of lines of communication and irrespective of the number of patients.[1] The 1881–82 Royal Commission had inclined to the view that all smallpox hospitals in the metropolis shared the apparent ability of the Fulham institution to spread smallpox 'by some means or other' over the neighbourhood around them.[2] Dr. George Buchanan, Chief Medical Officer of the Local Government Board at the time, collected reports from health officers in the hospital districts and continued to study the situation in the vicinity of the M A B Fulham Hospital. In 1885, he affirmed that all the experiences then on record formed a very strong corroboration of the Royal Commission's view. The hospitals' supposed evil power appeared to remain undiminished by improvements in institutional administration and the restriction of personal communication with patients. Dr. Buchanan concluded, therefore, that during the years leading to the investigations of the Royal Commission the M A B smallpox hospitals should be held responsible for London's consistently high death rate from smallpox relative to that obtaining in the provinces.[3]

By the time this indictment was published, the M A B had completed the sweeping changes initiated in 1882, following immediately on the issue of the Royal Commission's report, and all but the most severe cases of smallpox were being isolated in hospital ships and riverside encampments seventeen miles below London Bridge. During 1886, the year following the completion of the changeover, only twenty-four smallpox deaths were recorded in London, a dramatic contrast to the 1,057 a year which had been the metropolitan average to date since the inception of death registration in 1838.[4] Commenting on smallpox in London during 1886, the Registrar-General, Sir Brydges P. Henniker, pointed out

---

[1] Supplement to the *Tenth Report of the LGB*, 1881–82: BPP, 1882, vol. xxx, Part II, 1 [Cmd. 3290].

[2] *Report of the Royal Commission on Smallpox and Fever Hospitals*, 1882 [Cmd. 3314].

[3] Sir George Buchanan, MO to the LGB, illustrated (in his 1885 Annual Report, p. xi) London's mortality from smallpox relative to the provinces as follows:

Smallpox mortality (per million) in London and the Provinces, 1838–84:

	a	b	c	d	e	f	g	h	i
	1838–42	1847–49	1850–54	1855–59	1860–64	1865–69	1870–74	1875–79	1880–84
London	755	460	300	237	281	276	654	292	244
Provinces	547	274	271	192	175	122	389	48	34

With provincial rates constant at 100, London rates would be:

a	b	c	d	e	f	g	h	i
138	168	111	123	161	226	168	608	718

[4] See Appendix II, Table A.

that, since the establishment of the M A B hospitals in 1871, London's annual death rate from smallpox had averaged 380 per million. This was lower than that of Sunderland, Newcastle-upon-Tyne, Norwich and Wolverhampton, and only very slightly higher than the rates in Liverpool, Salford and Portsmouth. In the decennium immediately preceding the opening of the M A B hospitals (1861–70), the London rate had been higher than any of these towns, with the exception of Liverpool, with which it was nearly equal. Despite the disadvantages it suffered from its perpetually shifting population and comparative neglect of vaccination, London had thus improved its position among the great towns, so far as death from smallpox was concerned, between 1870 and 1885. When, however, London was compared with the provinces generally, the Registrar-General was obliged to admit that the metropolitan record of smallpox mortality appeared less satisfactory. He was obviously at pains to repudiate the suggestion that the M A B hospitals had aggravated rather than controlled the frequency and intensity of smallpox outbreaks during their earlier years. He went on to explain that, in the decennium immediately preceding the advent of the hospitals (1861–70), to every 100 deaths from smallpox in the provinces, there had been 191 in London, and for the period 1851–60, there had been 130, while in the first decennium following the establishment of the M A B hospitals (1871–80), this had risen to 218. As the increase from 191 to 218 was less absolutely, as well as relatively, than the pre-hospital increase from 130 to 191, the Registrar-General concluded that 'whatever . . . may be the cause why London does not improve in its relation to smallpox to the same extent as the provinces, it is something that came into operation long before the hospitals were opened.'[1]

This statistical rationalization of the M A B hospitals' experience was readily accepted by the Board's chairman as 'conclusive testimony of the advantages to the metropolis . . . of the Board's hospitals'; and in May 1887—on the twentieth anniversary of the Board's creation—Sir Brydges Henniker's comments were quoted at length.[2] This unique expression of official commendation was, however, shortly followed by disenchantment. In his next annual report, Dr. George Buchanan refuted the reasoning of the Registrar-General in citing metropolitan and provincial smallpox mortality rates in three successive decennia as proof that the M A B hospitals were blameless concerning the continued rise in metropolitan mortality from smallpox. In his turn, Dr. Buchanan cited mortality rates for the periods 1873–82, 1874–83 and 1875–84, which excluded the exceptional years of the great epidemic (1871 and 1872). To every 100 deaths in the provinces in these three decennia, London had 461, 538 and 700 deaths respectively. 'On these later decennia', he affirmed, 'the influence of smallpox hospitals upon the death rate of the metropolis has been most undisturbedly seen.' He echoed his earlier assertion that 'a hypothesis of atmospheric convection over considerable distances is wanted, not for Fulham alone, but for London generally, in order to explain the observed behaviour of smallpox in . . . the metropolis.'

[1] *Registrar-General's Annual Summary of Births, Deaths and Causes of Death in London and Other Great Towns*, 1886, p. vii.
[2] M A B *Mins.* vol. xxi (21 May 1887), p. 222.

Dr. Buchanan hesitated to rejoice in the sudden fall in metropolitan mortality from small-pox during 1886. He required, he said, 'further time to show how far the duration of smallpox epidemics in London may be affected by the new plan of taking to Long Reach every case of smallpox that can possibly be removed out of London.'[1]

As records for subsequent years have shown, the unprecedented decline in metropolitan smallpox deaths immediately following the exodus was maintained until the end of the century, when the rate was negligible.[2] The reduction in the number of cases notified in London and admitted to hospital[3] suggests that the disease became less prevalent, as well as less lethal, during the fifteen years from 1886 to 1900. It would seem that the 'evil in-fluence' referred to by the Royal Commission, and the undefined affinity of smallpox for the capital described by the Registrar-General, had been effectively overcome for the time being by the prompt removal of all cases out of London. The assumption that London's control of smallpox was entirely due to the changed location of treatment after 1885 would, of course, be in the nature of a *post hoc ergo propter hoc* argument. Even after the banishment of the stricken to the river hospitals, the disease attacked the capital on at least two further occasions,[4] and a number of secondary infections were reported among the inhabitants of Purfleet, about half a mile downwind from the Long Reach hospital ships.[5]

Historians of epidemiology have been unanimous in resisting attempts to define the causes of long-term trends in the behaviour of particular pathogens. The decline, or dis-appearance, of a disease is frequently attributed to a diminution of imperfectly known factors which favour epidemics. Estimates differ widely concerning the part played by inoculation and vaccination in controlling the decline of smallpox in this country. Any-thing less than compulsory total vaccination and re-vaccination is regarded as incompletely effective as a public health measure. In any case, practical difficulties would defeat such a scheme. The sudden decline in smallpox in the metropolis during the last fifteen years of the century can hardly be attributed, therefore, to vaccination, although the less rigorous practice of infant vaccination following the unprecedented years of relative immunity may well have contributed to the two subsequent outbreaks.

As far as compulsory notification was concerned, important as this measure proved during the last decade of the century, it was not in force when smallpox mortality first began to fall in 1886, immediately following the removal of patients out of London. Like-wise, the increasing availability of the Board's hospitals probably played a relatively minor role in the decline of smallpox in the capital at the end of the century. Improved environ-mental conditions in the country as a whole might have been expected to play some part in the increased immunity of town-dwellers. But when the 1889 Royal Commission on Vaccination reported in 1896, it was revealed that, although mortality from smallpox in

[1] *Annual Report to the MO of the LGB*, for 1886, pp. vii and xi.
[2] See Charts A and B following and Appendix II, Tables A and B.
[3] See Table 3 (i) following and Appendix II, Table B.
[4] Smallpox epidemics of 1893–95 and 1901–2.
[5] Ronald Hare, *Pomp and Pestilence* (1954), p. 20.

England and Wales had fallen between 1838 and 1894 from 216 to 2 per million, there had been no corresponding decline in deaths from measles. They concluded, therefore, that general sanitary improvements had played only a subsidiary role in reducing mortality from smallpox.[1]

Although difficult to substantiate, the view that smallpox changed in type after 1885, suddenly becoming less common and less lethal, has gained wide acceptance. The decline was not peculiar to the capital. For some unexplained reason, a sudden and sustained fall in mortality was recorded for the whole of England and Wales after this date.[2] When consideration is given to each of a number of possible reasons for the changed behaviour of major smallpox towards the end of the century, it is only possible to observe with certainty that, while mortality from smallpox in London had been maintained at a rate significantly higher than that in the provinces during the whole of the nineteenth century before 1885, its decline was more sudden and more pronounced than that obtaining in the rest of the country during the last fifteen years of the century (see Chart AB following). The extent to which the M A B smallpox hospitals affected the spread of the disease in London before 1885 must remain a matter of medical conjecture until the capability of smallpox infection to travel distances by aerial convection can be proved or disproved conclusively.[3] Recovery from smallpox relies to a high degree on vigilant medical attention and to an even greater extent on careful nursing. These prerequisites were available for Londoners on a scale unsurpassed elsewhere in the country. Once these were removed from the hazards of an urban environment, the ability of the M A B smallpox hospitals to reduce prevalence and mortality would seem to be well substantiated.

While the ebb of classical smallpox in nineteenth-century England is generally traced in the literature as part of a long-term decline punctuated by occasional peaks, the reasons for its final disappearance as a native disease have been variously and incompletely assessed. The experiences of the M A B in their assault on the historic scourge may throw some light on the process of its eradication and, in particular, suggest why London, formerly a focal area of attack, appeared to accelerate this triumph of man over virus.

III

During the Board's three pioneering decades, sanitary conditions in the metropolis had been improving but slowly, although the tendency was towards a better administration

[1] Cited by J. H. H. Williams in *A Century of Public Health in Britain, 1832–1929*, p. 252.

[2] During 1886, the first year of the dramatic fall in smallpox mortality in London following the removal of M A B patients away from the capital, only 275 people died from smallpox in the whole of England and Wales. Of these, 24 were in London and 29 in Liverpool. (Registrar-General's *Annual Summary of Births, Deaths and Causes of Death in London and Other Great Towns*, 1886, p. vii.)

[3] According to Professor Ronald Hare, the only infection capable of travelling any distance by air currents is smallpox. In severe cases of this disease, the eruption may release into the atmosphere large amounts of dried pustular material heavily charged with virus. Provided there is a sufficient number of patients in this condition, the air on the leeward side may become dangerous. (Ronald Hare, op. cit., p. 20.)

of the law. By the 1890s, public health functions still remained unco-ordinated and cumbrous. At local government level, prevention was in the hands of over forty sanitary authorities; thirty boards of guardians; the M A B; and what *The Times* described as 'that respectable if not very brilliant body, the new LCC'.[1] In addition to main drainage and the housing of the working classes, the duties of the LCC included infant life protection and control of contagious diseases in animals. It had no jurisdiction over the guardians, who were empowered to administer public vaccination, and no concern whatever with the rate-aided poor, sick or able-bodied. The LCC and the M A B each had their separate areas of public health responsibility, as laid down in the 1891 Act.[2] Under the London Government Act of 1899, the vestries were replaced by twenty-eight metropolitan borough councils, which became the new public health authorities.

Although London had lagged behind the provinces in local government reform,[3] and lacked co-ordination in public health administration, it could claim superiority in organized defence against infectious disease. By the end of the century, the M A B administered 2,486 smallpox beds in its country institutions, and 6,108 fever beds in its London establishments.[4] These were the hospitals from which the central authority had sought to exclude the stricken who applied for entry without a relieving officer's order. These were the institutions in which four out of every five fever patients were under fifteen years of age. These were the patients who had illegally occupied hospital beds because the poor law had precedence over public health in the priorities of Whitehall. Conceived in 1867 as a means of relieving overcrowding in the workhouses of London, the M A B 'asylums' for infectious diseases treated over 307,000 cases during their first thirty years, and entered the twentieth century as pioneers of public hospital provision in this country.

[1] *The Times*, 18 January 1889.

[2] Public Health (London) Act, 1891 (54 & 55 Vict. c. 76).

[3] As London was excluded from the 1835 Municipal Corporations Act and the 1875 Public Health Act which covered the rest of the country, local government reforms in the capital were delayed until the 1855 Metropolis Management Act and the 1888 Local Government Act, while codification of public health in London was deferred until the consolidating 1891 Public Health (London) Act.

[4] For details of the location and bed complement of the M A B isolation hospitals in 1900, see Table 7 following this chapter and Map II of London following Appendix IV.

TABLE 1

Mortality from the Diseases treated in the M A B Hospitals

Comparison of LONDON rates with those in ENGLAND and WALES during the decennia 1861–1870 and 1891–1900.

Diseases	MORTALITY (Average annual rates per million living)							
	LONDON				ENGLAND AND WALES			
	1861–1870	1891–1900	Reduction	Increase	1861–1870	1891–1900	Reduction	Increase
Smallpox	276	10	− 266		162	13	− 149	
Scarlet Fever	1,133	188	− 945		971	158	− 813	
Diphtheria	179	500		+ 321	187	262		+ 75
Typhus, Enteric and 'simple continued Fevers'	904	147	− 757		886	183	− 703	
			− 1,968				− 1,665	
			+ 321				+ 75	
			− 1,647				− 1,590	

Source: Registrar-General's Sixty-Third Annual Report (1900), Table 24, p. civ, and Table 25, p. cv.

TABLE 2

Admissions to the M A B Isolation Hospitals, and Metropolitan mortality rates for selected diseases in four periods between 1871 and 1900

Phases	Admissions to M A B hospitals (annual averages)					Metropolitan mortality rates per 1,000 of the estimated population (annual averages)				
	Scarlet Fever	Diph-theria[1]	Typhus	Enteric Fever	Small-pox	Scarlet Fever	Diph-theria[1]	Typhus	Enteric Fever	Small-pox
I. *1871–1878* Eight years during which admissions were legally limited to the destitute.	554	—	214	350	3,704	0·56	0·12	0·06	0·25	0·54
II. *1879–1886* Eight years during which admission regulations were slightly relaxed.	1,705	—	72	387	3,396	0·48	0·20	0·01	0·21	0·21
III. *1887–1891* Five years during which admission regulations were further relaxed.	5,325	992	19	487	42	0·24	0·32	0·00	0·15	0·00
IV. *1892–1900* Nine years during which all restrictive regulations were removed.	13,040	5,050	7	841	568	0·19	0·52	0·00	0·13	0·01

[1] Diphtheria cases were first admitted in October 1888.

Sources: M A B Statistical Reports and Registrar-General's Returns for the years indicated.

TABLE 3 (i)
**London notifications of the principal diseases admissible to the M A B Hospitals
from 1890–1900**

(Under the Infectious Disease (Notification) Act, 1889, and the Public Health (London) Act, 1891

Year	Scarlet Fever	Diphtheria	Enteric Fever	Typhus	Smallpox
1890	15,330	5,870	2,877	35	60
1891	11,398	5,907	3,372	27	114
1892	27,095	7,781	2,465	20	423
1893	36,901	13,026	3,663	22	2,813
1894	18,440	10,655	3,360	21	1,192
1895	19,757	10,772	3,506	14	979
1896	25,647	13,362	3,190	6	225
1897	22,848	12,803	3,103	4	104
1898	16,894	11,543	3,024	16	32
1899	18,089	13,346	4,453	13	29
1900	13,800	11,776	4,291	7	87

TABLE 3 (ii)
**Admissions to the M A B Isolation Hospitals between 1890 and 1900
expressed as *percentages* of the annual NOTIFICATIONS in Table 3 (i) above[1]**

Diseases	1890	1891	1892	1893	1894	1895	1896	1897	1898	1899	1900
	%	%	%	%	%	%	%	%	%	%	%
Scarlet Fever	42·9	46·9	48·8	39·7	64·0	58·2	62·7	67·0	73·2	74·3	75·2
Diphtheria	17·9	25·1	30·2	24·5	38·9	41·5	40·0	51·6	62·1	69·7	72·5
Enteric Fever	22·6	27·4	25·3	20·0[2]	20·2[2]	24·1[2]	27·0	30·4	36·7	40·8	47·7
Typhus	42·9	70·4	60·0	36·4	62·0	42·9	33·3	50·0	87·5	84·6	57·1
Smallpox	36·7	55·3	76·8	84·5	93·7	96·1	84·4	67·3	15·6[3]	62·1	75·9

[1] For the actual numbers of cases admitted to the hospitals in the years 1890 to 1900 see Appendix II, Tables B and D.

[2] Some cases of enteric fever were sent to general hospitals in the years 1893–95.

[3] Of the 32 London notifications of smallpox in 1898 (see Table 3 (i) above), only 5 were correctly diagnosed, and admitted by the M A B, thus accounting for the apparently low percentage for smallpox admissions relative to notifications in that year.

Sources: M A B Annual Reports for the years indicated.

Age Group	A	1871 to 1886[1] (15,480 cases)		B	1887 to 1889[2] (14,826 cases)	
	Admissions	Deaths	Case Fatality Rates %	Admissions	Deaths	Case Fatality Rates %
Under 5	4,112	950	23·1	4,415	840	19·0
5– 9+	6,051	582	9·6	6,294	388	6·2
10–14+	2,681	138	5·1	2,360	72	3·1
15–19+	1,300	54	4·1	904	35	3·9
20–24+	676	33	4·9	428	7	1·6
25–29+	336	21	6·2	202	4	2·0
30–34+	179	14	7·8	120	7	5·8
35–39+	86	10	11·6	54	1	1·9
40–44+	35	4	} 13·6	26	2	} 4·1
45–49+	10	1		13	—	
50–54+	10	1		10	—	
55–59+	2	1		—	—	
60 and over	2	1		—	—	
Totals:	15,480	1,810	11·7	14,826	1,356	9·1

[1] During the period 1871–86 patients required admission orders from a relieving officer (or a workhouse master) and from a poor law medical officer. (See Chapters 5 and 6.)

[2] During the period 1887–89 admission was granted on the certification of *any* registered medical practitioner. (See Chapter 7.)

D)

1871–1899

B Fever Hospitals from Poor Law to Public Health Status

Age Group	C 1890 *and* 1891[3] (*11,799 cases*)			D 1892 *to* 1899[4] (*107,020 cases*)		
	Admissions	*Deaths*	*Case Fatality Rates* %	*Admissions*	*Deaths*	*Case Fatality Rates* %
Under 1	101	29	28·7	1,037	245	23·6
1+	370	99	26·8	3,656	698	19·1
2+	781	181	23·2	6,778	933	13·8
3+	1,083	168	15·5	9,732	1,000	10·3
4+	1,213	141	11·6	10,802	721	6·7
Total under 5	3,548	618	17·4	32,005	3,597	11·2
5– 9+	5,078	206	4·1	43,556	1,212	2·8
10–14+	1,951	26	1·3	19,679	221	1·1
15–19+	653	6	0·9	6,236	78	1·3
20–24+	324	9	2·8	2,756	39	1·4
25–29+	123	2	1·6	1,436	19	1·3
30–34+	72	—	—	754	15	2·0
35–39+	28	—	—	319	6	1·9
40–44+	10	—		157	7	
45–49+	8	—		68	4	
50–54+	1	—	—	38	2	4·7
55–59+	—	—		11	—	
60 and over	3	—		5	—	
Totals:	11,799	867	7·3	107,020	5,200	4·9

[3] 1890 and 1891 were the first years of compulsory notification of scarlet fever and certain other infectious diseases under the Infectious Disease (Notification) Act, 1889. (See Chapter 7.)

[4] During the period 1892–99 the M A B fever hospitals were freely available to patients of all classes under the Public Health (London) Act, 1891. (See Chapter 8.)

Sources: M A B Statistical Committee Annual Reports for 1891, 1895 and 1899.

TABLE 5
Children in M A B Fever Hospitals, 1871–1899
Admissions and deaths compared with *total* admissions and deaths

Age Groups[1]	Scarlet Fever	Diphtheria[2]	Enteric Fever	Typhus	Combined Totals[3]
Admissions:					
Under 15 years	131,734	35,546	6,187	719	173,186
Over 15 years	17,397	5,107	8,365	1,481	32,350
Totals:	149,131	40,653	13,552	2,200	205,536
'Under Fifteens' as a percentage of total admissions	88·3	87·4	38·3	32·7	84·3
Deaths:					
Under 15 years	8,850	8,243	566	19	17,678
Over 15 years	383	202	1,765	421	2,771
Totals:	9,233	8,445	2,331	440	20,449
'Under Fifteens' as a percentage of total deaths	95·9	97·6	24·3	4·3	86·5

[1] The age-distribution of Fever Hospital admissions and deaths, of which this table is a summary, is analysed in greater detail in Appendix II, Tables H 1 (A) and (B), 2 (A) and (B), 3 and 4.

[2] Diphtheria cases were not treated before the end of 1888.

[3] Combined totals exclude the unspecified 'other diseases' treated in the M A B Fever Hospitals.

Sources: M A B Statistical Committee Annual Reports for 1891, 1894, and 1899.

TABLES 6 (A, B)
Mortality in London from 1881 to 1900
A: *From all causes*

Year	Estimated Population (mid-year)	Total Births	Total Deaths	Mortality per 1,000 living	Deaths of Infants under one year
1881	3,824,964	132,904	81,120	21·3	20,907
1891	4,221,452	134,484	90,595	21·0	20,776
1896	4,421,955	133,833	82,390	18·1	21,615
1897	4,463,169	134,187	81,119	17·7	21,286
1898	4,504,766	132,849	84,154	18·2	22,192
1899	4,546,752	133,134	89,705	19·3	22,287
1900	4,589,129	130,868	86,007	18·6	20,927

B: *From principal zymotic diseases*

Year	Total Deaths from Principal Zymotic Diseases	Small-pox	Measles	Scarlet Fever	Diph-theria	Whooping Cough	Enteric Fever	Diarrhoea	Cholera	Deaths from Principal Zymotic Diseases as Percentage of Total Deaths
1881	13,681	475	1,501	3,073	541	3,438	886	3,767	—	16·9
1891	9,839	8	1,807	598	1,135	2,872	613	2,435	71	10·9
1896	14,046	9	3,662	916	2,657	2,904	598	3,207	93	17·1
1897	11,674	16	1,909	782	2,273	1,839	594	4,146	115	14·4
1898	12,700	1	3,073	582	1,766	2,160	602	4,385	131	15·1
1899	11,394	3	2,134	398	1,951	1,720	811	4,225	152	12·7
1900	10,302	4	1,936	361	1,558	1,948	765	3,654	76	12·0

Sources: Registrar-General's Annual Returns for the years indicated.

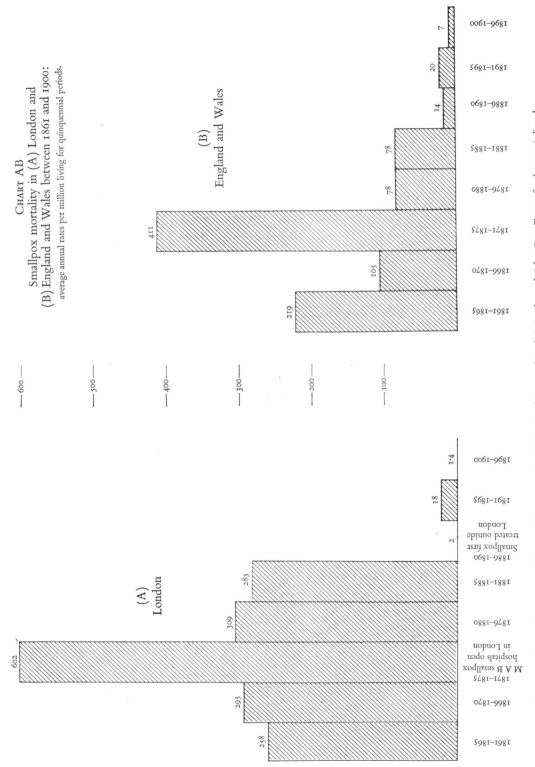

Chart AB

Smallpox mortality in (A) London and (B) England and Wales between 1861 and 1900: average annual rates per million living for quinquennial periods.

(B) England and Wales

411

105

219

78

78

14

20

7

1861–1865
1866–1870
1871–1875
1876–1880
1881–1885
1886–1890
1891–1895
1896–1900

600
500
400
300
200
100

(A) London

602

295

309

283

258

2

18

1·4

1861–1865
1866–1870
M A B smallpox hospitals open in London
1871–1875
1876–1880
1881–1885
Smallpox first treated outside London
1891–1895
1896–1900

Sources: Registrar-General's Annual Summaries of Births, Deaths and Causes of Death in London and Other Great Towns, for the years indicated.

TABLE 7
M A B Fever and Smallpox Hospitals in 1900

Hospital	Location	Date of Opening	Number of Beds
I. *Fever and Diphtheria*			
(a) *acute*			
North-Western	Lower Lawn Road, Hampstead	Jan. 1870	460
South-Western	Landor Road, Stockwell	Jan. 1871	366
Eastern	The Grove, Homerton	Feb. 1871	362
Western	Seagrave Road, Fulham	March 1877	450
South-Eastern	Avonley Road, New Cross (formerly Deptford)	March 1877	432
North-Eastern	St. Ann's Road, Tottenham	Oct. 1892	514
Fountain	Tooting Grove, Lower Tooting	Oct. 1893 (after 1911 used as a mental hospital)	402
Brook	Shooter's Hill, Woolwich	Aug. 1896	488
Park	Hither Green, Lewisham	Nov. 1897	548
Grove	Tooting Grove, Lower Tooting	Aug. 1899	522
			—— 4,544
(b) *convalescent*			
Northern	Winchmore Hill	Sept. 1886	764
Southern (later known as Queen Mary's Hospital for Children)	Carshalton, Surrey	(in course of construction in 1900)	800 —— 1,564
		Total 'Fever' beds existing and projected in 1900	6,108
II. *Smallpox*			
(a) *acute*			
Hospital Ships (abolished in 1904 on completion of Joyce Green Hospital with its adjuncts, the Orchard and Long Reach Hospitals)	Moored in Long Reach, near Dartford, Kent	July 1881 (*Atlas*) July 1881 (*Endymion*) July 1884 (*Castalia*)	300
Joyce Green	Dartford, Kent	(in course of construction in 1900)	986 —— 1,286
(b) *convalescent*			
Gore Farm (brick hospital and camp)	Darenth, near Dartford, Kent	Oct. 1890	1,200 ——
		Total Smallpox beds existing and projected in 1900	2,486 ——

PART TWO

Anatomy of the MAB Hospital System

'We owe it to the doctors not to hamper their beneficent work by clumsy administrative organization.'

Sidney and Beatrice Webb, *The State and the Doctor*, 1910.

'It is not so much knowledge . . . which a layman is expected to bring to his work in committees as sense, common sense. He is to check the excesses of bureaucratic and expert nonsense by the application of his own common sense. It is not enough for the layman to be interested, to be educable, or to be knowledgeable. He cannot make the best use of these qualities unless he has qualities of mind and temperament which mark him out as the sensible or reasonable man.'

Sir Kenneth Wheare, *Government by Committee*, 1955.

CHAPTER 11

Constitution, Functions and Structure
of the M A B

I

WHILE the Board's existing services continued to expand, the scope of its responsibility was extended to include the care of various categories of children and of tuberculous patients of all ages and classes. Before following the M A B into the twentieth century, however, it would seem useful at this point to examine its structure and mode of operation.

The constitution of the Board followed generally the traditional British principle of local government by amateurs. But, even if most of its members were initially unacquainted with institutional management, they brought specialized knowledge and experience from other fields, to produce, in Walter Bagehot's words, 'a due mixture of special and non-special minds—of minds which attend to the means and of minds which attend to the end'.[1] Those who were elected by the metropolitan parochial authorities—three-quarters of the total—invariably included a number of Justices of the Peace, chairmen of boards of guardians, a sprinkling of practising churchmen, an occasional ex-diplomat and a few retired army and naval officers. Elected medical men were usually a small minority but they often played a leading role in the Board's deliberations. One notable example was William Henry Brewer, MP, JP, MD, MRCS, whose fourteen years of dedicated and dynamic leadership have already been recorded. Formerly coroner and surgeon in Monmouthshire, he relinquished his appointments on election to the Board in 1867, secured a seat in Parliament the following year, and with deep religious fervour devoted himself to the Board's affairs until his sudden death in 1881.

The central authority nominees—one quarter of the total—usually included at least one medical man. The others were recruited mainly from other professions. The only qualification required by the 1867 Act for nominated members was that they should be assessed for the local poor rate at not less than £40 a year, the same as for poor law guardians.[2] Among the first members of the M A B to be appointed by the Poor Law Board were

---

[1] Walter Bagehot, *The English Constitution* (Nelson edn., 1872), p. 280.
[2] 30 & 31 Vict. c. 6 s. 11. Mr. Gathorne Hardy originally wrote into the 1867 Bill a rating of £100 as the qualification for PLB nominees, but in the Act, as passed, the figure was lowered to £40 p.a.

Mr. Timothy Holmes, FRCS, who had made an exhaustive survey of United Kingdom hospitals;[1] and Dr. Francis Sibson, FRCP, who, as a member of the Watson Committee, had studied the incidence of infectious disease in the metropolitan infirmaries and general hospitals.[2] The principle of appointing representatives of the medical profession was suspended for about five years following the creation of the Local Government Board in 1871. An anti-medical animus prevailed at this time due to differences between its first President, Mr. J. J. Stansfeld, and the head of the medical department, Sir John Simon.[3] Stansfeld publicly declared that he had 'no intention of committing the whole sanitary administration of this country to medical men'.[4] By the same token, it would seem that he had no intention of encouraging medical opinion to be voiced in the administration of London's new hospitals. At the triennial election of the Board which occurred during his term of office (1871–74), he replaced his predecessor's three medical nominees on the Asylums Board by laymen.

Within the compass of this study, it is impossible to refer to more than a very few of the many dedicated members who anonymously moulded history in the course of the Board's sixty-three years.[5] Their memorial remains enshrined in the prosaic records of its innumerable meetings. Those eminent members who also left their mark in other fields included a former infant pauper and a future prime minister. Will Crooks, who had made his way from workhouse to Westminster, presided over the Board's activities on behalf of deprived children early in the century.[6] He was the elected representative of his native Poplar, where he became London's first Labour mayor. For a time after World War I, a neighbouring poor law district, Stepney, was represented by Major C. R. (later Earl) Attlee. Following the establishment of the Ministry of Health in 1919, the nominated section of the Board regularly included well-known figures in the fields of social welfare, public health, clinical medicine and surgery.[7]

Early fears of friction between elected and appointed members were soon dispelled. The latter showed no tendency to act as central authority watchdogs. At first, an occasional jibe was made by an elected member against a nominated colleague, but, as time went on, an unwritten arrangement was established whereby elected members retired after a few years in favour of other local representatives and then offered themselves for nomination by the central authority. In this way, new blood was infused while a permanent nucleus of experienced members remained, making for unity of principles and continuity

[1] Bristowe and Holmes, *The Hospitals of the United Kingdom*, HMSO (1864).
[2] *Report of the Watson Committee on Metropolitan Workhouses*, 1867, op. cit. (Chapter 1, n. 67), Appendix XIII.
[3] R. Lambert, *Sir John Simon, 1816–1904, and English Social Administration*, Chapter XXII passim.
[4] *Hansard*, ccxii, col. 1268, cited by R. Lambert, op. cit.
[5] Chairmen and vice-chairmen of the M A B are listed in Appendix I, Document V.
[6] See Chapter 18.
[7] Among the Ministry of Health's nominees were: Dr. Ethel Bentham, JP, MP; Geoffrey Drage; Dr. H. L. Eason, CB, CMG, JP; Sir Francis Fleming, KCMG, JP; Sir Ernest Meinertzhagen, JP; Sir Shirley Murphy, KBE, FRCS; Sir d'Arcy Power, KBE, FRCS; and Dr. E. Lauriston Shaw, MD, FRCP.

in policy. Although most major issues gave rise to protracted debate, sectional and party politics were inconspicuous in the Board's deliberations.

An outstanding characteristic of many members was their attachment to the Board. Repeatedly, they offered themselves for re-election or nomination. Two members who died in 1924—Sir George Elliott, MP, and Sir Augustus Scovell, JP—each served for over forty consecutive years. Sir Edwin Galsworthy, JP, DL (uncle of the novelist-playwright, John Galsworthy, OM), held office from 1881 for twenty-one consecutive years and served altogether for well over three decades, as did the Board's last chairman, the Viscount Doneraile. Other leading and long-serving members, not recorded elsewhere, included Sir Michael Hicks Beach, John Bell Sedgwick, General Sir H. P. de Bathe, Dr. J. R. Hill, Earl Stanhope, Sir John Tilley and Sir William H. Wyatt.

The diversity of hospital managers was further broadened when, late in 1884, the central authority took the unprecedented step of nominating four women to the Board.[1] No marked enthusiasm for the newcomers was shown by their male colleagues, who had yet to discover the Whearian tenet of committee philosophy: 'The reasonable man is not enough; we need the unreasonable woman also.'[2] When, some twenty years later, the Clerk to the Asylums Board was questioned before the 1905–9 Poor Law Commission concerning the membership of women, he asserted emphatically and repeatedly that 'it was by no means a necessity'. On being pressed by a woman commissioner, he grudgingly conceded that 'there are particular things in which, of course, a lady manager is useful'.[3] There were then seven women on the Board. By 1930 they numbered eleven.

Who, or what, had inspired the Local Government Board in 1884 to appoint women to a statutory body? Circumstantial evidence strongly suggests that this innovation was related to another appointment made a few months earlier. In August 1884, the Local Government Board announced the nomination to the Asylums Board of Captain Douglas Galton, CB.[4] At this juncture in its development, a one-time army expert in barrack construction, ventilation, heating, water supply and drainage was of considerable value to the MAB. Captain Galton had been an administrator in various government departments, including the War Office. Furthermore, he had married Marianne Nicholson, cousin of

---

[1] A woman was first elected to the board of guardians of Kensington in 1875 without legal or official objection, although in 1850 the Poor Law Board had declared that 'the objections to the appointment of a female to an office of this nature upon grounds of public policy and convenience are so manifest that the Board cannot readily suppose that the question will become one of practical importance in the administration of the Poor Law'. R. A. Leach, *The Evolution of Poor Law Administration* (1924).

[2] Sir Kenneth Wheare, *Government by Committee* (1955), pp. 23–24. 'It is the quality', wrote Sir Kenneth Wheare, '—often associated, by men at least, with women—of the being unable to see the sense in what is being done, of questioning the whole basis of organization, of brushing difficulties aside, of ignoring logical argument, and of pressing a point beyond what most men consider a reasonable limit, which is required as part of the make-up of a good layman. It is against criticism of this kind that officials and experts should be required to justify their proposals and procedures in public administration'.

[3] Royal Commission on the Poor Laws: Minutes of Evidence, 23 July 1906 (BPP, 1909, vol. xi), QQ. 24434–39; Mrs. Bosanquet to Mr. T. Duncombe Mann.

[4] LGB letter to the MAB, 29 August 1884.

Florence Nightingale.[1] Following her Crimean experiences, it was customary for Miss Nightingale to use her powers behind the scenes, directing operations through her influential friends and family connexions to further those causes to which she had dedicated her life. 'I have thought I could work better . . . off the stage than on it', she once wrote to John Stuart Mill.[2] On a number of occasions, Captain Douglas Galton had been her ambassador. As Assistant Under-Secretary of State at the War Office in the early 'sixties (an appointment resulting from Miss Nightingale's intervention), all construction works were under his control, and almost all plans for barracks and hospitals were submitted to her.[3] At the time of the Franco-Prussian War, Miss Nightingale, declining to serve on the Executive of the National Society for Aid to the Sick and Wounded, had worked through Douglas Galton, whose appointment to the Committee she arranged.[4] He was also among those through whom she transmitted her ideas concerning the equipping of the 'new' St. Thomas' Hospital at Lambeth.[5]

And now, in 1884, when the building of new isolation hospitals outside London was to be undertaken, it could hardly be coincidence that the hospital reformer's emissary should be appointed to the Asylums Board. Miss Nightingale was now over sixty. The turbulent intolerance of earlier years had subsided with the onset of physical lethargy but the incisive mind remained alive to the need for improving standards of institutional care. She had regarded the 1867 Metropolitan Poor Act as only a partial victory for workhouse reform and had thereafter immersed herself in other causes.[6] Now, in the early 1880s, she was again free to contribute—albeit vicariously—to the betterment of institutions for the sick. Once her kinsman was on the Asylums Board, her aims, with his influence, could be implemented. To what extent she influenced the selection of the first four women members cannot now be determined. One of them, the Hon. Maude Amelia Stanley, pioneer of working girls' clubs, was very probably sponsored by Miss Nightingale, since the Stanley family was well known to her.[7] Of the other three women members, two resigned within months. Miss Stanley's remaining woman colleague on the Board was Miss Isabella Baker, who had been invited earlier in 1884 to organize the 1,000-bed emergency hospital camp at Darenth. In the role of 'lady superintendent', she had promptly created order out of chaos at the height of the epidemic through her remarkable drive and administrative ability, aided by her association with Dr. Bridges of the Local Government Board. Her appointment to the Asylums Board was unique; at no other time was a matron or

---

[1] C. Woodham-Smith, *Florence Nightingale, 1820–1910*, p. 243.

[2] Nightingale Papers, BM, Add. MSS., 45787. Letter from F. Nightingale to J. S. Mill, dated 11 August 1867.

[3] C. Woodham-Smith, op. cit., p. 303.   [4] Ibid., p. 376.   [5] Ibid., p. 383.

[6] After her dissatisfaction with the 1867 Act, Miss Nightingale devoted herself to new causes—the sanitary affairs of India; childbirth mortality statistics; French and German hospitals; and the reorganization of the Nightingale School for Nurses. (C. Woodham-Smith, op. cit., pp. 367–74; 356; 376; 383–98, passim.)

[7] The Hon. Maude A. Stanley was the sister of the second Lord Stanley of Alderley who, as chairman of the Indian Sanitary Commission, became well known to Florence Nightingale. (C. Woodham-Smith, op. cit., pp. 311–12 and 400.)

medical superintendent in the service of the M A B invited to participate in its counsels as a regular member. The contributions of Miss Baker and Miss Stanley alone would have vindicated the introduction of women to the Board's deliberations. Miss Baker served for thirty-five crowded committee years before retiring. Miss Stanley, who had been known to startle officials at the Local Government Board by appearing in person to enquire the reasons for their procrastination, died in office at the age of eighty-two, after thirty-one years of continuous service.

II

Although not an ardent feminist, Miss Nightingale had felt, no doubt, that on the all-male Asylums Board the distaff element might well serve a useful purpose, particularly concerning the more detailed and domestic aspects of institutional management. It soon transpired that there was ample justification for reasoning on these lines. Shortly after his appointment, Captain Galton was invited to sit on a committee of enquiry set up by the Asylums Board to look into excessive spending at one of its fever hospitals. An unwholesome and hitherto unsuspected state of affairs was revealed.[1] Not only was there evidence of negligent extravagance, but also misappropriation of public funds through collusion between officials, contractors and others. During one year, some £10,000 had been spent on structural projects when only £400 had been sanctioned by the Board. While some of these—such as laboratories and nurses' accommodation—were necessary improvements, other items—among them a swimming bath in the basement of the medical superintendent's official residence—were not. Although alcohol was generally considered of medicinal value at this time, records revealed what appeared to be excessive prescribing. Some dozen bottles of Beaune, with quantities of champagne, port and beer had been 'issued' to one ward on five consecutive days, and a children's ward at that! It transpired that diet sheets, compiled from medical officers' prescriptions on bed-cards, had been falsified, and then signed by an unsuspecting medical superintendent. In this manner, 2,500 chickens, lobsters and cigars had been 'consumed' by patients in six months, while more than £750 had been spent in three months on wines and spirits for the hospital staff.

In the course of the Board's enquiry, the management committee chairman disappeared, the committee clerk absconded, while the steward and others resigned. Although nothing elicited at the enquiry was regarded as in any way reflecting on the integrity of the medical superintendent, it was recommended that he should be suspended pending an independent investigation by the Local Government Board. This enquiry, which occupied thirty-nine protracted sittings,[2] added little of consequence to the Asylums Board's own findings, and similarly recognized that there were extenuating circumstances in favour of the medical superintendent. During the period in which the abuses had taken place, scarlet

[1] M A B *Mins.* (28 February 1885), vol. xviii, pp. 1347 *et seq.*
[2] M A B *Mins.* (7 December 1885), vol. xix, pp. 948 *et seq.*

fever and smallpox epidemics had made heavy demands on his hospitals. In addition, he had attended smallpox patients embarking for the river hospitals, and had been required, meantime, to investigate East London sites and buildings suitable for cholera hospitals. Nevertheless, his failure to detect errors on the diet sheets submitted for his signature and to check extravagance generally was severely censured by the Local Government Board, which also attributed blame directly to the Asylums Managers and their senior officials. Furthermore, the central authority declined to lift the suspension which had been imposed by the Asylums Board. This elicited strong representations from the Medical Defence Union and the Poor Law Medical Officers' Association. Written demands for the superintendent's reinstatement were followed by powerful deputations. These were received by the Board in plenary session. After heated discussions and numerous divisions, reinstatement was ultimately decided by a voting majority of one. The Local Government Board was thereupon urged to reverse its ruling, particularly as the medical officer in question had performed his clinical duties with zeal and efficiency. The central authority reluctantly conceded that 'the judgment of the body by whom Dr. *X* was suspended is entitled to consideration'. 'With considerable hesitation', therefore, the Local Government Board agreed to reinstatement on probation, with censure and loss of earnings for the period of suspension.[1]

III

These grave, but isolated, abuses had been made possible because 'top-level' control—legally vested in the Local Government Board but in effect assumed by the Asylums Board—had become more and more diluted as unit-level management had acquired increasing self-sufficiency. When the Asylums Managers initiated planning in 1867, one committee had been appointed for each of the three categories of patients for which the Board was required to provide—those suffering from fever, smallpox and insanity. These committees—and those for finance and general purposes—each comprised nine Board members, together with the chairman and vice-chairman *ex officio*. The system worked satisfactorily so long as the number of separate units controlled by each of the three management committees remained low. While day-to-day affairs in the hospitals were directed by individual visiting members of the committees, the Board at its fortnightly plenary sessions deliberated upon policy problems raised by the committees, and passed to the general purposes committee, for study and report, such issues as required further consideration. When, however, the fever and smallpox groups expanded, it became necessary for each unit to be controlled by a separate management committee. As these committees were composed exclusively of Board members merely 'wearing different hats', they had tended to assume an increasing measure of managerial power. Gradually a situation grew up in which the Board and its finance committee merely 'rubber-stamped' the decisions of the management committees.

[1] LGB letter to the M A B dated 18 December 1885.

IV

Following the corrupt practices resulting from this system, reforms were set afoot. Central authority sanction was sought, and obtained, for the enlargement of the Board from sixty to seventy-two members[1] and for the general purposes committee to include all members of the Board. Special committees were appointed for dealing centrally with supplies, building work and financial control.[2] One of the most important innovations was the formation in 1886 of a statistical committee.

The Board had already been concerned with statistics as tools of administration, mainly in the field of infectious disease. As early as 1872, a sub-committee had been formed to keep a continuous check on hospital admissions and deaths. One of its main functions during epidemics had been to serve as a centre for the allocation of beds. It also warned metropolitan local authorities when and where infectious disease was on the increase. In the course of its work, the committee kept in close touch with Dr. William Farr, superintendent of the statistical department of the Registrar-General's Office, who was always ready to advise.[3]

The new statistical committee was a high-powered, co-ordinating, policy-moulding body with rather wider functions, which included the study of organization and methods in the institutions. One of its main tasks was the publication of statistically-supported annual reports on all aspects of the Board's work. These included reasoned representations on matters deemed to demand administrative or legislative reform. For close on twenty years, records of the Board's deliberations had been given only a very limited circulation and had never been made directly available to the public.[4] The press was admitted to plenary Board meetings only with prior permission.

The creation of the new statistical committee had been recommended by a newcomer to the Board, Sir Vincent Kennett-Barrington, an eminent barrister internationally recognized for his services to the Red Cross and to a number of war commissions. Undoubtedly, he would have been known to Miss Nightingale, who had been instrumental

[1] Of the 72 members comprising the Board in 1886, 54 were elected and 18 nominated. One elective member was added in 1892; the total number thereafter remained at 73 until the dissolution of the Board.

[2] The work of these committees is dealt with in Chapter 13 on Finance.

[3] Among the statistical matters on which Dr. William Farr advised the M A B was the calculation of annual hospital fatality rates. In a letter of 23 April 1877 to the Board's chairman, he stated: 'Some divide the deaths in the year multiplied by 100 (1) by the admissions, A: others (2) by the discharges, including the deaths, D. It can be demonstrated that either method is less correct, as a general rule, than the division by $\frac{(1)+(2)}{2} = \frac{A+D}{2}$.'

This formula was used in all the M A B hospital returns, of which abstracts appear in the appendices to this study.

[4] Before 1886, periodical reports of the work of the M A B were included with the Board's minutes, which were circulated only to the central authority, metropolitan boards of guardians and M A B members. A proposal made at one of the first meetings of the M A B in 1867 that any ratepayer who so desired might obtain a copy of the minutes for the price of 1d. was overwhelmingly defeated. (M A B Mins., 16 November 1867, vol. i, p. 47.)

in the creation of a statistical section at the War Office in 1858.[1] Apart from the Registrar-General's Office, no other government department or public authority had hitherto devoted a special part of its establishment to statistical investigation. In 1886, the Asylums Board thus preceded the Ministry of Health by some seventy years in setting up a department for the express purpose of systematically assembling, processing and interpreting—as distinct from accumulating—statistical data on health and related topics, to enable administration to be based on facts, as opposed to common sense and conjecture.[2]

The twelve Board members constituting the statistical committee, with Sir Vincent Kennett-Barrington as its chairman, included a Member of Parliament, Mr. J. G. Talbot, JP; a Fellow of the Royal Society, Captain (now Sir) Douglas Galton, KCB; and two senior medical men: Deputy Surgeon-General J. A. Bostock, CB, and Dr. Edward Seaton, MD, an eminent authority on vaccination and successor to Sir John Simon as Medical Officer to the Local Government Board from 1876–79. For some thirteen years, this committee served as the nerve-centre of the M A B services until their operational structure was reshaped at the close of the century.

V

By this time, reform demanded bolder measures of devolution than had been attempted hitherto. The Board's functions[3] now fell into five separate departments—the isolation hospitals, mental institutions, ambulance services, a training ship, and the care of sick and defective children—a task which the Board had been assigned as late as 1897.[4]

Three of the Board's five departments were each managed by a central committee. When in 1875, the Asylums Managers had been instructed to administer a training ship, the work had been delegated to a special committee directly responsible to the Board. The ambulance stations, initially administered by the hospital management committees, were later placed under the control of a central ambulance committee which also administered the River Ambulance Service. As the Board embarked on the care of sick children, a central children's committee was formed and empowered to appoint institutional management committees. But, in respect of the isolation hospitals and mental institutions, the Board displayed a stubborn disinclination to relinquish the direct control which it had exercised since its creation over these branches of its work. Nevertheless, in 1898, the

---

[1] C. Woodham-Smith, op. cit., p. 243.

[2] The Guillebaud Committee, reporting on the cost of the National Health Service, recommended (Cmd. 9663, HMSO 1956, para. 699): 'the setting up of a Research and Intelligence Department which would devote the whole of its time to statistical investigations and operational research in general' and which would be 'constantly engaged in the search for facts and information which would enable administrators to make right decisions for the future of the Service; above all it should be looking out for the right sort of questions that ought to be asked' (para. 702). Not until 1958 was a statistical section set up at the Ministry of Health and then only on a minor scale.

[3] The functions of the M A B and the statutory instruments by which they were governed are set out in Appendix I, Document I.

[4] See Chapter 18 on Child Care.

Local Government Board announced that it had under consideration the appointment of central committees for these two services 'with a view to increasing the powers of supervision and strengthening generally the administration and financial control of the Managers over the institutions under their charge; of ensuring greater uniformity of administration; and, at the same time, economizing the time of the members'.[1]

When, in June 1899, these two additional central committees were created, the reformed operational framework of the Asylums Board was established for the next three decades. This three-tier structure—the Board at the summit, with central committees for each service and management committees for each institution—persisted until the outbreak of the First World War. By this time, the Board had established two additional services. In 1911 it was charged with the care of tuberculous patients[2] and the homeless poor of the metropolis.[3] It was also producing its own diphtheria antitoxin and maintaining bacteriological laboratories.[4]

After the war, expansion demanded further decentralization. As the base of the pyramidal structure broadened, the Board at the apex became a ratifying body, while all members, sitting as the general purposes committee, deliberated upon policy and matters affecting the Board's work as a whole. Eight sub-committees dealt with topics ranging from laundries to legislation and from statistics to sick children's education. In addition to the three main committees for administrative purposes—finance, contracts and works—the organizational structure comprised seven other standing committees, each in charge of a functional department of the Board's work. Of these, the four which governed the Board's hospital services—isolation, mental, tuberculosis and children's—were, in effect, subsidiary boards each comprising twenty-five to thirty-six members. Immediately responsible to each of these bodies was a 'central' sub-committee. Working under the immediate control and co-ordinating authority of these 'central' committees, were 'visiting' or 'house' committees for each unit. A substantial degree of latitude in matters of detail was accorded to these unit committees, which were empowered to give directions so long as they did not concern the service as a whole. The 'central' committees were enabled to delegate any of their own powers to their sub-committees, whose decisions, nevertheless, they retained the right to modify or reverse. In 1923, a scientific advisory committee was entrusted with general supervision over the work of the laboratories, antitoxin production, and research. Its seven members, mainly pathologists and epidemiologists, included the senior medical officer of the Ministry of Health, Sir George Buchanan, and the chief medical officer of the MAB isolation hospitals service, Dr. F. H. Thomson, the only committee member in the service of the Board.[5] Apart from this external body, the Board's operational network was manned entirely by its own members, most of whom sat on three or more committees. Following World War I, the Board's services were thus governed

---

[1] LGB letter to the MAB, 13 May 1898.   [2] See Chapter 19 on Tuberculosis.
[3] See Chapter 20 on the Homeless Poor.
[4] See Chapter 17 on, inter alia, Pathological Services.
[5] Members of the MAB scientific advisory committee are listed in Appendix I, Document V.

by a four-tiered hierarchy comprising eleven standing committees and fifty-three sub-committees.[1] One additional committee was created in 1928 to administer the Metropolitan Common Poor Fund.[2]

The Board claimed that its method of organization 'had been found by long experience to be thoroughly satisfactory; to retain the interest of members in the work allotted to them; and to produce the best results.'[3] In the last analysis, however, these results derived from the personal qualities of those who planned and managed the system. The unpaid, public-spirited members of the M A B were required to possess in a highly-developed degree those attributes which Miss Nightingale once cited as indispensable in those who administered services for the sick. 'They must not be sentimental enthusiasts', she asserted, 'but downright lovers of hard work . . . attending to and managing the thousand and one hard practical details which, nevertheless, plainly determine the question as to whether your sick shall live or die.'[4]

[1] For details of the committee structure of the M A B during its last decade, see Appendix I, Document IV. For systems of government of voluntary hospitals (general and special) in London at about the same time, see *Third Report from the Select Committee of the House of Lords on Metropolitan Hospitals, 1892*: BPP, 1892, vol. xiii, Appendix 3, p. 23.

[2] The Local Authorities (Emergency Provisions) Act, 1928 (18 & 19 Geo. 5 c. 9 s. 2) provided that metropolitan boards of guardians should submit to the M A B estimates of expenditure to be claimed from the Metropolitan Common Poor Fund, the administration of which was transferred from the Ministry of Health to the M A B under this statute. See note on the MCPF, Appendix IV.

[3] M A B Annual Report for 1929–30, p. 13.

[4] Florence Nightingale: an address delivered on 2 August 1870 to the Executive Committee of the National Society for Aid to the Sick and Wounded (subsequently the British Red Cross Aid Society).

CHAPTER 12

Administrative Organization and Personnel

I

HAVING surveyed the composition, functions and structure of the M A B, we may now consider it in action, with special reference to its roles as agent of a central government department and as employer of medical, nursing and lay personnel.

The substantial measure of 'delegated legislation'[1] which had been built into the 1867 Metropolitan Poor Act made it possible for the central poor law authority to issue dictatorial instructions to the M A B concerning any, or every, area of institutional administration, as it thought fit.[2] In practice, however, the extent to which the Local Government Board exercised its powers, and the effectiveness of its intervention, were appreciably attenuated with time, although the principle of central control over the activities of the M A B remained absolute in legal theory.

The friction between Whitehall and the hospital Managers during their first three decades stemmed largely from the anomalous and undefined role which the 1867 Metropolitan Poor Act assigned to the central authority in relation to the new State services. It was neither administrative nor supervisory but a jumble of the two. 'What is wanted', the *Lancet* suggested, 'is a better definition of the range of duties belonging respectively to the central and local authorities, and it will be a happy result of their quarrels if this should be attained.'[3] But it never was. Coupled with this imprecision was the imperfect adjustment of the central authority to the difference between the local hospital boards envisaged in the 1867 Act, and the body which resulted from Mr. Gathorne Hardy's decision to combine all the metropolitan localities into one large hospital region. The form of control and the type of regulations suitable for the small 'district asylum boards' provided for in the Act[4] were wholly inappropriate when applied to a hospital authority of a calibre vastly superior to that of an average board of guardians and larger than the Metropolitan

---

[1] What has come to be known as 'delegated legislation' was initiated during the last third of the nineteenth century, when the State was assuming responsibility for a greater measure of social administration than hitherto. The congestion of Parliament had perforce to be relieved by providing that the details of social legislation should be completed departmentally according to the discretionary powers of responsible ministers.

[2] 30 & 31 Vict. c. 6 ss. 4 and 15 (see Appendix I, Document II).

[3] *Lancet*, vol. ii, p. 225 (13 August 1870).

[4] 30 & 31 Vict. c. 6 ss. 8–37 (See Appendix I, Document II).

Board of Works (predecessor of the LCC).[1] To the Poor Law Board, and the Local Government Board in its early years, the M A B was just another metropolitan poor law authority and its institutions merely specialized workhouse infirmaries. The Asylums Managers, on the other hand, regarded their hospitals as an entirely new and separate system of institutional medical care, which they had no intention of administering on workhouse lines.

In the London general (voluntary) hospitals, the chief executive officers were laymen. At the endowed hospitals, the treasurer had always wielded great power. Generally, a voluntary hospital was controlled by a board of governors, often of enormous size, working through various sub-committees. The most important of these were the powerful house committee, composed of lay governors, and the medical staff committee. The lay group met frequently and usually reported to the full board once a quarter. In the general hospitals, the medical staff were seldom represented on the board, although in the special hospitals they played an active part in government. The lay chief executive officer, while answerable to the house committee for the general running of the hospital, exercised no authority over the nursing staff. The fully-trained matron, as distinct from the earlier housekeeper type, was generally accepted as *de facto* head of an independent department.[2]

While the Asylums Managers were not anxious to assign sole responsibility to any one officer, they favoured the voluntary hospital system of relieving the chief medical officer of administrative duties, in order that he might devote his time and skills exclusively to the patients. During the days when the M A B hospitals were under construction, members of management committees attended personally to the numerous day-to-day problems which beset their new venture. Once the institutions were in operation, their experimental character encouraged the Managers to continue their vigilance and to remedy such defects as became apparent. One committee member, for instance, invented a disinfector 'which caused a constant stream of chlorine to be generated below the surface of the sewage flowing through the drains'. Another recommended the use of portable disinfectors inside the hospital in order that 'the continuous gentle odour of chlorine gas should be maintained in the wards'. When Dr. Brewer saw nurses lifting heavy patients lying in beds only a few inches from the floor, he advised the use of 'Tinsley's elevating bedsteads'. The emergencies and need for quick decisions occasioned by the large-scale epidemics of their early days, led the Managers in more normal conditions to continue their personal supervision,[3] while day-to-day administration was conducted by the

[1] The membership of the Metropolitan Board of Works was 45 (W. A. Robson, *The Government and Misgovernment of London*, p. 58), whereas that of the M A B was originally 60 and ultimately 73.

[2] *Select Committee of the House of Lords on Metropolitan Hospitals, 1890–93*, Third Report, Appendix 3, p. 23; p. lxxxii; paras. 49, 297 and 462. See also B. Abel-Smith, *The Hospitals . . .*, op. cit., p. 155.

[3] The degree of control by different management committees varied. One chairman disagreed altogether with personal supervision by his committee and acted solely through the medical superintendent. In this case, there occurred, without direct proof of cause and effect, more complaints from patients and staff than in any of the other M A B institutions.

executive trio—the medical superintendent, the steward and the matron, each reigning over a separate department. Despite the categorical refusal of the Local Government Board in 1877 to sanction the 'principle of co-ordinate officers acting under the direction of the committee of management',[1] the practice of surveillance by peripatetic committee members continued unchanged, and apparently unsuspected by the central authority. During the 1885 Local Government Board enquiry into excessive spending already described,[2] the investigating committee commented on the constant visits paid to the hospital by the chairman of the management committee—'a practice which seemed to prevail at other asylums of the Board. . . .' The committee of enquiry 'doubted the legality or expediency of this arrangement' as 'it appeared to be calculated to weaken and invalidate the responsibility of the medical superintendent.'[3] The Asylums Managers contended that principal officers in their establishments 'should not be denied opportunities of consulting the chairmen of management committees and obtaining advice when dealing with emergencies'.[4] And the system continued unchanged.

The M A B came more and more to assert its independence. When the official regulations proved unworkable, protests were made. Sometimes these were successful, as in the case of the central authority's powers concerning personnel. The 1875 instructions had required that all appointments and scales of pay should receive the prior approval of the Local Government Board. This form of control had been introduced by the 'new' poor law in the interests of national uniformity, but it had little relevance so far as the M A B was concerned. By 1888, the M A B management committees had secured the right to appoint their own staff in accordance with conditions prescribed by the full Board and reported on periodically to the central authority.[5] Other unacceptable rules, if not revised by compromise, were moulded in practice to meet workaday requirements, or unobtrusively modified to extinction. Sometimes they were completely ignored. The administrative hierarchy—from the medical superintendent down to the gate porter—had been lavishly endowed by the official regulations with books in which to enter details concerning a variety of topics. The gate porter, for instance, was required to record particulars of all persons, including staff, entering and leaving the hospital, as well as of all packages they carried. This was never done. Even when the required records were kept, it seems they served no very useful purpose. In 1885, one M A B medical officer reported that, in the course of his fourteen years' service, 'no committee, auditor, government inspector or other person had ever called for the books, to which so much importance appeared . . . to be attached.'[6]

Provision for any form of systematic governmental inspection of the M A B institutions

[1] See Chapter 5.
[2] See Chapter 11.
[3] M A B *Mins.*, vol. xix, p. 940 (14 July 1885).
[4] Ibid., p. 957 (7 December 1885).
[5] LGB order to the M A B dated 23 March 1888, section xii.
[6] Letter from the Medical Superintendent of the M A B Eastern Hospital (Dr. Collie) to the M A B Chairman, 1 December 1885 (M A B *Mins.*, vol. xix, p. 927).

was conspicuously absent from the central authority's regulations.[1] These merely assigned to the Board's hospital committees a limited inspectorial role. It was laid down that the 'asylum committee' should 'visit the asylum from time to time, inspect the reports of the officers, examine the stores and investigate any complaints made by the paupers',[2] while clinical and administrative aspects of the institutions were not mentioned. In their own standing orders, the Asylums Managers prescribed that not less than two members of each hospital sub-committee should be deputed once between each fortnightly committee meeting to inspect specific parts of their establishment, such as the stores, kitchen or laundry, in addition to one or more wards and the administrative blocks, which they were obliged to visit on every tour of inspection. Reports on such matters as required investigation were communicated to the hospital committee, or higher authority if necessary, and, in very exceptional cases, to the Local Government Board. 'Are the beds turned up and every detail looked at?', the Clerk to the Asylums Board was asked when giving evidence in 1906 before the Poor Law Commission. 'I believe that is so', he guardedly replied, 'but some have a faculty for minute examination; others have not.'[3]

Inspection of the M A B mental institutions was conducted annually by the Commissioners in Lunacy under the Lunacy Acts. In addition, the M A B management committees held fortnightly meetings in the institutions and inspected them at least once between each meeting. Medical superintendence as a principle of government in mental hospitals had been accepted almost everywhere in the United Kingdom since about 1845.[4] In the Board's establishments for the insane, the medical superintendent had always been regarded by the Managers as the chief responsible officer. The location of these institutions some distance outside London rendered impracticable the same detailed supervision by management committees as was exercised over the infectious disease hospitals.

When, early in the twentieth century, the Board established institutions for sick children,[5] superintendence was vested in the visiting consultant—dermatologist or ophthalmologist—while his functions were delegated to a resident assistant medical officer in his absence. Later, when tuberculosis sanatoria were added to the Board's empire,[6]

---

[1] Even as late as 1909 there was neither systematic governmental inspection nor central audit of the 700 municipal hospitals by then established in various parts of the country with an aggregate of nearly 25,000 beds. Beyond sanctioning the loans for these hospitals under the Public Health Acts, the Local Government Board appeared to have no other official knowledge of this branch of civic activity than could be gleaned from the local taxation returns and from the annual reports of the 1,800 medical officers of health. There appeared to be no official statement to show how many sanitary authorities, or what proportion of the whole, maintained their own hospitals, or made arrangements to use other hospitals, or made no provision at all. (Minority Report of the Royal Commission on the Poor Law, BPP, 1909, vol. xxxvii (Cmd. 4499), p. 877, n.)

[2] LGB order, 10 February 1875, article 26.

[3] *Royal Commission on the Poor Law*, 1905–9, Vol. II [Cmd. 4684], Q.24365 (BPP, 1909, vol. xi).

[4] Alexander Walk, 'Mental Hospitals', in F. N. L. Poynter (ed)., *The Evolution of Hospitals in Britain* (1964), p. 132.

[5] See Chapter 18.   [6] See Chapter 19.

the principle of medical superintendence was extended to these institutions, the chief executive officer being also a clinician.

In 1906, a 'medical investigator' was appointed to the Board's isolation hospitals service. His duties included the study of complaints and 'return' cases. This post later broadened into that of 'medical officer for general purposes' and carried with it the duties of abstracting and commenting on medical superintendents' reports; keeping abreast of advances in the treatment of disease; and investigating outbreaks of infection in poor law and other metropolitan institutions. During the Board's later years, functional groups of hospitals, as well as the research and pathological services, were placed under the general supervision of medical directors, on the lines of the North American 'chiefs of service' system. All these appointments were initiated by the Asylums Board and accepted without demur by the central authority.

By the end of the century, relations between the Local Government Board and the Asylums Board had begun to improve significantly. Personalities had played an important part in this *rapprochement*. Dr. John Henry Bridges, 'the only progressive doctor in the Local Government Board',[1] had retired by this time, but he had been succeeded in the Poor Law Division by Dr. (later Sir) Arthur Downes, a close associate of Charles Booth, pioneer in scientific social investigation. In Dr. Downes, the M A B found a sympathetic and co-operative ally. Further, Dr. Bridges had been nominated to the Asylums Board shortly after retiring from his office in 1892. To the end, his position as sole medical inspector in a department of lay administrators had been a difficult one. During his last years in the Poor Law Division, he wrote in a personal letter: 'The LGB . . . will use me as a sort of skirmisher if they can, and then fail to support me when they find it inconvenient. But I . . . intend to walk warily.'[2] Although his role as hospital manager offered to his humanitarian and creative qualities the scope they had been denied in the Civil Service, he was never wholly reconciled to the principle of hospital control by the State, the results, in his estimation, being 'wholly disproportionate to the labour and the cost'.[3] Despite the experiences of the sensitive Dr. Bridges, however, a more enlightened regime had been slowly developing at the Local Government Board since the middle 1880s. In 1882, Sir Hugh Owen (jr.), 'a model of all that a civil servant should be',[4] had succeeded Sir John Lambert as permanent head of the Local Government Board. On retiring in 1899, Sir Hugh Owen was succeeded by Sir Samuel Provis, who, with Dr. Arthur Downes, served on the 1905–9 Poor Law Commission.

[1] R. Lambert. *Sir John Simon, 1816–1904*, p. 420, n. 55.

[2] Letter, 28 December 1888, from Dr. J. H. Bridges to his wife, cited by S. Liveing in *A Nineteenth-Century Teacher*, p. 211.

[3] In an article in the *Positivist Review* (February 1895, p. 203), Dr. J. H. Bridges, revealing his personal views on State hospitals, wrote: 'Every society has to heal its sores and uproot its diseases. In default of the organized voluntary enterprise to which work of this kind properly belongs, the State has to step in and do the business, inefficiently and clumsily, with results wholly disproportionate to the labour and the cost . . .'.

[4] Viscount Long, *Memories* (1923), pp. 94–95. Sir Hugh Owen had served as temporary Clerk to the M A B before the first permanent appointment in 1867.

This period of more harmonious relations between the Asylums Board and the 'parent' department witnessed the tacit waiving of those impracticable minutiae which had persisted unrevised in the 1875 Local Government Board regulations. Giving evidence before the Poor Law Commission in 1906, the M A B Chairman, Sir Augustus Scovell, was able to affirm that 'the general supervision of the Local Government Board has undoubtedly proved helpful' although 'many of their orders are more or less obsolete and demand revision.'[1] The Clerk to the Board, Mr. Duncombe Mann, who corroborated the chairman's assessment, added: 'I do not pretend that the Local Government Board press their detailed supervision in the least.'[2]

In 1900, after thirty years of hospital management, it was recognized that the time had come to revise the obsolete, and often conflicting, instructions which the Managers had received from the central authority during that time. The work of reducing into reasonable compass the four hundred printed pages of official regulations was begun, and at the end of 1903 the Local Government Board consented to the Clerk to the Asylums Board preparing a comprehensive draft order setting out the Managers' powers and duties.[3] In 1907 the draft consolidated order was submitted to the Local Government Board with the suggestion that it should be brought into force experimentally for a year, subject to modification or revocation in the light of experience.[4] It was neither accepted nor rejected, remaining indefinitely in abeyance, while the Asylums Managers proceeded, as in the past, on their own momentum.

In 1909, the tripartite system of administration in the M A B isolation hospitals came to an end. After considerable correspondence and prolonged consideration, the Local Government Board acquiesced in the Managers' proposal that stewards in their service should no longer rank as principal officers.[5] The main reason urged by the Managers in support of this change was that there should be only one recognized head at all the Board's establishments with general authority and control over the entire staff, thereby removing all doubts as to the semi-independence of other officers. The earlier preference of the Asylums Managers for co-ordinate authority had been motivated by no desire to subordinate the medical superintendent, whom they had always acknowledged as the most senior member of the tripartite partnership. The submergence of the chief medical officer in 'a variety of topics relating to the stores, farm, water and gas supplies, the engineering and laundry management and the judicious dealing with the nurses and servants in their domestic relations' would, the Managers reasoned, deprive the hospital of his medical skills. The alternative was to entrust these duties to other chief officers in their special departments. 'The difficulty of divided authority', they had concluded, 'seems to consist in the demand for greater supervision from the committees. This the committees are willing to submit to. . . .'[6] In this way the Managers in their early days rationalized their

---

[1] *Royal Commission on the Poor Law, 1905–9*, Vol. II, op. cit., Q.24670 (6).   [2] Ibid., Q.24210.
[3] LGB letter to the M A B, 12 November 1903.   [4] M A B letter to the LGB, 15 October 1907.
[5] LGB order to the M A B, 22 September 1909; M A B Annual Report, 1909, p. xxiv.
[6] M A B *Mins.*, 1876, vol. ix, p. 668.

undoubted preference for active participation in the executive work of hospital management, in the belief that their medical superintendents would be able to devote the greater part of their time to clinical duties. In practice, the contrary was the case. Their clerical work was always so onerous that they had far too little time to devote to their patients. A well-known hospital administrator of the day suggested that 'in order to relieve the resident staff of M A B hospitals, visiting physicians and surgeons should be appointed, assisted by efficient juniors and aided by a staff of clinical clerks, dressers, sisters and nurses'.[1] Not until 1920, some forty years later, were visiting consultants employed on a regular part-time basis.

Despite the zealous assumption of detailed supervision by individual members of management committees, the system appears to have worked without friction at the institutional level. The Managers co-operated closely with their medical superintendents, whose functions, according to Local Government Board regulations, included the monthly reporting of 'any defect in the diet, drainage, furniture, ventilation, warmth . . . or any excess in the number of the inmates. . .'.[2] The traditional suspicion which professional expertise arouses in administrators was inconspicuous in the deliberations of the Asylums Managers. Medical members of the Board were usually elected as chairmen of management committees and superintendents' recommendations were invariably acted upon. Medical counsel had provided the thrust behind the Board's representations to the central authority on a number of important public health issues. Stricter enforcement of the Vaccination Acts;[3] universal compulsory notification of infectious disease;[4] the inauguration of London's first ambulance services; clinical instruction in the M A B isolation hospitals;[5] and free admission for patients of all social classes to these institutions, were among the reforms which had been persistently advocated in M A B medical reports before reaching the Statute Book.

The principle and practice of overall medical superintendence, combined with supervisory control by management committees, continued in the M A B hospital services until their appropriation by the LCC in 1930; but, thereafter, administration on the executive level showed signs of reverting to the earlier tripartite system of responsibility.[6]

[1] H. C. Burdett, 'Is it desirable that hospitals should be placed under State supervision?' *Trans. NAPSS*, 1881, p. 508.

[2] LGB order, 10 February 1875, op. cit., article 72 (6).

[3] Vaccination Acts in relation to smallpox: see H. Williams, *A Century of Public Health in Britain*, Part VI, Chap. 2, pp. 245–50 and 258; and Ministry of Health Special Report No. 62, 1931, *Smallpox: prevention in relation particularly to the Vaccination Acts*.

[4] Several large provincial towns had been empowered by special Acts of Parliament to make prompt notification of infectious disease compulsory. The authorities could not, however, be prevailed upon to apply the same protection to the far more densely populated metropolis.

[5] See Chapter 17.

[6] In the 1930s the position of the medical superintendent in local authority hospitals showed signs of becoming modified by a tendency to give a measure of direct responsibility to the clerk, or steward, and matron for their respective duties and to give these officers direct access on their own initiative to their opposite numbers at the Town or County Hall. See Bradbeer Report on the *Internal Administration of Hospitals*, HMSO, 1954, p. 6.

II

Although the medical profession had been regulated by the Medical Act of 1858, the recruitment of hospital superintendents in the Board's early days presented acute problems, particularly in the fever and smallpox establishments. There were few specialists in infectious diseases at this time and almost none combining a specialty with administrative experience of public institutions. M A B superintendents were recruited mainly from among medical officers of prisons, asylums and poor law districts. Once appointed, they frequently remained until superannuated, as remuneration for posts under the M A B was slightly superior to that in other branches of the Poor Law Medical Service.[1]

The salary scale for medical superintendents in the Board's earliest isolation hospitals in 1870 ranged from £350 to £450 a year and included a house, with coals and gas. With the same additional emoluments, the scale varied only slightly during the next thirty years, reaching £400–£600 in 1900, by which time salaries were supplemented by fees for clinical instruction.[2] Salaries paid to senior medical officers of metropolitan infirmaries at this period averaged £422 a year, added to which were fees for vaccination and certification.[3] Medical superintendents of M A B smallpox institutions originally received less than their opposite numbers in the fever hospitals, as remuneration was based on the size of the establishment, but later, when the infection risk of smallpox was considered greater than that of fever, they received £100 a year more than their colleagues. In the Board's 2,000-bed mental institutions, medical superintendents in 1870 received £500 a year with accommodation. By 1910, £800 was the highest point on the salary scale, being £100 above that for the corresponding grade in the isolation hospitals. By 1925, remuneration for medical superintendents in the fever hospitals and children's institutions ranged from £770 in the smallest establishments to £1,250 in the largest; while in the mental health service, the minimum salary had increased to £850 in the small Fountain Hospital, and to £1,250 in the four large institutions at Darenth, Tooting Bec, Leavesden and Caterham. The medical superintendent's unfurnished house, which was worth £70 a year in 1900, was valued at £110 in 1925.

In 1870, resident assistant medical officers began with £120 a year in the isolation hospitals and £150 in the mental institutions. By 1900, salary scales for this grade in the two services had reached £180–£240 and £180–£300 respectively. These rates compared not unfavourably with those in metropolitan poor law infirmaries, where the average annual salary of a junior assistant was about £100. In the LCC asylums, however, an assistant medical officer could reach £400 during the early years of the century.[4] While

---

[1] Among a large medical staff, the following are recorded as having given the M A B a lifetime of devoted service: Drs. R. A. Birdwood, R. M. Bruce, F. Foord Caiger, H. E. Cuff, W. Gayton, E. W. Goodall and F. N. Hume. For salary scales of M A B medical staff at various dates, see Appendix IV, Table J.

[2] Fees for clinical instruction received by medical superintendents totalled between 26 and 46 guineas a year, two of the three guineas charged for each student being paid to the instructor. See Chapter 17.

[3] *Royal Commission on the Poor Law, 1905–9*, op. cit., p. 306, para. 14 (evidence of Mr. Spurrell).

[4] Ibid.

in the London infirmaries there was an average of 233 beds per medical officer at this time, the number in the M A B isolation hospital service was roughly 100 per medical officer (exclusive of the superintendent).[1] Not until 1908, were assistants permitted to apply for M A B medical superintendentships prior to public advertisement. Before that date, aspiring practitioners had scant opportunities for promotion. Turnover was rapid, as young men stayed for short periods merely for experience. Much more was expected of the junior medical officer in the care of the hospital patient in the days before standards of nursing were improved by an organized profession.

III

In the diseases and disabilities treated in the M A B institutions, nursing played a vital role, and there was never a time in the Board's history when staffing the wards was not a major problem. Mr. Gathorne Hardy had said during the passage of his 1867 Act: 'I know that we cannot, by paying, get trained nurses. Miss Nightingale says no such thing exists as a body of trained nurses at present: we must train them.'[2] The Asylums Managers recognized this situation all too soon and would have been powerless to deal with the early epidemics had the nursing nuns not come to their aid.

The era of 'scientific cleanliness' and the systematically trained nurse began with the opening in 1860 of the Nightingale Fund School at St. Thomas' Hospital. During the early years of the M A B hospitals, most of the 'assistant nurses' were former domestic servants, who applied for the nursing vacancies advertised by the Board in the national press. Previous experience was hardly expected. The only qualification required of a nurse in the Poor Law Service was the ability to read directions on medicine.[3] Her duty was 'to obey orders', and she was expected to pick up the work as she went along.

When the Board's hospital at Deptford was opened during the 1876–78 epidemic for male smallpox patients, it was decided, in view of the shortage of suitable women, to staff the wards entirely by men. The medical superintendent later affirmed that they were far preferable to women as ward attendants, despite the extra vigilance required from medical officers during the early stage of the disease. He found the male staff 'better fitted to maintain order among the patients, who were from the lowest class of the population'.[4] The medical superintendent at Hampstead, on the other hand, found that 'ill-behaviour' was restrained in his hospital by the mere presence of the lady-sisters[5]—

---

[1] Ibid., para. 12.   [2] *Hansard*, vol. clxxv (third series), 8 February 1867.

[3] LGB order, 10 February 1875, section xi, article 45.

[4] Report of Dr. C. W. Waylen, Medical Superintendent of Deptford Smallpox Hospital, for 1877–78. M A B *Mins.*, vol. xi, p. 634.

[5] For the origin and training of nineteenth-century 'lady' nurses, see B. Abel-Smith, op. cit., pp. 19–24 and 30, and E. S. Haldane, *The British Nurse in Peace and War* (1923), p. 95 *et seq.* Even before the emergence of 'lady' nurses from the Nightingale training school, which opened in 1860, 'lady-sisters' were noted in the literature: e.g. Bristowe and Holmes' 1863 survey of UK hospitals records their inclusion on the staffs of University College and King's College Hospitals (Sixth Report of the MO to the Privy Council, 1864,

a particular feature of the Hampstead smallpox hospital. 'There is', he reported, 'a tone of refinement, a quiet industry, and an absence of frivolity to be observed, both among nurses and patients, in a ward under the superintendence of a lady, which is usually wanting in one under the control of the ordinary nurse.' He urged the advantages of 'bringing the lower classes during the impressionable period of sickness into contact with the sweetness and light that are ever diffused around her by the cultured gentlewoman.'[1] Besides brute force and feminine refinement for maintaining discipline, however, the hospitals badly needed adequately trained staff for nursing. The medical superintendents constantly reminded the Managers that 'in no department is parsimony more dangerous, for bad or inefficient nursing may more than neutralize all the efforts of the rest of the staff.'

By 1890, developments arising out of the Poor Law Act of 1889 rendered nursing reforms imperative. Treatment had become legally available in the M A B infectious disease hospitals to patients of all social classes,[2] and medical students were being admitted for clinical instruction.[3] This latter innovation had led to classes in elementary anatomy and physiology for the nurses—the first attempt at formal training which had been undertaken by the Board. The most important reform, however, was the change in the matron's status. The Managers had persuaded the Local Government Board that the time had come for her to be placed in authority over the nurses while on duty and be given responsibility for the patients in the wards. By now, a number of London and provincial voluntary hospitals and infirmaries employed matrons of the new type, who had been trained in the Nightingale school.[4] While M A B matrons hitherto had been disciplinarians with some administrative ability, the Managers decided that in future they must be fully trained nurses. In the order specifying the new responsibilities of M A B matrons, the Local Government Board included the words: 'subject to the control of the medical superintendent'.[5] As the Managers had come to regard the matron as one of the executive trio, they ingeniously waived this limitation by invoking the 1875 definition of the medical superintendent's sphere of authority, which decreed that it was unnecessary for him to interfere with the departments of other officers.[6]

Table on p. 488). See also C. Dainton, *The Story of England's Hospitals* (1961), p. 113. Concerning seventeenth-century lady-sisters, the Receipt Book of St. Thomas' has an entry: 'D . . . V . . . did her dutie from 1618 to 1621 . . .' and a note explaining that 'at about this time, or a little later, hospital sisters received a salary of eleven shillings a quarter if they were in charge of a large ward and ten shillings and sixpence for a small ward, plus wages of about three shillings and sixpence. They earned their money the hard way and it was only in the middle of the seventeenth century that "helpers"—later called nurses—were appointed to lighten their work'. (*The Times*, commenting on an exhibition of documents from the archives of St. Thomas' Hospital: 'Nearly a thousand years of service', 27 November 1961.)

[1] Report of Dr. Samuel Bingham, Medical Superintendent of the Hampstead Smallpox Hospital, for 1878 (M A B *Mins.*, vol. xiii, p. 284, *et seq.*).

[2] 52 & 53 Vict. c. 56 s. 3. See Chapter 6.

[3] 52 & 53 Vict. c. 56 s. 4. See Chapter 17.

[4] Concerning matrons of the new type, see B. Abel-Smith, op. cit., pp. 24–29, passim.

[5] LGB order to the M A B, 9 May 1890.

[6] LGB letter to the M A B, 18 February 1875, op. cit.

The attempts initiated in 1890 to improve the Board's nursing service proved unequal to the demands imposed by the rapid growth of isolation accommodation during the terminal decade of the century. In two years, over £1,200 was spent on advertising for nursing and domestic staff, but with little success. Early in 1892, the Managers consulted Dr. J. H. Bridges of the Local Government Board. In the course of a detailed study of the nursing situation in the Board's institutions, he found a general lack of trained staff. In one fever hospital, out of nineteen 'charge nurses', only one was fully trained and a number were under twenty years old. Some had served previously in workhouse sick wards, though untrained, and relatively few had passed through a regular course of instruction at a hospital or at one of the eighteen poor law infirmaries in the country which could be called schools for nurses.[1] Dr. Bridges' investigation[2] resulted in a number of reforms. Nursing staff, he recommended, should rank as a class separate from, and superior to, the other female subordinate staff, and be boarded and lodged apart from them; separate, comfortable, roomy sitting rooms should be provided; where possible, every nurse should have a separate bedroom; the Board's nursing staff should be centralized and an irreducible nucleus fixed. Generally, the Managers would do well to spare neither trouble nor expense in making their nursing service as attractive as possible.

In the 1870s, M A B assistant nurses had received £20 a year, with board and uniform—£2 more than the ward servants. London workhouse nurses a few years earlier were paid between £12 and £30 a year (averaging about £21).[3] The pay of M A B 'charge nurses' in 1870 had been £27 a year, while superintendent nurses, of somewhat higher social class, received at this time between £36 and £42 annually. In order to augment the supply of fever nurses in the 1880s, rates were increased to £22–£26 for assistants; £34–£36 for 'charge nurses'; and £40–£46 for superintendents.[4]

Following Dr. Bridges' recommendations in 1892, a standing committee was formed to keep nursing conditions under review. Pay was immediately increased and two grades of assistant nurse created, with annual cash emoluments fixed at £20–£24 and £24–£28 respectively, with three weeks' annual leave, 12 hours off duty weekly and 24 additional hours monthly. Future recruits to grades higher than second assistant were required to produce certificates of training—one year for first assistants and three years for 'charge nurses', whose scale was raised to £36–£40. The minimum age for nurses, fixed by the Committee at 22, had to be lowered later.

A genuine effort was made by the Asylums Board to promote the welfare and status

---

[1] In 1871, the poor law institution at Highgate was the first in London to open an infirmary and the first to be used as a training school for nurses under the 1867 Metropolitan Poor Act. Miss Nightingale supplied the matron and nurses from St. Thomas' Hospital. The next infirmary nursing school to be opened was in 1873 at the Central London Sick Asylum. (Elizabeth M. Ross, 'Women and Poor Law Administration, 1857–1910', MA unpublished thesis, Chap. VIII, p. 19; and Glen's *Poor Law Orders*, 11th edn., p. 749, *et seq.*)

[2] Dr. J. H. Bridges' report enclosed with LGB letter to the M A B, 4 March 1892; and M A B general purposes committee report, 3 March 1893, M A B *Mins.*, vol. xxvi, p. 893, *et seq.*

[3] B. Abel-Smith, op. cit., pp. 14–15.

[4] For salary scales of M A B nursing staff at various dates, see Appendix IV, Table K.

of nurses. When approached in 1904 by the newly-formed Society for the State Registration of Trained Nurses, the Managers expressed the hope that they might be represented on the General Nursing Council envisaged in the Bill which the Society had drafted for submission to Parliament.[1] Although invited to comment on the issues embodied in the draft Bill, the Managers sedulously abstained, as they did not wish to become involved in the politics of opposing pressure groups. To the brief communication of the Asylums Board, the Society petulantly replied: 'When the Board has come to a decision as to the principle of registration, the Council will take into consideration the question of representation of the Board on the General Nursing Council which is proposed in the Bill now before Parliament.'[2] This the Board ignored. Miss Nightingale had been averse to the registration of nurses, but since the death of her friends on the Board, her influence no longer pervaded its counsels.[3] The need for further consideration of the registration question did not arise until sixteen years later, when the General Nursing Council was eventually appointed.[4] By 1923, however, it was agreed that members of the M A B medical and nursing staffs should be permitted to serve on the board of examiners for the Council in connexion with the State examinations.

Training in the M A B hospitals had been deferred until 1909, when the Board opened an 800-bed establishment at Carshalton.[5] This was designed originally as a fever hospital, but when the Board was asked to provide urgently for sick children from the London workhouses, it was opened as a children's infirmary, and the opportunity was taken to equip it as a school for nurses. It was now more than forty years since Miss Nightingale had successfully lobbied for the new public hospitals to be used for training nurses under the 1867 Act.

The first probationers at Carshalton received £10–£18 annually, with board residence and uniform. This was rather less than probationers were paid in other sectors of the Poor Law Service early in the century[6] and on a par with the pay of the earliest probationers at St. Thomas' Hospital in 1860.[7] By 1920, the annual salary scale for first-year probationers in the Board's isolation and children's hospitals had reached £30–£34 while senior probationers received £42–£48. These rates were considerably above those for the same grades in all other types of hospital.[8] Training in the Board's mental institutions was made compulsory in 1919 for both male and female nurses. In mental nursing it was customary for patients to be cared for by 'attendants' of their own sex. Before 1919, 'proficiency

[1] Correspondence between the Society for the State Registration of Trained Nurses and the M A B of February 1904, M A B *Mins.*, vol. xxxvii, p. 131.

[2] Reply of the Society for State Registration to the M A B, 31 March 1904. M A B *Mins.*, vol. xxxvii, p. 225.

[3] By 1904, Miss Nightingale was relinquishing her hold on active life and her supporters on the Asylums Board had vanished from the scene. Sir Douglas Galton died in 1899 and Sir V. Kennett-Barrington was killed in a balloon accident in 1903.

[4] Concerning the registration of trained nurses, see B. Abel-Smith, op. cit., Chapter VII.

[5] See Chapter 18.

[6] See B. Abel-Smith, *A History of the Nursing Profession* (1960), App. III, Table 1 (p. 281) and p. 55.

[7] Ibid., p. 280.   [8] Ibid., Table 2 (p. 282).

pay' was given to those who acquired a diploma in mental nursing by voluntary effort. Probationer scales in 1920 reached £83–£104 (females) and £104–£130 (males), but no additional emoluments, apart from uniforms, were allowed in the mental institutions.

By the mid-twenties, despite improved rates of pay and living conditions for nurses in the service of the M A B, the staffing problem remained as acute as ever. More alternative openings for women, competing demands of hospital development throughout the country, and increasing severity and scope of nursing examinations restricted the choice of candidates. Although nursing in the Board's institutions was considered less strenuous than in general hospitals,[1] hours of duty and annual leave were improved to compare favourably with the majority of hospitals elsewhere. In order to attract and improve the prospects of better educated probationers, the salaries of the senior nursing grades were increased; staff nurses were placed on a £60–£70 annual scale, and the rate for 'charge nurses', now known as 'sisters', was raised to £80–£95. Following the changed status of matrons in 1890, their salary, which had averaged about £100 annually in the 1870s, remained almost unchanged until 1909, when they were all placed on a £100–£150 scale, with board-residence. By 1930, matrons' salaries ranged from £160 a year in the smallest sanatoria to £340 in the largest mental institutions and children's hospitals. By this time, remuneration was graded according to the size and type of institution.

When the earliest M A B hospitals opened, they had no fully trained matrons and hardly a nurse with hospital experience, apart from the temporarily engaged nursing nuns. For nearly four decades, the lack of fully qualified senior staff had made it impossible to embark on any scheme of training. At the close of the Board's sixty years of administration in 1930, however, probationers were being instructed in twenty-three approved M A B training schools,[2] and about one in five of the Board's 4,475 nurses was entered on

---

[1] The strenuousness of the work of M A B nurses is difficult to assess objectively. Patient-staff ratios fluctuated considerably, particularly in the Isolation Hospitals Service. In the mental hospitals service, totals for staff in existing records represent the aggregate for all types of institution—for senile dements, feeble-minded children, congenital mental deficients and sane epileptics—all of which would have varied concerning patient-staff ratios. Despite their limited value, the following patient-nurse ratios have been calculated on the basis of the total of patients and the *total* of nurses (day and night) in each of the M A B services at the end of 1929: isolation hospitals, 4 to 1; mental hospitals, 7 to 1; TB sanatoria, 5 to 1; and children's hospitals, 9 to 2. By this date, the hours of duty per week worked by M A B nursing staff were as follows—in all institutions other than mental: probationers, 56 (day duty) and 60½ (night duty); staff nurses, 58; ward sisters, 55. Mental nurses worked a 50-hour week. Nurses in all M A B services had four weeks' annual leave; matrons had six weeks. For average hours worked in other hospitals in 1937, see B. Abel-Smith, op. cit., Appendix II, Table 11.

[2] The 23 M A B training schools for nurses comprised: 1 for children's diseases, 10 for fever, 7 for tuberculosis and 5 for mental diseases. The number of probationers required at any one time during the late 1920s was about 1,420, distributed as follows: children, 160; fever, 550; tuberculosis, 170; and mental, 540. The period of training for M A B probationers was three years in the mental hospitals and the children's general hospital, and two years in the fever and tuberculosis services. Probationers at the children's and fever hospitals were trained for the State examinations; those in the tuberculosis sanatoria entered for the examination held by the Society of Superintendents of Tuberculosis Institutions; and those at Princess Mary's and St. Luke's Hospitals (mainly tuberculous children) were examined by an outside examiner. At most of these hospitals the probationers who completed the prescribed period of training and obtained certificates could obtain a

the State Register.[1] The vicissitudes of the M A B nursing service, in effect, mirrored the trend of change which had taken place in the character, status, conditions and organization of the nursing profession generally during the six most crucial decades of its development.

IV

The first public service of hospital administrators was a totally spontaneous development, undreamed-of by the creators of the M A B in 1867. Soon after the Board was formed, a Clerk, Mr. W. F. Jebb, was appointed at an annual salary of £500.[2] Until the hospitals came into being, Mr. Jebb was the Board's sole administrative officer. After working single-handed for some months, he was allowed an assistant 'at wages not to exceed thirty shillings a week'. Later, a 'temporary' copying clerk was appointed at £1 1s. a week.

When the institutions were first staffed, stewards were appointed at a salary of £100 per annum with residence. By 1909, stewards' minimum remuneration had risen to £150.[3] According to the official 1875 regulations, the province of the steward's duties included responsibility for the grounds, gardens, farms, livestock, the discipline of male staff and, in the mental institutions, the care of male patients on outdoor or domestic occupations. To assist him in these multifarious duties, the steward was allowed one clerk. No clerical assistance was provided for the medical superintendent until after the turn of the century. The central authority suggested that, when necessary, he should share the steward's clerk.

---

remission of one year at certain general hospitals if they went on for general training, without which the higher posts in the profession were closed to them. The best appointment which the Asylums Board offered to probationers trained in its own services was that of staff nurse. Nurses above this grade were required by M A B regulations to possess a certificate of general training. Probationers at the mental hospitals were trained for the State examinations or the diploma of the Royal Medico-Psychological Association.

[1] Of the total M A B nursing staff of 4,475 in 1930 (581 male and 3,894 female), 846 were on the State Register, distributed as follows:

General	General and Fever	Mental	Sick Children	Tuberculosis	Total
269	82	77 (F)	16	183 (F)	627 (F)
		218 (M)		1 (M)	219 (M)
					846

In 1937, 18 per cent of ward staff in the voluntary hospitals were trained. Of the aggregate of all hospitals participating in the pre-war Athlone Committee enquiry, 31 per cent of ward staff were trained. (See Abel-Smith, op. cit., Appendix II, p. 272.)

[2] Comparable salaries in 1871 of civil servants and others are listed by Professor R. K. Kelsall in *Higher Civil Servants in Britain* (1955), Table 27, p. 183. These include: Professor of Moral Philosophy, Edinburgh University, £502 p.a.; Headmaster, City of London School, £1,000 p.a.; Permanent Secretary to the Board of Trade, £1,500 p.a.

[3] Stewards' remuneration was fixed in 1909 at £150–£200 p.a., with residence, in both the mental and isolation hospitals. Twenty years later, salary scales ranged from £275–£325 p.a. in the smaller isolation hospitals to £400–£450 p.a. in the larger mental hospitals.

When, in 1891, Mr. Jebb retired, the salary and status of the Clerk to the Board were comparable with those of a Higher Division Clerk (third grade) in the Civil Service.[1] During the decade following the appointment of Mr. Duncombe Mann, who succeeded to the office of Clerk to the Board, the M A B empire expanded rapidly; personnel was considerably increased; and administrative organization was in a state of flux. In 1909, a central establishment committee was appointed to recruit staff and increase efficiency throughout the Board's services. Grades approximating to those in the Civil Service were established, while superannuation schemes and conditions of work were negotiated with the workers' unions.

When Sir Duncombe Mann retired in 1922 (he was knighted on retirement), he was succeeded by Mr. Allan Powell, CBE, barrister-at-law, who had entered the service of the Board in 1894 and had been Deputy Clerk since before World War I. On the dissolution of the Board, he too was knighted and appointed Chief Officer of Public Assistance under the LCC. By this time (1930), the status and responsibilities of the Clerk to the M A B were roughly equivalent to those of a Permanent Secretary of a government department.[2] At the M A B Head Office on the Embankment, departments under Principal Clerks dealt centrally with all the Board's institutional and other services, for the operation of which the Clerk was ultimately responsible to the Board.

At the end of 1929, the Board's labour force of nearly 10,000 was about twice as large as it had been at the turn of the century.[3] Nearly half was concerned directly with the care

---

[1] The maximum salary of a Civil Service Class I Clerk (3rd grade) was £500 p.a. in the 1890s. In 1890, two orders-in-council were issued based on the reports of the Ridley Commission on the civil service establishment (1887). These constituted two divisions of civil servants—Lower Division and Higher Division clerks. These were sub-divided into salary grades. (*Enc. Britannica*, vol. xxvii (MCMII), article on the Civil Service.)

[2] The salary of a Permanent Secretary of a government department in 1929 was £3,000 p.a. (R. K. Kelsall, op. cit., p. 183.)

[3] The following distribution of M A B staff in 1901 and 1929 suggests the growth of the various services of the Board in the intervening period:

Institution or Dept.	No. of Staff	
	1901	1929
Isolation Hospitals, River Ambulance and Laboratories	3,486	4,884
Mental Hospitals	1,023	2,294
Tuberculosis Sanatoria	—	1,069
Children's Institutions and Training Ship	173	1,082
Ambulance Stations, Casual Wards and Central Stores	280	409
Head Office	102	211
Totals:	5,064	9,949

of some 19,000 patients and other dependants.[1] In addition to the 4,500 nursing staff, 200 medical and dispensary staff were resident in the institutions, and a score or so consultants attended part-time. About 150 teachers were employed full-time in the children's institutions, while nearly 100 chaplains and ministers had permanent appointments on the staff of the Board. Of the remaining 5,000 employees, domestic, laundry and porter staff, farm hands and other ancillary grades accounted for nearly 4,000. The remaining 1,000 comprised mainly engineering staff (about 600) and clerical staff (about 400, of whom 200 were attached to the Head Office). By the end of 1929, the annual cost of wages and salaries in all the Board's services amounted to £938,000. This was 35 per cent of its total annual expenditure. At the turn of the century some £137,000 had been spent on wages and salaries, but this item then represented only 18 per cent of the Board's total annual outlay.[2]

The power of the central authority under the 1867 Act to control the salaries of M A B personnel remained in abeyance after the early ineffective attempts at regulation. As time went on, the Local Government Board intervened in the affairs of the M A B hospitals only when invited by the Asylums Board to do so. The absolute powers of compulsion and prohibition with which the central authority was endowed 'on paper' were in any case unworkable as a mainspring of administrative control, since they were wholly unsupported by practical sanctions for enforcing compliance. As will be seen from the following chapter on finance, the M A B was not dependent on any centrally controlled source of revenue which could have been used as an instrument of coercion. Although in legal theory it remained an agent of the central poor law department, to all intents and purposes the M A B functioned for the greater part of its lifetime as a quasi-independent authority.

[1] The daily average of M A B patients and other dependants in 1929 was 19,232. The total bed complement of the Board's institutions at the time of their transfer to the LCC in 1930 was 22,572 (see Appendix I, Document VI).

[2] See Appendix IV, Table D. Total annual expenditure on salaries and wages in the M A B *institutions for the sick*, exclusively, was £790,000 in 1929, being 39 per cent of the total; and £110,000 in 1899, being 22 per cent of the total.

CHAPTER 13

Finance: Revenue, Expenditure and Control

I

'THE main principle of the measure, which stood the test of time, was that it threw improvements on a common fund.'[1] In these words, written some twenty years after the passing of the 1867 Metropolitan Poor Act, Gathorne Hardy (by this time, Viscount Cranbrook), focused the essential feature of his State hospital scheme for London. A consolidated metropolitan rate for maintaining the poor law hospitals had been urged by both Miss Nightingale and Dr. Hart of the *Lancet* Commission; and during the debates on the 1867 Bill, Gathorne Hardy's introduction of this device had been ardently supported by John Stuart Mill and Sir Harry Verney, 'Member for Florence Nightingale'. Though not new in principle, the Metropolitan Common Poor Fund for financing the poor law medical reforms of 1867 had been wider in application than any previous attempt to distribute the burden of relief.[2] Gathorne Hardy, however, had done more than extend the principle of collective responsibility; he had used the fund to serve both as an instrument of central control over the metropolitan guardians and a means of ensuring their participation in the schemes which they had originally suspected of undermining local self-government.

So far as the guardians were concerned, the operation of the fund was relatively simple. The parochial boards contributed to it, on the basis of rateable value, as instructed by the central authority, and made claims upon it in respect of such relief expenditure as was specified in the Act.[3] But the role of the fund in the financial arrangements of the M A B was more complex. When Gathorne Hardy included among the items to be borne by the fund the cost of maintaining the infectious sick and insane in the new institutions, it would have been reasonable to expect that the Asylums Board would be authorized to draw on the fund direct. Instead, Gathorne Hardy involved the local guardians in the procedures for admitting and maintaining their parishioners in the district 'asylums'. Originally, it was intended that the M A B should receive patients only through the poor law authorities, thus enabling them to maintain their functional association with their sick poor. Under the 1867 Act, the M A B was empowered to call upon the guardians for contributions to

---

[1] A. E. Gathorne-Hardy (ed.): *Gathorne-Hardy, First Earl of Cranbrook—a Memoir* (1910), vol. i, p. 194.
[2] See Chapter 2.
[3] 30 & 31 Vict. c. 6 s. 69. See also Note on the Metropolitan Common Poor Fund, Appendix IV.

meet the cost of running the hospitals,[1] while the guardians were entitled to make claims on the fund for the reimbursement of their payments to the M A B.[2]

M A B charges were of two kinds—'maintenance' (or 'direct'), and 'common' charges. Patients' food and clothing were the main items included in the former, while the latter covered all other expenses.[3] 'Common' charges were levied by the M A B on the same rateable-value basis as the central authority precepts for guardians' contributions to the Common Fund.[4] 'Maintenance' charges were based on the number of patients received from each locality,[5] and these amounts could be claimed from the Common Fund by the destitution authorities, regardless of the number of patients sent from any one parish. The *total* running costs of the hospitals were thus, in effect, distributed throughout the metropolitan area. The end result of equalized incidence could, of course, have been obtained more readily and directly if the Common Fund had been by-passed, so far as M A B expenditure was concerned, and the Asylums Board had been empowered to raise the *whole* of its expenditure direct from the guardians on a proportional basis by precepts for inclusive amounts. As it was, each head of 'common' charges had to be assessed for each poor law district according to rateable value, and accounts kept for each in respect of individual patients' 'maintenance' charges, a procedure which involved some eight hundred calculations every half year.

When invited in 1902 to give evidence before the Departmental Committee on Workhouse Accounts, the M A B finance officer suggested that the Board's accounts would be simplified by the aggregation of 'direct' and 'common' charges. He also pointed out that, as about two-thirds of M A B expenditure was in respect of non-pauper patients, its inclusion in the Local Government Board's computation of metropolitan poor relief was somewhat anomalous.[6] By this time, the M A B isolation hospitals had been open to the general public for over a decade, following the Public Health (London) Act of 1891, which empowered guardians to recover charges for non-pauper patients from the Common Fund.[7] In its report of 1903, the Departmental Committee on Workhouse Accounts endorsed the suggestions of the M A B finance officer. The Asylums Managers thereupon appealed to the central authority to promote amending legislation which would enable them to raise the *whole* of their expenditure on a proportional basis.[8] The request was repeated over the years without success until 1916, when war-time conditions necessitated simplification. The Local Government (Emergency Provisions) Act of that year[9] em-

---

[1] 30 & 31 Vict. c. 6 s. 31. [2] Ibid., s. 69 (2).
[3] Ibid., ss. 31 & 32. [4] Ibid., s. 64.
[5] Statistical disadvantages resulted from the classification of patients according to poor law districts for accounting purposes, since notifications of infectious disease were made to the MOH of the sanitary districts, which were not co-terminous with the poor law districts. This made it difficult to compare notifications of disease and confirmed cases in the M A B hospitals.
[6] *Report of the Local Government Board Departmental Committee on Workhouse Accounts*, 1903: BPP, 1903, vol. xxvi [Cmd. 1440], p. 567.
[7] 54 & 55 Vict. c. 76 s. 80 (3).
[8] M A B *Mins.*, vol. xxxvii, 1903, pp. 217 and 423.
[9] 6 & 7 Geo. 5 c. 12.

powered the Asylums Board to drop the distinction between 'common' and 'direct' charges and to assess the total proportionally on the parochial authorities. The guardians were then no longer permitted to make claims on the Metropolitan Common Fund in respect of any of their contributions to the Asylum District Fund—as the M A B account was known. As to the anomalous inclusion of M A B expenditure in official returns of metropolitan pauper relief, this practice died quietly. The cumulative table of such expenditure in the Local Government Board's annual report for 1901-2 omitted M A B costs, while a footnote merely indicated that, prior to the year 1900-1, such M A B expenditure had been included.[1] In 1906—fifteen years after the M A B infectious disease hospitals had been legally divorced from the poor law—the footnote added: 'Patients treated in the smallpox, fever, etc. hospitals provided by the Managers of the Metropolitan Asylum District are to be understood as excluded from the term "paupers" and the hospitals referred to as excluded from the term "poor law institutions"'.[2] Belatedly, the changed status of the M A B hospitals for infectious diseases was thus officially, if unobtrusively, announced.

II

While accounting complexities bedevilled the collection of M A B revenue, problems of another order beset the Board's initial attempts to raise and allocate capital funds. Insufficient provision had been made in the 1867 Act for security in respect of loans for hospital building. Consequently, the Board found it impossible to negotiate for the purchase of the first five sites which had been carefully selected at Leavesden, Caterham, Hampstead, Stockwell and Homerton. The Asylums Managers urged the Poor Law Board to introduce a Bill immediately to rectify the deficiencies of the 1867 Act. Meantime, they were refused loans by the Bank of England and other bodies they approached. Eventually, the Public Works Loan Commissioners were persuaded to lend a limited amount but at an unusually high rate of interest.

In the absence of central authority action, Dr. Brewer, M A B chairman, called at the Poor Law Board, where he was informed that 'the difficulties attending the borrowing powers of the Asylums Board had been occupying the President's attention'. Weeks passed: then, in one frustrated body, the M A B finance committee descended upon Mr. Goschen, the President, and urged that a clause be inserted into the pending Metropolitan Board of Works Loans Bill to enable the Treasury to include in the monies to be borrowed by the Board of Works the sums required by the Asylums Board. After a further lapse of time, Dr. Brewer went direct to the Treasury, where he saw the Parliamentary Secretary, Mr. Ayrton, who had been an ardent supporter of Gathorne Hardy's hospital scheme. The outcome of the interview was the insertion into the Bill of a clause providing for the borrowing powers of the Metropolitan Board of Works to be extended by a sum not

[1] LGB Annual Report, 1901-2. BPP, 1902, vol. xxxv, p. lxxiii.
[2] LGB Annual Report, 1905-6. BPP, 1906, vol. xxxv, p. cxlviii.

exceeding half a million pounds. This was to be advanced by the Board of Works to the Asylums Managers, who would repay it by annual instalments with interest in sixty years. During the debates on the amended Bill, three Members of Parliament displayed outstanding energy in successfully defending the inclusion of the new clause. They were Dr. Brewer and two of his M A B colleagues, Mr. John G. Talbot and Mr. W. H. Smith, who had secured seats in the House since the creation of the Board.

Out of the £500,000 provided by the 1869 Metropolitan Board of Works Loans Act, the Asylums Board was authorized to borrow some £460,000. This loan was negotiated with the Board of Works at the rate of 3¾ per cent, which represented for the hospital authority an annual saving in interest alone of over £5,000. Thus, after two years' delay, the Asylums Managers were able to secure their first hospital sites.[1] Following the arrangement under the 1869 Act, future borrowing was secured by the Loans Act of 1870 and subsequent legislation.[2]

In 1907, the Asylums Managers adopted the policy of consolidating all outstanding loans, of which there were then over a hundred at twelve different rates of interest, and liquidating the whole by equal half-yearly payments of principal and interest. These loans, amounting to some £3 million, were all paid off by March 1922. After 1908, the M A B followed the practice of charging to current (rate) account as much capital expenditure as possible. During its last twenty-two years, over £900,000 of capital expenditure was provided for in this way.

The total sum expended by the M A B on land, buildings and equipment between 1867 and 1930 amounted to some £7·8 million. About £200,000 of this sum represented government grants towards the cost of building tuberculosis sanatoria under the National Insurance and Finance Acts of 1911.[3] Of the £6·7 million raised by loans, only £304,000 remained outstanding at the time of the transfer to the LCC. An indication of the deployment of M A B capital funds during the six decades of the Board's administration is given in Appendix IV, Tables A(I) and A(II). It will be seen that £3,620,325 (46·7 per cent) was devoted to the infectious disease hospitals; and £1,872,956 (24·1 per cent) to the mental and epileptic institutions; while £1,007,712 (13 per cent) was spent on tuberculosis sanatoria; £674,154 (8·7 per cent) on children's institutions; and £355,329 (4·6 per cent) on ambulance services. When the capital costs of all the institutions and services for infectious patients are aggregated, it will be seen that they amounted to over £5 million, representing 65 per cent of the Board's total capital outlay.

One of the most costly of the M A B establishments was the Queen Mary's Hospital for Children at Carshalton, opened in 1909. By 1930, the capital outlay on this 800-bed

---

[1] The actual sums paid by the M A B for the first hospital sites were as follows: £8,651 for 80 acres at Leavesden; £5,846 for 72 acres at Caterham; £15,544 for 8 acres at Hampstead; £11,812 for 8 acres at Homerton; and £15,075 for 7 acres at Stockwell.

[2] 33 & 34 Vict. c. 24; 38 & 39 Vict. c. 65; 39 & 40 Vict. c. 55; 40 & 41 Vict. c. 52; 41 & 42 Vict. c. 37. The M A B was eventually empowered to raise loans up to an amount not exceeding one-fifth of the rateable value of the Metropolitan Asylum District.

[3] See Chapter 19, section III.

institution, including land, buildings and equipment, had totalled £325,696. In 1895, when the Board first considered purchasing the extensive Westcroft Farm estate at Carshalton, the price for the entire site was £12,000. When it became known that the M A B was interested in the site for hospital building, the vendors raised the price to £100 per acre. Since the location proved suitable in every other way, the Board paid £13,550 for a portion of approximately 136 acres. Of the M A B mental institutions, the most expensive was the Tooting Bec Hospital, opened in 1903. By 1930, after it had been extended to accommodate 2,230 patients, inclusive capital costs totalled £629,152. By this time, the Board's country institutions had been accommodating harmless chronic patients for sixty years. During this period, £387,596 had been spent on the 2,159-bed hospital at Leavesden; £272,277 on the 2,068-bed institution at Caterham; and £392,432 on the 2,260-bed Darenth Colony.

Comparisons between capital costs at different types of hospital in different locations, however, have little meaning unless the unit—the bed—is defined. The bed in an M A B fever ward represented 156 square feet of floor space (2,028 cubic feet); in a ward for diphtheria and enteric cases, the floor space occupied by a bed was 195 square feet (2,535 cubic feet). In the largest smallpox institutions, floor space per bed was also 156 square feet (but 2,000 cubic feet), although in the smaller wooden buildings it was only 120 square feet (1,350 cubic feet). In the mental hospitals, floor space per bed averaged 62 square feet (739 cubic feet).

At the Leavesden and Caterham mental institutions, costs per bed—based on the original capital outlay during their first decade—averaged £86 and £89 respectively, while at the later and better equipped Tooting Bec institution the cost per bed averaged £328. At the Brook fever hospital (opened in 1896) and the Park fever hospital (opened in 1897), costs per bed reached £566 and £505 respectively. These later figures were comparable with capital expenditure at the 'new' St. Thomas' Hospital in Lambeth, which had cost £374,000 by the time it opened in 1871, averaging £530 per bed. This, however, contrasted markedly with bed-costs at the M A B Homerton and Stockwell isolation hospitals, which opened earlier in the same year. Capital outlay per bed in these smaller institutions averaged £281 and £339 respectively.[1]

III

Within its first decade in Lambeth, the Governors of St. Thomas' Hospital found it necessary on economic grounds to institute paying beds, a practice which was followed three years later by Guy's Hospital.[2] In 1902, the M A B first considered admitting paying patients to its isolation hospitals and mental institutions,[3] but the proposal was rejected

[1] See Appendix IV, Table B, for details of capital expenditure on the early M A B hospitals built between 1869 and 1878.
[2] E. M. McInnes, *St. Thomas' Hospital* (1963), pp. 144–45; and *The Hospital*, vol. 59, No. 8, p. 511.
[3] M A B *Mins.*, vol. xxxvi (1902), p. 606.

on this and subsequent occasions. No public complaint was ever made concerning the lack of M A B pay-beds. The Board was not pressed by economic necessity to exact direct payment for admission, since there was no statutory limit to the total amount of revenue which it might raise from the poor law districts of London, provided precepts were levied proportionally upon each.

The revenue of the M A B was thus more readily expandable than that of the endowed and voluntary hospitals. With population growth, London's ratepayers increased in number and each quinquennial rating assessment augmented the value of the property comprised in the Metropolitan Asylum District.[1] During the financial year 1870–71, when the Board's first hospitals were opened, the rateable value of the metropolis was upwards of £20 million, yielding about £83,000 from a rate of 1d in the £. During the first year of the LCC (1889), the penny rate produced nearly £130,000. Of the central rate of nearly 3s. in the £ in that year, the LCC required 1s.; education (then under the School Board), 9d.; the police, 5d.; and the M A B, 2d. The remainder was raised for the equitable distribution of local poor law burdens. In 1913, the year before the outbreak of World War I, the main items covered by the central rate of 5s. 7d. in the £ were: education, 1s. 11d., the police, 7d.; and the M A B, 5d., the remainder being allocated to special needs and the equalization of poor relief.[2]

Annual precepts levied by the M A B on the metropolitan poor law authorities in selected years are shown in Appendix IV, Table C. As will be seen, total revenue requirements for 1871 were estimated at some £130,500, which called for a rate of about 1¾d. in the £. By 1901, annual estimates had reached £852,500, requiring a rate of 5½d. in the £. The highest demand levied by the M A B was for nearly £2·9 million in 1921, when scarlet fever and diphtheria epidemics were in progress. This represented a rate of over 1s. 2d. in the £.

IV

The manner in which the Asylums Board allocated its revenue is shown in the analysis of annual expenditure at five decennial periods between 1889[3] and 1929, set out in Appendix IV, Table D. Viewing the entire scope of the Board's activities (items 1–12), it will be seen that total annual expenditure ranged from £330,000 in 1889 to nearly £2·4 million in 1929. Up to 1919, between 60 and 70 per cent of the total was devoted to its institutions for medical care, the remainder being spent on ambulance services, non-medical establishments and administration. By 1929, the Board's hospitals absorbed 85 per cent of total expenditure, the proportion for each of the four branches being: isolation hospitals, 38 per cent; mental institutions, 27 per cent; children's hospitals, 9 per cent; and tuberculosis

[1] See Appendix IV, Table C, col. 1.
[2] Sir I. G. Gibbon and R. W. Bell, *History of the LCC, 1889–1939* (1839), pp. 188–90.
[3] Expenditure during the Board's earlier years is not included in comparative tables since there was a lack of uniformity in the financial records of the various institutions during that period.

sanatoria, 11 per cent. During the Board's lifetime, very little was generally known concerning the extent of its work. Consequently, its *total* annual expenditure was often erroneously assumed to relate solely to the infectious disease hospitals, and charges of excessive spending resulted. The authors of the Minority Report of the Royal Commission on the Poor Law (1909) did not escape this misconception.[1]

Considering that part of the Board's expenditure which was devoted *exclusively to the hospitals* (Table D, items 1–5), it will be seen that in 1889, of a total of some £208,000, £66,450 (32 per cent) was absorbed by 'maintenance' costs for some 6,400 patients. Of the other heads of expenditure, the two largest were salaries and wages amounting to £43,000 (21 per cent), and daily maintenance of buildings amounting to some £57,700 (28 per cent). By 1929, patients' maintenance (£319,500) represented about 16 per cent of the annual total; salaries and wages (£789,000), 39 per cent; and daily upkeep of buildings (£369,000), 19 per cent. Expenditure on drugs and surgical appliances never exceeded 2 per cent of total hospital expenditure in any year, but this item is interesting chiefly on account of its steady absolute increase. In 1889, less than £1,200 was spent on drugs for a daily average of nearly 6,500 patients. By 1899, when the antitoxin treatment for diphtheria was in general use, the drugs bill rose steeply to nearly £6,000 (for 10,225 patients). Ten years later, it reached some £10,000 (for nearly 13,000 patients), and by 1919 it was £17,000 (for 12,000 patients). In 1929, it exceeded £37,000 (for 18,000 patients). About 58 per cent of this sum was incurred by the infectious disease hospitals, with their daily average of over 5,000 patients.

The credit items in this analysis (Table D, column 10) are not without interest. The produce of the work of mental patients, mainly the higher-grade defectives at Darenth, was either sold or consumed in the institutions and the accounts credited accordingly. By 1929, the value of work done by patients employed in the workshops and on farming, agriculture and domestic occupations exceeded £28,000.

Current expenditure, in terms of average weekly costs per patient in the M A B infectious disease hospitals and mental institutions between 1886 and 1929, is shown in Appendix IV, Table E. The wide disparity between the relatively high average cost of infectious patients and the modest cost of mental patients reflects the dissimilarities of the two types of institution—differences of location, size, bed-space, staff-patient ratio, length of patient-residence and patients' capacity to contribute their services. It will be seen that in 1886 the average weekly cost per fever patient ('maintenance' and 'common' charges) totalled 38s. 5d., while the corresponding cost per mental patient totalled 8s. 4d. a week. There was no significant movement in patient-costs during the generation preceding World War I. By 1919, however, the average weekly cost per fever patient had risen to

---

[1] The authors of the Minority Report of the 1905–9 Royal Commission on the Poor Law referred to the '3,000 to 6,000 patients in these [M A B isolation] hospitals, costing nearly £1,000,000 a year...' (BPP, 1909, vol. xxxvii [Cmd. 4499], p. 877). The actual cost of the M A B fever and smallpox hospitals in 1909 was less than £400,000, representing about 37 per cent of the £1 million of *total* M A B expenditure (See Appendix IV, Table D).

53s. 6d., reaching nearly 68s. five years later and falling to 59s. 6d. in 1929. The average weekly cost per mental patient during these post-war years remained below 25s. In the smallpox institutions, the average cost per patient fluctuated with the incidence of the disease. During the relatively mild outbreak of 1894, the total average weekly cost per patient exceeded 74s., while during the more serious epidemic years of 1902 and 1928, when overheads were distributed among a larger number of cases, patient-costs per week averaged approximately 54s. and 58s. respectively. During quiescent periods, overhead expenditure was maintained almost at epidemic level; consequently average patient-costs at these times were abnormally high. In 1889, the Local Government Board created a sensation by quoting, in an official return, a figure of nearly £2,000 as the average annual cost of a smallpox patient in the M A B hospital ships.[1] This figure, based on only five smallpox admissions during the year, brought the average cost per patient in the whole of the infectious hospitals service up to nearly £500 a year. The three fever hospitals functioning at this time were in fact each treating a daily average of 257 patients at an average annual cost of £78 per patient. Deploring the unwisdom of deriving general averages from very small numbers and very limited periods, Mr. R. M. Hensley, M A B chairman, explained that the cost of maintaining the hospital ships in constant readiness averaged £10,000 a year, which represented a metropolitan rate of only 0·077d. in the £— a modest premium for insuring London against economically crippling epidemics.[2]

A more realistic illustration of the total burden sustained by metropolitan ratepayers as a result of a large-scale smallpox epidemic is given in Appendix IV, Table F. This shows all relevant costs, including those of the Board's ambulance services, incurred in providing for the 11,060 victims of the 1884–85 outbreak, when, for the first time, M A B smallpox patients were removed out of London for treatment. As will be seen, expenditure for the two-year period totalled £257,165, resulting in an inclusive average cost of £23 5s. 0d. per patient.

V

While estimates of M A B revenue expenditure were regularly submitted to the central authority, they were rarely, if ever, questioned after the early years. Like the official regulations concerning hospital management, those issued to the Asylums Board in 1870 on accounting[3] were never revised during the ensuing sixty years, despite the eccentricity and eventual obsolescence of some of the items. Central authority sanction, for instance, was required before a porter could be given a gratuity or a copying clerk be paid more than one shilling an hour. In the main, the central authority's intervention in financial

---

[1] LGB return relating to accommodation in workhouses and infirmaries in the metropolis and in the Poplar and Stepney and Central London Sick Asylums, 1888: BPP, 1889, vol. lxxxvii, p. 741; and M A B *Mins.*, vol. xxvii (1893), p. 183.

[2] M A B *Mins.*, vol. xxvii (1893), pp. 183–85.

[3] PLB order to the M A B, 28 November 1870.

matters was limited to sanctioning the raising and allocation of M A B loan capital, and to appointing an auditor to the Asylum District.

The most powerful check on M A B expenditure of public funds was through the audit. Centrally appointed but independent district auditors were empowered—as they are still—to disallow illegal or improper expenditure on the part of local authorities, either on their own initiative or on the complaint of ratepayers, and to surcharge it upon the individual members of the offending authority.[1] Metropolitan ratepayers were accordingly invited, by a notice posted on the outer door of every London workhouse, to inspect the books of the Asylums Board before each audit and, if they wished, to prefer any objections to the Asylum District Auditor. Within one month of the audit, each board of guardians in the metropolis received an abstract of the M A B accounts.[2] Thus, was the doctrine of public accountability upheld.

The Board's internal system of control evolved with the growth of its responsibilities. In the early days, spending in each hospital was regulated and authorized solely by the institution management committee, guided by M A B standing orders, while the Board as a whole remained unaware of the detailed allocation of resources. Following the revelations of excessive spending in 1885, controls were tightened and centralized. A vigilant finance committee took every possible precaution to ensure that funds were not improperly spent. Convinced of the need to hold all the purse-strings in its own hands, the committee made it clear to the full Board that, if it desired

> ... to have security, such as in national matters is furnished by the existence of the Treasury and the Auditor-General, that none of its expenditure is extravagant and unjustifiable, the Managers must make up their minds to give to their finance committee powers not only to audit past expenditure, but to report and recommend as to proposed expenditure, and must supply that committee with the necessary staff and machinery for the purpose.[3]

The finance committee was accordingly granted full powers to decide upon the amounts to be raised for current and capital spending. It also regulated the work of the head office accounts department and the financial procedure of committees empowered to incur expenditure. Periodically, it presented estimates of expenditure to the full Board, after consultation with the central committees; otherwise it reported to the Board only on such financial matters as it deemed necessary.[4] While it was constitutionally possible for a

[1] Although appeal by a local authority from an auditor's decision lay to the central authority, the general policy of the Local Government Board prior to 1887 was in practice to relieve the members of the authority from the consequences of their illegal action in the particular instance but to warn them that such relief would not be given again. In 1887 the Local Authorities Expenses Act (50 & 51 Vict. c. 72) empowered the central authority to authorize expenditure by local bodies which otherwise would be disallowed by the auditors.

[2] 30 & 31 Vict. c. 6 ss. 33–35.

[3] M A B finance committee report to the full Board, dated 17 June 1899 (M A B *Mins.*, vol. xxxiii, p. 164).

[4] See Appendix I, Document IV (M A B committee structure) for details of the functions of the M A B finance committee and its sub-committee.

member of the Board to propose a modification of any finance committee recommend-ation, a tacit relationship developed analogous to that existing between a major local authority and its statutory finance committee.[1]

The centralization of internal control was further consolidated by the establishment of a works committee for the supervision of all matters relating to building projects, and a con-tract committee for the provision of all articles required in the Board's institutions. The works committee was responsible for obtaining tenders for all building schemes and for general supervision while construction work was in progress. The erection of a new establishment was never sanctioned by the Board until reports had been received which showed, not only the estimated cost of the projected building, but also the approximate cost and methods of working the institution. A central warehouse was established for all non-perishable goods. Located first in 1896 in Mermaid Court, Borough High Street, it was transferred in 1908 to Peckham Rye. Here an expert staff received and examined all supplies which were purchased in bulk. Drugs and food, also purchased in bulk, were delivered direct to the institutions. Of £800,000 expended on supplies during the Board's last year, £430,000 represented the cost of foodstuffs for its daily population of nearly 30,000 patients and staff. By this time (1929), substantial economies were being effected by the direct purchase of goods from manufacturers and producers, a practice which began in 1917. When, for example, a broker was employed to buy tea on the open market, the cost was reduced by £1,000 during the first year; while £3,500 a year was immediately saved on coal when contracts were first competed for by the collieries.

For the acquisition of goods not included in contracts, each item was entered in the 'requirements book' of the institution steward and ordered through the head office after it had been sanctioned by the hospital sub-committee and the group central committee. Sub-committees were discouraged from authorizing local expenditure by an M A B standing order which required that three prices should be obtained before any item costing more than £2 was purchased. Accounts for exceptional and non-recurring payments were submitted to the central committee concerned before being passed with all routine accounts to the finance committee. A list of all the accounts for payment was forwarded to each member of the Board with the agenda for each plenary meeting, and even at this stage any member might object to the payment of a bill. Finally, all the books and accounts of the hospital finance officers were subject to a running audit by travelling inspectors from the M A B accounts department. These internal procedures appear to have supplemented meticulously the merely formal statutory controls, and to have assured, after the initial experimental period, that resources were economically and efficiently directed towards providing adequate, if not lavish, institutional care and treatment for the ever-increasing sick and deprived dependants of the Asylums Board.[2]

[1] See, e.g., the London County Council (General Powers) Act, 1934, Section 20 (1).
[2] See Appendix I, Document III, for a list of the categories of persons for whom the M A B was responsible.

VI

By the time the responsibilities of the Board passed into the hands of the LCC, metropolitan ratepayers had been supporting London's public hospitals for sixty years. This financial burden had been equitably distributed throughout an extensive region embracing a wide disparity of needs and means.[1] In 1929, the scope of the common fund system was further extended and consolidated in the capital. The Local Government Act of that year placed upon the London County rate the whole cost of administering the poor law, as well as of maintaining the M A B institutions and the metropolitan infirmaries, which were brought under municipal management by the Act.[2] This, the largest measure of collective responsibility for social services which had been achieved in this country up to that time, pointed the way towards the relief of poverty and sickness on a national scale. If Gathorne Hardy could re-appraise today the mainspring of his Act, he might well claim that the common fund principle had so effectively 'stood the test of time' that it had successfully survived a century to serve this end.

[1] Following the London Government Act of 1899, the items for which rates were raised uniformly over the whole area of the County of London were: (1) county contributions for general county purposes; (2) contributions to the London School Board; (3) guardians' contributions to meet expenses chargeable upon the Metropolitan Common Poor Fund (excluding the proportion of such expenses as were chargeable upon the Common Fund of the Metropolitan Asylum District; (4) guardians' contributions to the Metropolitan Asylum District Fund in respect of M A B services (including the proportion of such expenses as were chargeable upon the Metropolitan Common Poor Fund; and (5) contributions to the Equalization Fund formed under the London (Equalization of Rates) Act, 1894. (See LGB Annual Report for 1902–3, p. 658.)

[2] See Chapter 22.

PART THREE

The MAB—1900 to 1930: Three Decades of Twentieth-Century Development

'. . . in every country as civilization advances and the public conscience is aroused, not only is public health work in its limited sense increasingly developed, but there is also a corresponding increase in communal effort towards satisfactory and complete medical care for the sick.'

Sir Arthur Newsholme, *International Studies on the Relation between the Private and Official Practice of Medicine* (1928–32).

CHAPTER 14

Mental Deficiency

THE dawn of the twentieth century launched the M A B infectious disease and mental health services into the second half of their life span. Behind them were the three pioneering decades of battles against pestilence, public hostility and obscurantist bureaucracy. The new era, marked by the marriage of science and medicine; a modified man-microbe economy; changing attitudes towards mental defect; total war; and socio-economic readjustment, made fresh demands upon the Asylums Board as new categories of dependants were committed to its care.

Arrangements for the inclusion of one new group of patients within the M A B mental health service were being completed as the century opened. The Asylums Board had been instructed by the Local Government Board in 1897 to provide for poor law children who, by reason of defective intellect, could not be trained in association with children in ordinary schools. As a group, these children were less severely handicapped than those who had been separated in the early days of the M A B from the chronic adult residents of Leavesden and Caterham and who were now being trained in the Darenth schools.

At this time, 'feeble-mindedness', as a condition distinct from 'imbecility', had only recently become a subject of medico-psychological study, although as early as 1847 the Lunacy Commissioners had cited the 'weak-minded' as one of four grades into which they divided congenital mental defectives in poor law institutions.[1] The distinction was made more explicit by Dr. P. M. Duncan, physician to the Eastern Counties' Asylum for Idiots and Imbeciles at Colchester, when he classified his patients as 'simpletons, imbeciles and idiots'. 'The first,' he wrote, 'are those feeble-minded who have not been able to receive instruction in the ordinary manner and who do not possess the experience in life peculiar to those of their age and social position. . . .'[2] Later, problems which had been brought to light by the introduction of compulsory education in the 1870s, promoted a number of studies of intelligence in school children. From these, it was evident that the concept of defect would have to be extended to include a group of children whose mental

---

[1] The Lunacy Commissioners, in their Second Report, 1847, divided the insane in workhouses into three classes: the demented, the deranged and the defectives from birth. This last group they sub-divided into four grades: 'the weak-minded, the imbeciles, the idiotic, and the idiots proper'.

[2] P. M. Duncan, *First Report of the Eastern Counties' Asylum for Idiots and Imbeciles* (1860).

capacities lay between the level of the imbecile and the normal range and who were ineducable with children of average intelligence. In 1888, a committee of the British Medical Association investigated the development and condition of brain function among children in London primary schools, and emphasized the distinction between the feeble-minded and the imbecile.[1] The following year, evidence was given by this committee before the Royal Commission on the Blind, Deaf and Dumb.[2] In 1892, the London School Board established special schools for handicapped children. The prime mover in this pioneer project was General Moberley, vice-chairman of the London School Board and a member of the Charity Organization Society, which had been actively concerned since 1876 with promoting the cause of the mentally defective.[3] In its surveys of physically and mentally handicapped children in London elementary and poor law schools, the Society had collaborated with the British Association for the Advancement of Science. In 1892, the British Association appointed a committee with terms of reference resembling those of the 1888 British Medical Association committee. Under the chairmanship of Sir Douglas Galton, a member of the Asylums Board, the British Association committee worked with a similar group appointed the year before by the International Congress on Hygiene and Demography. Of the 100,000 children studied, nearly 10,000 were in metropolitan poor law schools. Of these, 8 per cent were found to be mentally dull.[4] Provision for the education of this group became one of the main preoccupations of the departmental committee which was set up in 1894 to study the systems of maintenance and education of children in the care of the London poor law authorities. Although there was conflicting evidence on the subject, it was unanimously concluded by the departmental committee that the aggregation of backward children in large numbers would be specially harmful; and that separate arrangements should be made for their tuition.[5]

As a result, the Local Government Board instructed the M A B to provide for these children from the metropolitan poor law schools. After considering the evidence submitted to the departmental committee, the Asylums Managers adopted, as an alternative to institutional care, the system of 'scattered homes' which had been introduced by the Sheffield guardians in 1893.[6] A few ordinary dwelling houses were accordingly acquired in Pentonville, Fulham, Wandsworth and Peckham. In each of these, from twelve to twenty children were grouped according to age and sex. They resided in the homes in the care of foster-parents and were encouraged to lead as normal a life as possible. By arrangement with the London School Board, the children, who were between the ages

[1] *Brit. med. J.*, 1889, II (27 July), p. 187 *et seq.*, 'A report on investigations in fourteen schools in London'.
[2] Cmd. 5781 (1889).   [3] Kathleen Jones, *Mental Health and Social Policy, 1845–1959*, pp. 45–47.
[4] *Annual Report of the British Association for the Advancement of Science*, 1893, pp. 614–20.
[5] *Report of the Departmental Committee on Metropolitan Poor Law Schools*, 1896: BPP, 1896, vol. xliii, I [Cmd. 8027, Cmd. 8032, Cmd. 8033]. The antecedents of this committee are discussed in Chapter 18 on child care.
[6] *Poor Law Conferences*, 1895–96. Paper read by J. Wycliffe Wilson at the Yorkshire Poor Law Conference of 1895; and the paper by the Clerk to the Sheffield Board of Guardians, A. E. Booker, included in the volume *Poor Law Conferences*, 1903–4, relating to the Sheffield 'scattered homes' experiment.

of seven and sixteen, attended its special schools for the handicapped. These were within easy reach of the homes, which had been specially selected with this object in view.

The scheme worked well until the children attained school-leaving age, which was sixteen for physically and mentally handicapped children, that is, two years beyond that of their contemporaries who were more fortunately endowed.[1] As the future of the defective poor law children had not been considered by the departmental committee, and as they were still incapable at the age of sixteen of taking up ordinary occupations without supervision, the Asylums Managers suggested to the central authority that the children should remain in their care. Four years later, the Local Government Board provisionally authorized the Asylums Board to retain these adolescents up to the age of twenty-one.[2] A working colony for male patients was opened at Witham, Essex—The Bridge Training Home—and the older feeble-minded girls were sent to an institution known as High Wood School at Brentwood, Essex, built on the cottage home principle. In 1907, further temporary authority was secured by the Asylums Managers to retain these cases after the age of twenty-one, as they were still unfit for discharge.

By this time, the Board had completed the plans at Darenth for the education and occupational training of subnormal children, which had been begun and suspended some twenty years before. In addition to the schools, the Board now maintained a flourishing training colony, where higher-grade mental defectives were taught industrial skills and crafts. The original project, which had required a substantial capital outlay and the services of specialist teachers, had appeared to the Local Government Board to be too costly and ambitious. But in 1903, after modified plans had been discussed personally by the Managers with the President, the work was begun, and the colony was inaugurated in 1904. During the first year, about 400 males and 300 females were employed, some for forty-one hours a week, on a variety of occupations, including engineering, farming, plumbing and the production of every kind of requirement for the Board's institutions, from clothing to bedding and domestic equipment. The Darenth Industrial Colony—as it came to be known—eventually employed up to 1,200 patients at one time—men and women in approximately equal numbers—and produced goods and services to the value of over £10,000 a year.[3]

The hesitation of the Local Government Board to give more than temporary authorization for the retention of the feeble-minded children, and the lack of whole-hearted support for the Darenth training colony, were related to the prospect of a full-scale investigation of the care of the feeble-minded. The extent of subnormality among school children, which the independent enquiries had revealed, had aroused public concern. This had grown into alarm with the advance of genetic studies, the development of intelligence

[1] The Elementary Education Act of 1876 declared that it was the duty of the parents of every child between five and fourteen to cause such child to receive efficient elementary education in reading, writing and arithmetic. The Elementary Education (Blind and Deaf Children) Act of 1893 raised the school-leaving age of handicapped children to sixteen years.

[2] LGB letter to the M A B, 7 November 1905.

[3] M A B Annual Report for 1929–30, p. 71 (col. 20).

testing, and the publication, mainly in America, of family studies which associated the effects of a morbid inheritance with social deterioration.[1] As a result of public pressure, a Royal Commission to examine the care and control of the feeble-minded was appointed in 1904; the Earl of Radnor was its chairman during the greater part of its existence. In the course of its report, issued in 1908, the Commission commended the M A B colony at Darenth, together with the older charitable institutions and the more recently founded voluntary colony at Sandlebridge, Cheshire, which, like Darenth, represented a 'complete experiment for providing permanently for the feeble-minded'.[2] The Commission advocated the education of feeble-minded children from an early age in colonies of the Darenth and Sandlebridge type in preference to 'scattered homes'. 'The special school or class', the Commission declared, 'is to be regarded rather as incidental to a general organization of industrial or institutional training than as of main or ultimate importance in itself.'[3] This was completely at variance with the views of the departmental committees which a decade before had studied defective children in elementary schools throughout the country[4] and in poor law schools in the metropolis.[5] As a result of the Royal Commission's disapproval of small-group training, the Asylums Managers disposed of their foster-parent London homes. The higher-grade feeble-minded adolescents were transferred to the Darenth colony, while the remaining occupants of the 'scattered homes' were integrated into the children's institution at Darenth. Final authorization to retain these young feeble-minded patients indefinitely was received by the Board in 1911.[6]

A few years later, the Asylums Managers undertook to receive epileptic children, and in 1917 they were empowered to provide for both juvenile and adult epileptics admitted through poor law channels.[7] A colony was established at Edmonton for some 300 male patients, and a similar number of female epileptics was accommodated at a home at Brentwood, by arrangement with the Hackney Board of Guardians.

Meantime, a further attempt had been made to classify the younger patients. In 1911, the Fountain Hospital at Tooting was detached from the isolation hospitals service and allocated for the use of the lowest grade of severely subnormal children. At this time, the tower age-limit of children admissible into the Board's institutions was five years, despite the efforts of the Asylums Managers to lower it to three. As late as 1903, the Local Government Board had insisted that it was not prepared to depart from the view it had held hitherto that children under five should be retained in the workhouse, although it was

[1] Kathleen Jones, op. cit., pp. 49–50.
[2] The Sandlebridge Colony later became known as the Mary Dendy Homes. Miss Dendy of Manchester had founded the institution early in the century. (See C. P. Lapage, *Feeble-Mindedness in Children of School Age* (1920), Appendix by Mary Dendy (1855–1933)).
[3] *Report of the Royal Commission on the Care and Control of the Feeble-Minded*, 1908: BPP, vol. xxxix, 1908, 159 [Cmd. 4202].
[4] *Report of the Departmental Committee on Defective and Epileptic Children*, 1898: BPP, vol. xxvi, 1898 [Cmd. 8746].
[5] *Report of the Departmental Committee on Metropolitan Poor Law Schools*, 1896, op. cit.
[6] M A B (Mentally Defective Persons) Order, 29 December 1911.
[7] M A B (Epileptics) Order, 26 March 1917.

aware that 'the detention of imbecile children under five years old in workhouses might be a source of inconvenience'.[1] The Asylums Managers were concerned with the effect on the young child of the workhouse environment and lack of systematic training. The results obtained at the Fountain Hospital—the only institution in the country at this time devoted exclusively to the training of severely subnormal children—had convinced the Asylums Managers that, the younger the patients were when first received, the greater were the chances of improvement. Eventually, they were able to persuade the central authority to lower the admission age to three years. After a period of progress in teaching these severely handicapped children to feed and dress themselves, a school was started in 1917 where very simple instruction in play and handwork was given by teacher-nurses. Suitable children's nurses were recruited and trained under the supervision of qualified sisters. Some of the Fountain children even graduated to industrial training at the higher-grade Darenth institution.

While the needs of the young subnormal patients had been provided for in educational establishments and training colonies, the bed-ridden and infirm had not been left to languish in the country institutions where they were originally accommodated. An 'infirmary for imbeciles' had been erected on the land at Tooting Bec which the Board had acquired at the end of the nineteenth century. This was opened in 1903. It was intended to bring in about a thousand patients from Caterham and Leavesden, so that the sick and elderly could be within easier reach of their relatives. The experiment was also based on practical considerations. It was found that the increasing number of infirm patients in the existing establishments interfered with their economical administration. The original plan was suspended, however, as the M A B was called upon to accommodate patients displaced from the County Asylum at Colney Hatch by a disastrous fire in February 1903. Eventually, Tooting Bec was freed for its original use as an infirmary. It also served as a children's receiving home. Later, it became a hospital exclusively for senile dements, and was eventually extended to accommodate two thousand residents. Between 400 and 600 patients over seventy years of age were admitted annually. All had to be certified under the Lunacy Acts in order to qualify for the institutional care they required. Thus, patients had to be stigmatized as 'lunatics' when suffering only from mental weakness due to infirmity of age. The Asylums Managers appealed to the Local Government Board for the abolition of certification in these cases. Finally, in August 1924, the Minister of Health, Mr. Neville Chamberlain, responded to the Board's twenty-year-old plea, and authorized the Asylums Managers to admit without certification rate-aided Londoners over the age of seventy who had not been certified previously and who required institutional care or treatment solely by reason of mental infirmity due to advancing years.[2]

By this time, the needs of the mentally defective, as distinct from the mentally ill, were being recognized by public opinion and provided for by legislation. The Mental Deficiency Act of 1913 had reached the Statute Book after a protracted struggle. While

[1] LGB letter to the M A B, 11 November 1903, and M A B *Mins.*, vol. xxxvii, 1903, p. 716
[2] Ministry of Health order to the M A B, 20 August 1924.

the Royal Commission on the Feeble-Minded (1904–8) had been deliberating, the Vice-Regal Commission on Poor Law Reform in Ireland (1902–6) and the United Kingdom Royal Commission on the Poor Law (1905–9) also had been considering the care of the mentally defective. All were agreed that the presence of such handicapped people in poor law institutions should be discontinued. The Church and the medical profession supported the agitation for legislative reform sponsored by the Eugenics Education Society and the National Association for the Care of the Feeble-Minded.[1] The main purpose of the 1913 Mental Deficiency Act was to ensure systematic provision for the mentally deficient under the major local authorities, the existing lunacy units.[2] The mentally defective described in the Act as 'subject to be dealt with' comprised four categories: idiots, imbeciles, the feeble-minded, and moral defectives.[3] For nearly half a century before the passing of the 1913 Act, the Asylums Board had been responsible for patients who would have fallen within the first three of these grades, and there was no immediate change in the Board's policy.

In May 1914, however, the LCC, as the mental deficiency authority for London, requested the Asylums Board to provide accommodation for LCC patients under the Act. With the outbreak of World War I, and demands for military and other accommodation, the Board reluctantly declined to enter into an agreement. Two years later, however, the decreased demand for mental hospital beds, which had been noted generally all over the country, became manifest in London.[4] During the war years, there was a steady decline in the total numbers on the registers of the M A B mental institutions. Admissions, which did not diminish significantly, ranged from 900 to 1,400 a year, but more patients were being discharged relative to earlier years, most of them in the 'not improved' category. There was also a rise in death rate, mainly as a result of tuberculosis and influenza. In the absence of any scientific study of the cause of the reduced demand for mental hospital accommodation at this time, it is only possible to suppose that it was associated in some way with wartime conditions, as, for example, the greater opportunities for employing the subnormal and the resulting willingness of relatives to accord them 'community care'. At the instance of the Board of Control[5] and the LCC, negotiations were resumed, and it was arranged that five of the M A B institutions should be certified for the treatment of cases under the 1913 Act, and that the group should be known as the 'M A B Certified

---

[1] The National Association for the Care of the Feeble-Minded, inaugurated in 1896, was a development of the movement which aimed to promote the proposals of the Charity Organization Society for government intervention concerning provision for 'improvable idiots'. The influence of the Association was due largely to the work of Miss Mary Dendy and Mrs. Hume Pinsent. (Kathleen Jones, op. cit., p. 48).

[2] 3 & 4 Geo. 5 c. 28 ss. 27–33.   [3] 3 & 4 Geo. 5 c. 28 s. 1.

[4] The diminution in the demand for mental hospital beds, noted during the First World War, recurred during the Second World War.

[5] The Mental Deficiency Act, 1913, established a Board of Control, consisting of 15 commissioners, including at least 5 lawyers and 4 medical practitioners of 5 years' standing, to be responsible for mental deficiency and lunacy. In 1948, many of their duties were transferred to the Minister of Health, those remaining with them being connected mainly with the preservation of the liberty of the subject. The Board was dissolved under the Mental Health Act, 1959.

Institution'. The Darenth Training Colony and the Bridge Training Home were to receive improvable juveniles; Leavesden and Caterham hospitals, unimprovable adults from sixteen years; and the Fountain Hospital, 'idiot' children.

The M A B, concerned that its normal work should not be jeopardized by its new responsibilities, reserved the absolute right to accept or reject LCC patients and to transfer them within the 'Certified Institution' without consulting the Board of Control. The Asylums Managers also insisted that Mental Deficiency Act cases should be treated in precisely the same way as poor law cases received under the Lunacy Acts. The first 1913 Act patients were admitted in 1918. It was then agreed that, for a period of five years, up to 500 cases might be accommodated by the Asylums Board from the LCC area and from the Home Counties, with possibly a few from the provinces. The five-year arrangement was renewed in 1923, by which time the Board was providing for nearly 2,000 subnormal patients under the 1913 Act, and again in 1928, when this category totalled nearly 2,500. M A B poor law patients now numbered about 6,500.[1]

Hitherto, the Board had always declined to admit patients suffering from permanent mental defect coupled with strong vicious or criminal propensities, and it refused to accept moral defectives[2] under the 1913 Act. During the middle 1920s, however, the Board's policy in this connexion was modified to some extent. About this time, there came into prominence an epidemic disease of the central nervous system known as encephalitis lethargica, or 'sleepy sickness'. In 1924, when the incidence of the disease had reached its peak, applications were made to the M A B by hospital almoners and boards of guardians for the admission of children suffering from its after-effects. The Board sought, and obtained, the consent of the Ministry of Health for the admission of a selected group of 125 children in whom the disease had been followed by behavioural deterioration. The 1913 Act provided only for patients whose deficiency had existed from birth or an early age, but this limitation was remedied by the Mental Deficiency (Amendment) Act of 1927, which defined 'mental defectiveness' as 'a condition of arrested or incomplete development of mind existing before the age of eighteen years, whether arising from inherent causes or induced by disease or injury.'[3] This regularized the acceptance of the post-encephalitis lethargica patients, who were accommodated in a special unit in the M A B Northern Hospital at Winchmore Hill. As some of these patients were certified under the Lunacy Acts, some under the Mental Deficiency Acts and others not at all, this group cut right across the Board's general classification of admissible categories.

Apart from the post-encephalitis lethargica cases, the population of the M A B mental hospitals could be classified broadly as follows. The *certified* comprised, first, those admitted under the Lunacy Acts—the chronic harmless cases of all forms of insanity and certain congenital cases described as 'idiots' and 'imbeciles'; and secondly, those admitted under

[1] Appendix III, Table D.
[2] 'Moral imbecile', the term used in the 1913 Mental Deficiency Act, was changed to 'moral defective' by the 1927 Mental Deficiency (Amendment) Act.
[3] 17 & 18 Geo. 5 c. 33 s. 1 (2).

the Mental Deficiency Acts—'idiots', 'imbeciles' and feeble-minded persons. The *uncertified* groups were: first, the sane epileptics; secondly, feeble-minded schoolchildren and others under 21 years when admitted; and thirdly, the mentally infirm 'over-seventies' who had not been certified previously.

During the Board's earlier years, no statistical distinction was made between congenital mental deficiency and other forms of mental disorder. The first available record of M A B cases classified according to mental disorder relates to patients resident at the end of 1889. At this time, all were certified under the Lunacy Acts. This classification (see Appendix III, Table G (a)) shows that, of a total of some 5,000 cases, roughly 48 per cent (about 2,400) were classified as demented; and 44 per cent (some 2,200) as 'idiots', 'imbeciles' and 'of weak mind'; while the remainder were regarded as suffering from mania, melancholia or general paresis. The figures for 1929 (ibid., Table G (b)) record that about 2,700 of the 4,400 Lunacy Acts patients then in the care of the M A B were suffering from congenital or infantile mental deficiency, and about 1,700 from mental disorder acquired later in life. Of these, roughly 81 per cent (about 1,400) were classified as dements (primary, secondary and senile), while the remainder suffered from various specialized forms of insanity.[1] Although about 4 per cent of all patients admitted during the Board's first thirty years (1870–1900) were discharged as 'recovered', by the end of the second thirty years, when the distribution of patients between the County mental hospitals and the Board's institutions was somewhat less faulty, the prospect of complete recovery was deemed to be unfavourable in all cases.

Where two local authorities in the same region were responsible for the institutional care of the mentally disordered, it was almost inevitable that there should be some overlapping. While the M A B managed institutions for imbeciles and the feeble-minded, the LCC controlled asylums for 'lunatics', each body having an asylum committee with a complete set of administrative machinery. When giving evidence before the 1905–9 Poor Law Commission, Mr. Duncombe Mann, Clerk to the M A B, explained that the line between the two classes was not precise and definite. The M A B, he affirmed, had admitted every case for which application had been made, but the LCC constantly alleged that the Council was providing for many cases which should properly be the responsibility of the Board. In his opinion, the distribution of mental cases depended very much upon the application of those who set the machinery in motion. It was partly a medical question and partly an administrative one. With the existing dichotomy, he did not think any amount of administrative genius would provide a scientific division between the inmates of a 'lunatic asylum' and the inmates of an 'imbecile asylum'.[2] When the Chairman of the M A B, Mr. Augustus Scovell, was asked whether he thought

---

[1] Classification was on the basis of the Board of Control's official scheme, which was very imprecise and generally admitted to be out of date; for instance, patients suffering from schizophrenia might be registered as suffering from 'primary dementia', 'mania' or 'imbecility'.

[2] Royal Commission on the Poor Law, Minutes of Evidence: BPP vol. xi, 1909, Q.24155, paras. 93–95, p. 344.

the care of chronic imbeciles should be handed over to the lunacy authority, he asserted that it would be better for both chronic and acute cases if they could be given the undivided attention of one authority, preferably an *ad hoc* body.[1]

While the earliest residents of the M A B 'imbecile asylums' were mainly from the habitually destitute class, patients who had not had recourse previously to poor relief were later admitted in increasing numbers. Records of admissions, classified according to employment on entry, ceased to be included in annual reports after 1909. Up to that time, the occupation of at least 50 per cent of patients received each year was entered as 'none' or 'not known'. Of those whose last occupation was ascertainable, however, about 75 per cent were unskilled labourers, casual workers and domestic servants, while about 20 per cent were of the artisan class. 'White-collar' workers were regularly received, but they rarely exceeded 5 per cent of the 'ascertainable' group in any year. Occasionally, a clergyman, doctor, or other professional worker, was admitted, but their numbers were statistically negligible.[2] The range of occupations represented continued to widen throughout the period in which they were recorded; but no legislative change in the status of the M A B mental health service resulted from the extended scope of admissions, as in the case of the infectious disease hospitals. Before 1913, no alternative provision existed outside the poor law for mentally subnormal patients whose relatives could not, or would not, pay for care in private or charitable institutions.

Except for local authority cases received under the Mental Deficiency Acts, M A B mental patients were maintained from the poor rates. By 1929, patient-costs averaged 22s. 1d. per week, compared with 8s. 8d. forty years earlier. Of these sums, 5s. 11d. was spent on 'maintenance' in 1929, and 3s. 9½d. in 1889.[3] The dietary scale set out in Appendix III, Table D, indicates how the greater part of this money was spent.[4]

During the six decades of the Board's administration, the 'imbecile asylums' admitted some 46,000 Lunacy Acts cases.[5] Following World War I, about 10,000 other cases were received. Approximately half of these were certified under the Mental Deficiency Acts, while most of the remainder fell into the three uncertified groups—feeble-minded children, sane epileptics and senile dements.[6] By the end of 1929, the M A B mental health service, with a total of 9,742 beds—including 355 for epileptics—was providing for patients of

---

[1] Ibid., QQ., 24733–39, p. 366.

[2] Incomplete data during a limited period, and the fact that a patient's last occupation was not always indicative of his habitual calling, makes it impossible to offer more than a very broad outline of the occupational structure of the M A B mentally disordered population.

[3] See Appendix III, Table E, and Appendix IV, Table E.

[4] The dietary of M A B mental patients was originally prescribed by the LGB in its 1875 regulations which, however, empowered medical superintendents to modify diet in special cases. This latitude led to such a lack of uniformity in the various units that in 1887 a special M A B committee was set up to formulate a revised dietary on the advice of the senior medical staff. Central authority approval was obtained the following year (LGB letter, 31 March 1888). No later communication on the subject can be traced. It is possible that this diet was improved by the M A B without further reference to the central authority.

[5] For statistical details of these admissions, see Appendix III, Tables A and C.

[6] For statistical details of these admissions, see Appendix III, Table D.

all ages from three years upwards. The Fountain Hospital (670 beds) admitted unimprovable boys up to nine years and girls up to sixteen, together with a few adult females as working patients. Caterham Hospital (2,068 beds),[1] devoted primarily to physically healthy adults of both sexes, received untrainable boys over nine years as they left the Fountain Hospital, as well as other children of unimprovable type and semi-educable cases not up to the standard required at the Darenth Training Colony (2,260 beds).[2] This institution provided facilities for educable children and working patients, whether certified or not. Leavesden Hospital (2,159 beds) was in the nature of an infirmary accommodating adults of both sexes suffering from chronic infirmity not principally due to old age, while the elderly uncertified cases were cared for at the Tooting Bec Hospital (2,230 beds).

Despite obstacles and obscurantism, the M A B unhesitatingly sought means to replace the old practice of undifferentiated custodial segregation by treatment designed to salvage and develop such potentialities as its mental patients might possess. The younger and more malleable minds were separated from the chronic and incurable; children were classified and instructed according to their educability, even the most deeply defective being trained to the extent of their capacity; the young feeble-minded were spared from institutional life by foster-parent care in small homes; higher-grade defectives were trained and given sheltered employment; while the senile were rescued from isolation and certification.

For nearly half a century, the M A B led the way as the only public authority in the country providing specialized institutional care for the mentally defective, as distinct from the mentally ill.[3] But pauperization continued to be the price of admission, despite the advances made in the socio-medical approach to mental deficiency following World War I. Apart from the Metropolitan Poor Act of 1867 and the Local Government Act of 1929, which brought mental and other hospitals together under local authority management, public health and welfare legislation differentiated mental illness and mental defectiveness from the general concept of ill-health until the National Health Service Act of 1946 integrated mental health into the national scheme.[4] By this time, the M A B institutions had been functioning for upward of two decades as part of the LCC mental health service.[5]

[1] Caterham Hospital was later re-named St. Lawrence's Hospital.
[2] Darenth Training Colony was later re-named Darenth Park Hospital.
[3] In 1897, the Chorlton and Manchester poor law unions provided a workhouse for the reception of imbecile paupers. This was the only other public institution in the country which was devoted exclusively to the care of such patients before 1913, apart from the M A B institutions. This was a voluntary arrangement on the part of the unions and not the result of statutory direction.
[4] 9 & 10 Geo. 6 c. 81, Part V.
[5] The transfer of the M A B services to the LCC is described in Chapter 22 following.

CHAPTER 15

Epidemic Diseases

I

By the end of the nineteenth century, the M A B fever and smallpox hospitals had earned a unique reputation, both at home and abroad. It was not unfitting, therefore, that this country should be invited to send a contribution to the 1900 International Exhibition in Paris, which would show to the world something of England's State services for infectious patients. Models of M A B isolation establishments, ambulances and hospital ships[1] were accordingly commissioned by the Asylums Board and eventually displayed in the Social Science Section of the Exhibition, accompanied by explanatory literature. Revealing the national flair for fusing ostensibly unblendable elements into a working unity, the M A B brochure depicted a *de jure* poor law system functioning as a *de facto* public health service, administered by elected and nominated managers, financed from local poor rates, and controlled by the central government. In retrospect, the international publicity accorded at this time to England's first State hospitals may be regarded as symbolic of the progress of English State medicine. From an age in which public health controls had grown out of an ever-present fear of pestilence, it was emerging into an epoch in which welfare legislation came to be framed increasingly on preventive lines, with special reference to the individual in his social setting.

For the M A B infectious disease hospitals, the period 1900 to 1930 was marked by two important trends: first, the new emphasis which the State was placing on the health of the individual, especially of mothers and children; and secondly, the changing pattern of infectious disease. The new science of bacteriology was bringing greater precision to measures of control; but, while the old 'crowd' diseases were being overcome, other forms of infection were replacing them. Further, the concept of isolation was acquiring a new meaning, as old theories of infection were being rejected. It became recognized that most of the epidemic diseases assumed more than one form, and also that different diseases required varying types and degrees of isolation. Formerly, the rationale of isolation had related primarily to the protection of the community. Now, it equally emphasized therapeutics for the benefit of the individual. Out of preventive measures, new concepts of 'positive health' were born.

---

[1] Models of the hospital ship *Castalia*, the hospital pier at Long Reach, the Brook Hospital and a horse-drawn ambulance are at present in the possession of the Greater London Council at County Hall.

Of the diseases originally admitted to the M A B hospitals, typhus occurred very exceptionally after the turn of the century; smallpox in its virulent form faded from the scene after a final flare-up in 1901–2; scarlet fever, though still prevalent, became less fatal; the death rate of enteric fever, which had remained constant from about 1885, began to fall after 1900; while the steady decline in the death rate of diphtheria, following the introduction of antitoxin, was generally maintained. With periodic ebb and flow, this downward trend in the mortality curves of the old pestilential diseases continued until, by the middle of the century, they had virtually disappeared from this country and, to a lesser extent, from Europe generally.[1] The prelude to this dramatic improvement is illustrated, with reference to London, by Graphs A and B (Appendix II), which show the incidence and case mortality rates of the principal diseases treated in the Board's hospitals during their last seventeen years (1913–29).[2]

A comparison of Tables D and E (Appendix II) will show the increasing use made by scarlet fever and diphtheria patients of the M A B isolation hospitals after they became generally accepted as public health institutions. Between 1900 and 1929, upward of 400,000 scarlet fever cases were treated, compared with 162,000 during the previous three decades. Even in relatively normal years after 1900, annual admissions of scarlet fever rarely fell below 10,000, while three times this number would be treated in the course of an epidemic year. By 1929, scarlet fever and diphtheria admissions to the M A B fever hospitals represented 93 per cent of the total number of cases of these diseases notified in the London area.

II

The first serious encounter with disease which the M A B experienced in the twentieth century was the 1901–2 smallpox epidemic. This had been anticipated by the Board's medical staff, as the metropolitan community had been relatively free from smallpox since

[1] A. H. Gale, op. cit., pp. 140–43 and passim; and WHO, *Epidemiological and Vital Statistics Report*, 4 (1951), p. 71 (scarlet fever); p. 53 (typhoid fever); and p. 108 (diphtheria).

[2] The principal trends emerging from Graphs A & B (Appendix II) of the incidence and mortality of scarlet fever, diphtheria and enteric fever in London during the period 1913–29 (extracted from M A B Annual Report for 1929–30) may be summarized as follows:

Scarlet fever: Incidence between 3 and 4 cases per thousand of the population of London for most of the period, with epidemic peaks at about 7-yearly intervals, compared with an incidence rate of 5 per thousand during the decennium 1890–99 (the first decade of compulsory notification). Annual case mortality rates remained at 1 per cent or less for most of the period, compared with 5 per cent, the annual average for the period 1890–99. General trends: steadily becoming less prevalent and far less lethal.

Diphtheria: Incidence well below 3 per thousand for most of the period, except during 2 major epidemic periods—1921–22 and 1928–29. Annual case mortality rates fell steadily after 1919 from 8 per cent to below 3 per cent in 1929. During the terminal decade of the nineteenth century the case mortality rate for diphtheria was sometimes as high as 24 per cent. General trends: an increase in prevalence but a steady diminution in mortality.

Enteric fever: Apart from epidemic peaks, case mortality rates showed a steady decline but remained relatively high, i.e. above 11 per cent for most of the period, compared with an average annual case mortality rate of 17 per cent for the period 1890–99.

the 1893–95 outbreak. The five-year battle with the Local Government Board concerning the size of the projected Joyce Green Hospital came to an end only when the epidemic had firmly established itself in London in 1901. It was then too late for the institution to be of immediate use, and temporary structures—the 'Long Reach' and the 'Orchard' hospitals—had to be erected on the riverside nearby at Long Reach. The outbreak continued throughout 1901 and 1902 and gradually died out during the next two years. Graph C (Appendix II) illustrates the course of the epidemic week by week during its worst year, 1902, when the M A B smallpox hospitals treated nearly 8,000 patients, of whom some 1,300 died.

This outbreak, which cost London ratepayers about £500,000, proved to be the last occasion on which the capital experienced a large-scale visitation of smallpox in its virulent form. When the epidemic had died down, steps were taken to reorganize the smallpox establishments. The 986-bed Joyce Green Hospital was opened at the end of 1903, and in 1904 the hospital ships, which had accommodated approximately 20,000 patients during their twenty years' service, were disposed of. The 2,000 beds in the Joyce Green, Long Reach and Orchard hospitals were then considered adequate accommodation for smallpox. After 1910, only the Long Reach Hospital was held permanently in reserve for this purpose. It had become apparent that months of high incidence of smallpox were generally those of low incidence of scarlet fever, and *vice versa*, so that the riverside institutions could be used for either disease as required.

III

With smallpox on the wane, the Asylums Board turned its attention once again to London children suffering from measles and whooping-cough. Since the early years of the nineteenth century, these two diseases had replaced smallpox as killers of young children. In London, epidemics of measles had been occurring with almost biennial regularity,[1] but no provision existed for the institutional treatment of measles or of whooping-cough because it was felt that, as they were so highly infectious in their early stages before diagnosis, isolation was less likely to affect their prevalence than was the case in the notifiable diseases. In 1910, however, the M A B 'medical officer for general purposes', Dr. H. E. Cuff, studied the problem and urged that measles and whooping-cough had strong claims to hospital treatment on curative and social grounds, if not as a preventive measure. Their mortality was high, and their sequelae were more serious to the patient's future efficiency than, for instance, were those associated with scarlet fever.[2] In 1888, the Local Government Board had ignored the offer of the M A B to receive cases of measles, but by 1910 the chances of obtaining legal sanction for the admission of measles and

---

[1] Table 6 (b), Chapter 10, shows the number of deaths in London from measles and whooping-cough between 1881 and 1900. See also A. H. Gale, op. cit., Chapter 9, passim.

[2] Memorandum by Dr. H. E. Cuff, 5 July 1910 (Medical Supplement to M A B Annual Report, 1910, pp. 279–82).

whooping-cough appeared to the Asylums Managers to be more favourable than ever before.

During the first decade of the twentieth century, concern for child welfare had been aroused by an accumulation of evidence which pointed to the need for urgent action to reduce infant mortality and to improve conditions for those who survived. By 1901, the rate of infant mortality in England and Wales—about 150 deaths per thousand live births—had remained almost constant since the beginning of death registration (1838). Charles Booth's London studies (1889–97) had already exposed the effects of poor social conditions on schoolchildren's capacity to learn.[1] The poor physique of recruits for the South African War (1899–1902) had led, in 1904, to the investigations of the Inter-Departmental Committee on Physical Deterioration.[2] In 1905, the Committee on Medical Inspection and Feeding had confirmed the need for safeguarding the health of the schoolchild, and its recommendations had led to the setting up of a medical service for all elementary schools in the country,[3] and to the provision of meals for needy schoolchildren.[4] At the Local Government Board, Sir Arthur Newsholme, principal medical officer, had been concentrating since his appointment in 1908 on research into child mortality with a view to improving child health services.[5]

In this more auspicious climate, the Asylums Managers proposed to the Local Government Board that measles and whooping-cough should be treated in the M A B hospitals. They proposed to make beds available by reducing the length of stay in the acute fever hospitals,[6] now that vacant smallpox accommodation was free for convalescent fever cases. In July 1910, the Local Government Board offered to consider the suggestion. The legal aspect of admitting non-pauper cases of measles and whooping-cough preoccupied the Department until the end of the year. Meantime, in advance of statutory sanction, the Asylums Managers ordered the admission into the fever hospitals of poor law children suffering from these diseases. Their action was legalized by a Local Government Board order in February 1911,[7] by which time more than three hundred cases of measles and about one hundred cases of whooping-cough had been treated. Three months later, the central authority found it possible, by invoking the Public Health (London) Act of 1891,

---

[1] Charles Booth, *Life and Labour of the People in London* (3rd edn. 1902–3).

[2] *Report of the Inter-Departmental Committee on Physical Deterioration*, 1904, Cmd. 2176.

[3] Education (Administrative Provisions) Act, 1907.

[4] Education (Provision of Meals) Act, 1906.

[5] The results of Sir Arthur Newsholme's investigations concerning infant mortality during the years 1911–14 are recorded in *Reports of the Medical Officer of the LGB*: Cmd. 5263, 1910; Cmd. 6909, 1911; Cmd. 7511, 1914; Cmd. 8085, 1915; and Cmd. 8496, 1917; and commented upon in Chapter XVIII of Sir A. Newsholme's *The Last Thirty Years in Public Health* (1936).

[6] The average length of stay of scarlet fever patients in the M A B hospitals for the three years 1907–10 was nine weeks. At other large fever hospitals in England and Scotland at this time the length of stay was reported to be as follows: Leeds City Hospital, 63 days; Liverpool City Hospital, 7–8 weeks; Ruchill Hospital, Glasgow, 54·4 days; Edinburgh City Hospital, 48·6 days; Monsell Fever Hospital, 56 days. (Medical Supplement to M A B Annual Report, 1910, p. 279.)

[7] LGB order to the M A B, 18 February 1911.

to authorize the admission of non-pauper cases of both diseases.[1] Already, for the past seven or eight years, infants suffering from measles and whooping-cough, as well as their mothers, had been received by the municipal hospitals of Liverpool.[2]

During the next two decades, 45,000 cases of measles and 17,000 cases of whooping cough were admitted to the M A B institutions. Annual fatality rates in respect of both diseases ranged between 7 and 15 per cent. By comparison, the case fatality rate of scarlet fever patients during this period never exceeded 2 per cent and remained below 1 per cent after the mid-1920s.[3] While the death rate of measles declined, it seemed that its incidence remained relatively high. By the mid-1920s, it was known from education authority reports (these diseases were not generally notifiable until 1940) that during the recurrent seasonal high prevalence of measles, the number of cases amongst children attending LCC schools was about 30,000, and it was assumed that a similar number of children under school age would also have been affected. The Asylums Managers therefore arranged that, in times of pressure, the local Medical Officers of Health should select patients for admission to the M A B hospitals by reference to home conditions. Once admitted, most of the children remained for twelve or thirteen weeks.[4] A particular feature of measles mortality was its association with poverty. The rate of death from measles of children aged one in the Registrar-General's social class V was nearly twenty times that of children of the same age in class I.[5] In addition to its preventive and curative functions, therefore, the M A B hospital service for infectious diseases was contributing to the growing movement which aimed to eliminate by social action and technical medicine existing detriments to national health.

IV

Another field of infection in which the M A B hospitals were called upon to serve a socio-medical role was that of venereal diseases. New knowledge relating to aetiology and treatment,[6] and the findings concerning the effects of these diseases of both the 1904 Committee on Physical Deterioration and the 1905–9 Poor Law Commission, led the medical profession to press for an official investigation into their prevalence and methods of control. In November 1913, a Royal Commission was appointed, and in March 1916 its report was published.[7] Chief among the Commission's recommendations were that treatment of

[1] 54 & 55 Vict. c. 76 s. 80; LGB order to the M A B, 30 May 1911.

[2] S. and B. Webb, *The Break-Up of the Poor Law* (1909), p. 267.

[3] See Appendix II, Table E.

[4] See Appendix II, Table K, for length of stay of patients suffering from the infectious diseases treated in the M A B hospitals.

[5] Registrar-General's Decennial Supplement, 1931, p. 167.

[6] The gonococcus was discovered by Albert Neisser in 1879, and the spirochaete by Schaudinn and Hoffman in 1905. The Wassermann reaction for syphilis was introduced in 1906, and Ehrlich discovered salvarsan, a potent remedy against syphilis, in 1909. In 1913, Noguchi recognized the connexion between tabes dorsalis and general paralysis of the insane.

[7] *Report of the Royal Commission on Venereal Diseases*, 1916 (Cmd. 8189).

venereal disease should be readily available to the whole community; that the organization of the means of treatment should be in the hands of the county and county borough councils; that institutional treatment should, as far as possible, be provided at general hospitals by negotiation between them and the local authorities; and that this treatment should be free to all, subject to a Treasury grant of 75 per cent of the cost.

As this study has revealed a number of occasions on which the Local Government Board identified itself with Dickens' 'Circumlocution Office',[1] in fairness it should be noted that in this instance the recommendations of the Royal Commission on Venereal Diseases were implemented with unparalleled celerity. On a certain Friday morning when it was known that Mr. (later Lord) Long, then President of the Local Government Board, was about to leave London for the weekend, Sir Arthur Newsholme sent a summary of the Commission's recommendations urgently to his chief, with an intimation that proposals for immediate action would be following on the Monday. He received a red 'chit' with the instruction: 'Put forward your recommendations at once'. A major hurdle was to persuade the Treasury to contribute 75 per cent of the cost of treatment. Mr. Long thought that the entire cost should be paid from Exchequer funds, but was persuaded to adhere to the proposed 75 per cent. He walked over to the Treasury the same day, discussed the matter with the Rt. Hon. Reginald McKenna, Chancellor of the Exchequer, and returned with his sanction to the proposed expenditure.[2] Mandatory regulations were issued immediately to major local authorities requiring them to establish services for free diagnosis and treatment on the lines of the Commission's proposals.[3] Urgency arising from war conditions had expedited the launching of what was, in effect, the first gratuitous provision in this country of medical care on a national scale, mainly at the expense of the Exchequer.

As part of the prevention drive, the Asylums Board was instructed in September 1916 to provide special accommodation for the treatment of parturient women suffering from venereal disease in cases in which treatment could not be provided in the ordinary lying-in wards of metropolitan poor law institutions.[4] The Asylums Managers thereupon contracted with the City of London guardians to receive such cases into their Thavies Inn infirmary in Holborn. In 1919, the Board was asked to extend this provision to non-pregnant women,[5] and a small institution was acquired for this purpose in Sheffield Street, Kingsway.

---

[1] Charles Dickens, *Little Dorrit* (1857), Chapter X.   [2] Sir A. Newsholme, op. cit., p. 157.

[3] Public Health (Venereal Diseases) Regulations, July 1916. The important principles underlying the regulations were prevention of spread of the disease, provision of bacteriological aids to diagnosis and organization of treatment in such a way that no patient should be deterred from seeking it. London co-operated with the adjoining counties, Greater London being treated as one unit. The LCC negotiated with the voluntary hospitals and also invoked the help of the National Council for Combating Venereal Diseases (later the British Social Hygiene Council). The LCC also made grants to voluntary hostels on condition that they provided board and residence for women and girls attending VD clinics. (Sir I. G. Gibbon and R. W. Bell, *History of the LCC 1889–1939* (1939), Chap. 12.) The Public Health (Venereal Diseases) Act, 1917, prohibited the treatment of venereal disease by unqualified persons and the advertisement of remedies.

[4] LGB order to the M A B, 12 September 1916.

[5] LGB order to the M A B, 13 October 1919.

Some two hundred cases were dealt with annually in the two institutions. Meantime, the Board had been receiving infants infected with ophthalmia neonatorum, together with their mothers, in an institution known as St. Margaret's, in Kentish Town. This unit, which was opened in 1917,[1] was admitting about 150 mothers and 250 babies annually by 1929; but this was only one-third of all notified cases of ophthalmia neonatorum in London.

Other diseases which had become prominent during the war were admitted to the M A B hospitals following the cessation of hostilities. These included cerebro-spinal fever, dysentery, malaria and trench fever. First identified in Flanders in 1915, trench fever had been responsible for one-fifth to one-third of the total illness of the British armies in Western Europe.[2] During the next ten years (1919–29), other diseases which the M A B hospitals were empowered to treat included zymotic enteritis, puerperal pyrexia,[3] various children's infections[4] and tuberculosis.[5]

V

By 1928, it was generally assumed that smallpox would never again challenge the Board's accommodation. Nevertheless, the Long Reach Hospital was rebuilt with 250 beds, in case of need. No extensive outbreak had occurred since the 1901–2 epidemic of classical smallpox. Sporadic cases of this virulent form had appeared subsequently, but these were greatly outnumbered by cases of a much less severe, and relatively non-fatal, form of the disease known as alastrim, and, later, as variola minor.[6] The occurrence of the mild type of smallpox in this country began soon after the end of World War I, when international communications were resumed. The disease first became apparent in 1919, when outbreaks were reported in Suffolk and Norfolk. In 1920, fifty cases were admitted to the Board's hospitals when variola minor became prevalent in Essex and the outlying suburbs of London, at the same time as an outbreak of the more severe form of the disease in the east of London. During the following years, the line of spread of the disease was first directed towards the north midlands and the northern counties, where it attained a maximum incidence in the mining districts. Later, the disease became established in the mining districts of South Wales. Extension through the south midlands towards London was very slow and the metropolitan area remained relatively free from attack.[7]

[1] LGB order to the M A B, 29 September 1917. Ophthalmia neonatorum was made universally notifiable in February 1914, and preventive measures then became general.

[2] Sir A. Newsholme, op. cit., p. 229.

[3] All the diseases treated in the M A B hospitals between 1870 and 1929 are listed in Appendix I, Document III. The numbers of patients suffering from these diseases, notified and admitted, during the last complete year of the M A B (1929) are shown in Appendix II, Table J.

[4] See Chapter 18.   [5] See Chapter 19.

[6] The milder form of smallpox was first noted in South Africa in 1895 and again in Brazil in 1910, where it produced a quarter of a million cases. It was named 'alastrim' by the Brazilian natives, signifying a disease which spreads from place to place. R. Hare, *Pomp and Pestilence* (1954), p. 84.

[7] See Appendix II, Table C.

Late in 1928, however, minor smallpox at last gained a foothold in the capital. Londoners had lost their immunity during the generation of freedom from extensive outbreaks. By the end of 1928, three hundred cases had been treated in the new Long Reach hospital, but with only two fatalities. The epidemic gathered momentum throughout 1929 and, by the end of the year, over three thousand cases had been admitted. These included a number of extra-metropolitan patients, most of them poor law children from industrial schools. Nearly all the 1928–29 cases were of a type distinguished by a low fatality rate and a low degree of toxicity and infectivity; but the situation was complicated by the arrival in London in April 1929 of fourteen cases of the more deadly type, which had broken out on a large passenger liner from Bombay. Three of these died on admission to the M A B hospitals. Of the three thousand sub-toxic cases received in 1929, only six died.[1] An interesting feature of this epidemic was its relatively high incidence among children, probably due to neglect of infantile vaccination. Charts A, B, C and D, (Appendix II), prepared by the Board's medical staff, compare the age distribution of M A B smallpox cases in the epidemic years 1893, 1902, 1928 and 1929. It will be seen that, during 1893 and 1902, the years of toxic or major smallpox, the peak percentage of cases occurred in the 20–25 quinquennium, whereas, during 1928 and 1929, the years of the sub-toxic or minor type, the peaks occurred in the 10–15 and 5–10 quinquennia respectively, suggesting that smallpox was regaining its old-time position as a disease of childhood and adolescence. As no epidemic of comparable dimensions has since occurred in this country to make it possible to repeat such an analysis, this hypothesis must remain a matter of speculation. In the man-versus-virus conflict there is no finality, but it may be expected that, when the outbreak of the late 1920s subsided in 1934, it marked the close of an era in which London had cause to fear the ravages of epidemic smallpox.

In the course of their six decades of service, linking the Pasteurian age with that of the virologists, the M A B infectious disease hospitals treated more than 79,000 cases of smallpox, of which over 63,000 were admitted during the first thirty years. In addition, more than one million other cases of acute infectious disease passed through the M A B hospitals during their sixty years.[2] Three-quarters of these sought admission during the twentieth-century span of the Board's administration (1901–30), when the gratuitous

---

[1] See Appendix II, Table L.

[2] The total number of cases admitted into the M A B hospitals for infectious diseases, from the opening of the earliest institutions until the Board's dissolution, was 1,101,630, distributed as follows:

Type of Hospital	First Three Decades 1870–99	Second Three Decades 1900–29	Totals
Smallpox	63,634	15,473	79,107
Fever	244,206	778,317	1,022,523
			1,101,630

availability of the M A B isolation hospitals to patients of all social classes coincided with what has been described as 'the movement from fatalism to awareness in popular attitudes towards health and disease'.[1] The demands of the old diseases and the new attitudes had transformed a poor law system into a public health service.

[1] Richard M. Titmuss, 'Health', in *Law and Opinion in England in the Twentieth Century*, Morris Ginsberg (ed.) (1959), p. 318.

CHAPTER 16

Ambulance Services

I

THE M A B Land Ambulance Service, which had its rudimentary beginnings in 1881,[1] was still the only organized system of transport for the sick in London at the turn of the century. Most of the street accident cases at this period were removed by the wheeled litters which had been operating from the police stations since 1880, or by the St. John Ambulance Association, which manned a similar service from thirty-five voluntary first-aid posts in various parts of London. A few litters also remained of the system privately established in 1889 by the philanthropist, Mr. H. L. Bischoffsheim.

The M A B ambulances were based at six stations adjoining the Board's hospitals in Deptford, Fulham, Hampstead, Homerton, Stockwell and Woolwich,[2] so that the administrative area of London was almost completely covered by a three-mile radius from each station. The Board claimed that it was the largest user of civil ambulances in the world. By 1900, it was carrying 34,000 cases a year at an annual cost of £23,000. This covered the upkeep of the six depots, each of which provided residential accommodation for all necessary staff, coach houses, a forge, harness rooms and a laundry. The 'van'- and 'brougham'-shaped ambulance carriages for stretcher cases[3] were supplemented by omnibuses for convalescent patients. All vehicles were horse-drawn and the horses were hired by contract as required.

Mechanization of the ambulances began in 1902, when a steam vehicle, designed to carry eight stretchers, was introduced for the transport of patients to the Board's riverside hospitals. Although its road speed was only five miles an hour, it is recorded that a man

[1] See Chapter 6.

[2] For locations and dates of opening of the M A B ambulance stations, see Appendix I, Document VI, Section G.

[3] M A B ambulances at this time could be used with either one or two horses, and weighed $9\frac{1}{2}$ cwt. Lined with varnished wood and entirely free from absorbent upholstery, each vehicle was provided with two stretchers. The bed consisted of five air tubes placed lengthwise, with an air pillow. The stretcher was caned and fitted with telescopic handles each end. It had ball castors underneath, on which it rolled easily on 'tram lines' fixed on the floor of the carriage. The vehicle was warmed with hot water when necessary. The driver's seat contained duplicates of screws, nuts, etc., with rope and splints for broken shafts in case of need. A nurse and a male attendant accompanied each ambulance. Restoratives and refreshment were provided for the patient. (See figure 2.)

carrying a red flag walked in front.[1] The first ambulance driven by an internal combustion engine was manufactured in 1904. This carried one stretcher only and attained a speed of fifteen miles an hour. In 1907, the City Corporation inaugurated an electric motor ambulance to serve the City. By 1908, the M A B Western Ambulance Station in Fulham was completely equipped with motor transport. Gradually, horse-drawn vehicles were superseded throughout the service. When, on 14 September 1912, M A B horse ambulances were used for the last time, the familiar sight of urchins pursuing the slow-moving vehicles shouting 'fever!' was lost to the London scene.

On the river, the M A B continued to operate a service exclusively for smallpox patients. Although the hospital ships were dispensed with in 1904, the steamer service was continued. Patients were disembarked at Long Reach pier and conveyed by horse ambulances—and later by horsed tramcars—to the Joyce Green, Long Reach and Orchard hospitals nearby. The River Ambulance Service, which by 1900 cost approximately £8,000 a year to maintain, consisted of one screw steamer and three paddle-wheel steamers.[2] The largest, 143 feet in length, provided hospital accommodation for some fifty recumbent patients on the lower and upper decks on the outward journey, and space for about one hundred recovered patients on the bridge deck on the return trip. The sick were attended by doctors and nurses, and supplied with food during the two-hour journey down river to Long Reach. One of the smaller steamers was fitted up as a chapel. Miss Isabella Baker, when appointed 'lady superintendent' at Darenth during the 1884–85 smallpox epidemic, had been disturbed to find that no provision was made for religious services for the patients. She consulted her friend, Dr. Bridges of the Local Government Board, who at once arranged for the installation of the ship chapel and insisted on sharing the expenses with her.[3]

II

From the earliest years of the M A B Land Ambulance Service, the question of extending it for the removal of non-infectious patients had been considered from time to time. Hospital authorities and other interested bodies urged the need for special transport to carry medical, surgical and mental cases. But after two decades, the M A B service was still limited to conveying cases of dangerous infectious disorders; and no public provision existed for the transport of other patients. In 1903, in conjunction with the governors of the London general hospitals, boards of guardians and metropolitan borough and City councils, the M A B, therefore, studied the possibility of inaugurating a public ambulance service for non-infectious cases, and applied to the Local Government Board for authority to expand the scope of its ambulance service to meet this need.[4] Several weeks later, the

---

[1] Sir A. Powell, *The Metropolitan Asylums Board and its Work, 1867–1930*, p. 78.
[2] The *Maltese Cross*, the *Albert Victor*, the *Geneva Cross* and the *White Cross*.
[3] S. Liveing, op. cit., p. 197.
[4] M A B letter to the LGB, 30 November 1903.

central authority suggested that the M A B should contact the LCC, which, it was understood, was considering the question of London ambulance services.[1] During 1904 and 1905, the Council repeatedly deferred the invitation of the M A B to confer upon the matter, and at last definitely declined. Undeterred, the Asylums Board prepared special ambulances in differentiating colours for infectious and non-infectious patients. These were used by general practitioners who knew of the informal arrangement, but in the absence of legal sanction the Board was unable to announce the facilities which it wished to place at the disposal of the public.

In 1906, the LCC tried unsuccessfully to obtain from Parliament power to provide a motor ambulance service for the County. In the course of that year, M A B ambulances carried over four hundred medical and surgical cases to general hospitals and other places, as well as a thousand of its own non-infectious patients. The number of M A B non-infectious removals was doubled the following year and trebled in 1908.

Early in 1907, the metropolitan poor law authorities held a conference to consider the establishment of a general ambulance service for London. Shortly afterwards, the whole question of ambulance provision became the subject of a special enquiry by a Home Office departmental committee comprising three members. In his evidence before the committee, the Clerk to the Asylums Board, Mr. Duncombe Mann, referred to the conveyance of mental, medical and surgical non-infectious cases as 'a new departure, which, although not yet legally sanctioned, appeared to have the tacit approval of the Local Government Board'. He made it clear that the Asylums Board was fully equipped to carry out the rapid transport of cases of accident and sudden illness occurring in the streets.

In March 1909, two of the three members of the Home Office committee reported that 'under the circumstances at present prevailing in the metropolis, we think the most efficient and economical system would be found in an extension of the non-infectious service of rapid ambulances which has been initiated by the M A B. So far as relates to street cases, this service should be worked in close co-operation with the Metropolitan Police.'[2] When invited to express their views on the report, both the M A B and the LCC informed the, then, Home Secretary, Mr. Reginald McKenna, that they entirely concurred in this recommendation. In these circumstances, the Asylums Board was somewhat surprised when the Home Secretary subsequently supported, and Parliament passed, a private member's bill which empowered the LCC to establish, or aid in establishing, an ambulance service for dealing with accidents or illness (other than infectious disease) within the County of London. The private Member who introduced the bill was Sir William Collins, the dissenting member of the departmental committee and a member of the LCC.

It was felt by both the Asylums Board and the LCC that the new measure—the 1909 Metropolitan Ambulance Act[3]—would involve a costly and unnecessary duplication

[1] LGB letter to the M A B, 18 February 1904.
[2] *Report of the Departmental Committee on the Ambulance Service of the Metropolis*, 1909: BPP, 1909, vol. xxxi, p. 30, para. 108 [Cmd. 4563].
[3] 9 Edw. 7 c. 17.

of existing machinery in the metropolis. The LCC, therefore, deferred action for another four years, while the Board continued, illegally, to convey non-infectious patients, cases of accident and sudden illness in the streets, as well as LCC mental and ophthalmic cases. During the coronation festivities of King George V in June 1911, the M A B serviced the route with its new motor ambulances at the request of the Metropolitan Commissioner of Police.

In November 1913, the Asylums Board was invited by the LCC to prepare a scheme of co-operation with the Council, and other metropolitan authorities, for the establishment of a street ambulance service. The Board accordingly submitted a plan, but it proved unacceptable to the LCC. In 1914, tardily and reluctantly, the Council accepted its new obligation, and its ambulance service was established in February 1915 under the control of the chief officer of the Fire Brigade.

In March 1923, as a result of representations from the Metropolitan Commissioner of Police and others, the Minister of Health, Sir W. J. Joynson-Hicks, referred the question of street accident cases to the Voluntary Hospitals Commission, and a conference on the subject was held in July of that year, attended by representatives of interested bodies, including the M A B and the LCC. The question of setting up a central advisory committee was then fully considered, but the opinion of the conference was against it, as it was generally held that the separate transport functions of the M A B and the LCC were sufficiently clearly defined. The Council provided a free ambulance service to deal with street accident cases in the County, while the Board operated two road services in London and the surrounding area—one for patients with infectious disease, and the other for non-infectious cases. The latter involved the provision of ambulances and omnibuses for the removal of sick and invalid private patients, as well as all classes of persons coming under the public care. No charge was made for infectious patients to and from the Board's hospitals, as they were entitled by law to free transport.[1] A fee of ten shillings was charged for private infectious removals to destinations other than the M A B institutions, and for all non-infectious work. In cases of poverty, however, fees were waived. By 1929, the M A B was conveying over 100,000 patients a million miles a year at an annual net cost of £68,000.

On 1 April 1930, as a result of the abolition of the poor law authorities under the 1929 Local Government Act, ambulances owned by the metropolitan boards of guardians and the M A B were taken over by the LCC. Of the 46 parish vehicles, 10 were obsolete. The M A B fleet of 107 petrol-driven ambulances embodied the latest developments in what was then a comparatively modern branch of special transport. These, together with the Council's 21 ambulances, were welded together into one public transport system for all cases of illness and accident in London, and placed under the direction of the Medical Officer of Health for the County.[2] The M A B River Ambulance Service passed at the same time to the LCC but survived little more than a year. In 1932, it was disbanded,

[1] 52 & 53 Vict. c. 56 s. 6.
[2] *Ministry of Health Sixteenth Annual Report* (1934–35), p. 78.

having carried more than 45,000 patients to Long Reach since its inauguration in 1884. The old ships were sold to Russia to be broken up for the sake of the metal. The dossal and frontal of the ship chapel, however, were salvaged and preserved in the Joyce Green isolation hospital. Thus divested of their identity, the M A B ambulance services passed into history, unique as pioneers in this country of special transport for the sick.

CHAPTER 17

Medical Instruction, Pathological Services and Research

I

UNTIL the last decade of the nineteenth century, opportunities for medical students in this country to study at first hand the diagnosis and treatment of the acute infectious diseases were very limited. It was possible to qualify as a medical practitioner without any clinical experience of fevers and smallpox, although such cases formed a substantial part of private and poor law practice before the advent of the M A B hospitals. With this deficiency in mind, Mr. Gathorne Hardy had included clinical instruction in the new institutions for the London poor as part of his 1867 medical reforms. He regarded the attendance of clinical instructors and their students as a most effective form of inspection.[1] During the passage of the Metropolitan Poor Bill, he was strongly supported in this view; and the innovation accordingly became law.[2] Nevertheless, two years later, before it could be carried into effect, this provision was expressly repealed.[3] The ostensible reason was that the poor would object to it, but this view was not shared by medical men of long experience in treating the sick poor in the large voluntary hospitals, since it was known that the presence of a great many 'doctors' attending to his case was nearly always of positive satisfaction to the patient.[4] The Asylums Managers were not consulted beforehand, nor were they given the reasons for the amending legislation. Only the year before, at the 1868 Annual Congress of the National Association for the Promotion of Social Science, medical contributors had deplored the insufficiency of opportunities for clinical instruction in this country and had urged that public hospitals and dispensaries should be better utilized for this purpose.[5] Such suggestions continued to be made during the next fourteen years, for it was feared in medical circles that a race of half-educated practitioners would arise.[6] In accordance

[1] *Hansard*, vol. clxxxv (third series), 8 February 1867, col. 165.

[2] Metropolitan Poor Act, 1867 (30 & 31 Vict. c. 6 s. 29).

[3] Metropolitan Poor Amendment Act, 1869 (32 & 33 Vict. c. 63 s. 20).

[4] *Third Report of the House of Lords Select Committee on Metropolitan Hospitals*, 1892: BPP, 1892 vol. xiii, p. lxxv, para. 427.

[5] *Trans., NAPSS*, 1868. Elizabeth Garrett *et al.*, 'Public Hospitals and Dispensaries', pp. 464–67 and 482–94.

[6] Ibid., 1882. T. Gilbart-Smith, 'What Reforms are desirable in the Administration of Hospitals?', p. 426.

with a resolution passed at the 1882 Annual Congress of the National Social Science Association, the Council of that body addressed to the Home Secretary a series of recommendations which included an urgent plea that

> ... more use should be made, in the education of medical students, of the material contained in the numerous hospitals and dispensaries administered by the Poor Law Department and the M A B, and that there should be more intimate communication between these and the general hospitals.[1]

Like earlier recommendations, this appeal fell on stony ground. Within two years, poor law infirmaries became less accessible than ever to medical students. In 1884, the Local Government Board definitely declined to sanction the use of the Kensington poor law infirmary for clinical instruction.[2] It may be assumed that this was on grounds of poor law policy and not with the acquiescence of the principal medical officer of the Board, who was strongly in favour of the admission of students.[3]

At the end of 1884, a plenary meeting of the Asylums Board resolved, on the motion of two medical members, that consideration should be given to the advisability of making the M A B isolation hospitals available for clinical instruction to students 'in accordance with section 29 of the Metropolitan Poor Act of 1867'.[4] It would seem that the members and staff of the Asylums Board were unaware that this provision had been repealed. A special M A B committee was convened to study the matter. In February 1886, it recommended that registered medical men should be invited to apply for clinical assistantships in the Board's fever and smallpox hospitals. These appointments would be residential and tenable for three months, during which the assistants would work under the medical superintendents, from whom they would receive instruction on payment of a fee.[5] After seeking the central authority's approval and being informed of the change in the law concerning clinical instruction in poor law hospitals, the Asylums Managers urgently represented that they should be re-empowered to admit students to their hospitals.[6] In reply, the Local Government Board suggested that, if clinical assistants were considered necessary, they should be appointed with specified duties, but their emoluments should be limited to 'residence and rations' and they should pay no fees.[7] A few such appointments were accordingly made; but the Asylums Managers were not satisfied. Supported by the medical

---

[1] Ibid., 'Memorial of the Council of the National Association for the Promotion of Social Science to the Secretary of State for the Home Department', Resolution VI, p. 438.

[2] *Selections from the Correspondence of the Local Government Board*, vol. iii, 1888, p. 224.

[3] It is possible that the principal Medical Officer of the LGB was never consulted concerning the use of poor law infirmaries for clinical instruction. The duties of a later principal MO to the LGB, as set out in his letter of appointment in 1908, definitely excluded poor law work from the areas in which he was expected to advise. Sir Arthur Newsholme, *The Last Thirty Years in Public Health* (1936), p. 27.

[4] M A B *Mins.*, vol. xviii, 1884–85, p. 1093.

[5] M A B *Mins.*, vol. xix, 1885–86, p. 1202.

[6] M A B letter to the LGB, 1 March 1886; LGB reply dated 26 March 1886; M A B letter to the LGB, 10 May 1886.

[7] LGB letter to the M A B, 30 July 1886.

press,[1] they continued to urge the need for admitting students to the M A B fever hospitals. The required sanction was eventually granted by the Poor Law Act of 1889,[2] the measure which opened the doors of the M A B isolation hospitals to patients of all social classes.

As the use of the M A B 'asylums' for fever and smallpox courses was to be governed under the Act by regulations to be made by the Local Government Board, the M A B appointed a special committee to discuss this provision with the Fever Committee of the Royal College of Physicians. The College's committee undertook to draft the regulations and these were eventually accepted by the central authority and issued as a statutory order.[3] No student was to be admitted before the completion of his third year nor until he had held the offices of clinical clerk and dresser. Courses of not less than two months' duration were made available to qualified medical men as well as to students.

When the 1889 Infectious Disease Notification Act came into force, errors of diagnosis became increasingly apparent,[4] and in April 1891, the Society of Medical Officers of Health recommended the General Medical Council to make clinical instruction of medical students in infectious diseases compulsory. Reporting in 1892, the House of Lords Select Committee on Metropolitan Hospitals deplored 'the ignorance of infectious fevers which hitherto has prevailed among young practitioners. . . .'[5] In the same year, the Conjoint Board of the Royal Colleges of Physicians and Surgeons made a certificated course of instruction at a fever hospital a requirement of the five-years curriculum of all students entering the profession.

Classes began in the M A B institutions at Homerton, Deptford and Fulham in 1891, and by 1897 all the M A B fever hospitals were open for teaching. In 1893, the regulations for instruction in smallpox establishments were amended.[6] The course was altered to one of not less than two, and not more than four, weeks involving residence on the hospital ships. Later, the residence obligation was suspended, and, during the rare smallpox epidemics which subsequently occurred, special demonstrations were arranged for general practitioners and Medical Officers of Health. The fee for the three-months' fever course was three guineas; that for the two-weeks' smallpox course was two guineas; while qualified visitors paid one guinea for three demonstrations. The medical superintendents acted as clinical instructors and were permitted to receive two-thirds of the fees, the remainder being placed in a fund for ancillary expenses. No part of the cost of medical instruction fell upon the rates. Upwards of 3,000 students had passed through the M A B fever and

[1] The Hospital, vol. i, 13 November 1886, p. 116: 'Surely students . . . need to have a knowledge of fevers, and seeing that nearly all fevers in London go to the hospitals under the Board's authority, where are they to get it except at these hospitals . . .?'

[2] 52 & 53 Vict. c. 56 s. 4.   [3] LGB order to the M A B, 10 October 1890.

[4] In 1891, the M A B statistical committee reported that errors in the diagnosis of patients sent to the M A B hospitals had increased during the preceding five years from 2·4 per cent to 6·2 per cent (M A B Annual Report for 1891, p. 13).

[5] Third Report of the House of Lords Select Committee on Metropolitan Hospitals, 1892, op. cit., p. lxxii.

[6] LGB order to the M A B, 30 October 1893.

smallpox hospitals by 1900. From that time until the outbreak of World War I, attendance averaged about 250 annually. Numbers doubled after the war, ranging between 500 and 800 a year; about one quarter were women.

In 1903, the General Medical Council made it obligatory for candidates for the Diploma of Public Health to reside for three months in a fever hospital which provided opportunities for the study of methods of administration. The Asylums Board, which had not been consulted, found it difficult to comply with this requirement, and the Council could not see its way to modify it. The Board agreed to co-operate only if the DPH candidates entered as residential clinical assistants. This arrangement began in 1903. By 1911, however, non-residential classes in hospital administration were made possible in the Board's institutions, and from then on between fifty and eighty DPH candidates attended annually.

II

The era of the scientific approach to the treatment and study of infectious diseases in the M A B hospitals may be said to have dawned shortly after the opening of their doors to medical students. It began with the introduction in 1894 of the newly-discovered methods of diagnosing and treating diphtheria. In 1883, Klebs observed that a bacillus with certain characteristics occurred regularly in the throats of diphtheria patients. In 1884, Löffler demonstrated the aetiological association between diphtheria and what became known as the Klebs-Löffler bacillus.[1] During the ensuing decade, the diagnostic value of this discovery was developed. In the hospitals of the Asylums Board the detection of the diphtheria bacillus was regarded as a matter of prime importance. Hitherto, it had been impossible for medical practitioners to diagnose with certainty the existence of diphtheria. Seven thousand patients who had been certified and reported as suffering from diphtheria were admitted to the Board's hospitals between 1890 and 1893, but six hundred of them were not cases of diphtheria in the opinion of the Board's medical officers; and many other cases, where negative evidence was not sufficiently clear to warrant their being sent home, were perforce treated in the diphtheria wards.

The Asylums Board accordingly decided in 1894 that on scientific and economic grounds a central bacteriological laboratory was an essential adjunct to the work of the fever hospitals. Pending the erection of such a diagnostic and experimental centre, the Conjoint Board of the Royal Colleges of Physicians and Surgeons was asked whether its Laboratories Committee could provide the Asylums Board with facilities for the bacteriological investigation of doubtful cases of diphtheria. It was agreed that such tests could be undertaken, provided they were conducted by bacteriologists especially appointed by the Laboratories Committee under the superintendence of the Director, Dr. (later Sir) German Sims Woodhead, and provided the M A B defrayed the expenses of testing, including the salaries of those occupied in the work. The Board accepted these terms. The work, which

[1] F. Löffler, *Mitt. Reichsgesundheitsamt*, 2 (1884), 421.

began on 1 January 1895, included the examination of cases on discharge as well as on admission, and greatly exceeded the daily average of twenty tests which was originally anticipated. When, in January 1897, the arrangement lapsed, it was decided that the routine diagnostic work should be conducted in the Board's fever hospitals. Medical superintendents were then assisted by bacteriologists in the service of the Royal Colleges and provided with supplies of Löffler's culture medium.

At the time of enlisting the help of the Royal Colleges in diagnostic testing, the Board had also requested their assistance in the new treatment for diphtheria. The production by von Behring of an antitoxin serum from immunized horses had been reported in 1892.[1] In June 1894, when this discovery had made some advance in Germany and France, the Asylums Managers decided to introduce it into their hospitals. This step was met by strong opposition on the part of certain sections of the public and by a number of metropolitan boards of guardians. Notwithstanding, the Board proceeded with its plan. At first, the antitoxin serum was obtained from Paris, but later the bulk of it was supplied by the British Institute of Preventive Medicine. As early as November 1894, the Board realized that it would be both difficult and expensive to maintain a regular and sufficient supply for the treatment of all its diphtheria cases. The Royal Colleges were accordingly asked whether they would be prepared to supply sufficient antitoxin serum for use in the M A B hospitals. As the work could be carried out in conjunction with the bacteriological examination of the Board's diphtheria cases and thereby lead to research into improved methods both of serum production and its application in treatment, the Royal Colleges acceded to the Board's request. The stabling and upkeep of the ten horses required were undertaken by the Board, which also agreed to defray laboratory expenses. This arrangement came to an end in 1904. The Asylums Board then decided to undertake the work of serum production. An agreement was made with the Royal Colleges for the use of their laboratories on the Victoria Embankment and of their stables at Balham. The staff previously employed by the Colleges in connexion with the preparation of the serum was taken over by the Board, and the Director, Sir German Woodhead, was retained as the Board's adviser. Soon, it was decided that more extensive accommodation for both serum production and pathological investigations was essential. After protracted discussions with the central authority, which placed a limit of £6,500 on the capital cost of the projected laboratories, these, with stables, were erected at Belmont, near Sutton, Surrey, and opened in 1909.

III

Systematic research into the diseases treated in the M A B hospitals began shortly before the outbreak of World War I. A comprehensive survey of this aspect of the Board's activities is beyond the scope of this non-technical study, and reference is made here only to the principal fields which engaged the attention of the Board's research staff. Papers on

[1] Behring and Wernicke, *Dtsch. Med. Wschr.*, 39 (1892), 873.

organized projects and independent investigations were published in the annual reports of the Asylums Board, and an index to these contributions is appended to this study (see Medical Supplement).

At the end of 1912, the Board was reminded by its hospitals committee (which included three medical men and four women) that, since the opening of its institutions in 1870, nearly half a million fever patients had been treated; that fatalities numbered 40,000; that nearly £15 million had been spent in providing and administering the isolation hospitals; but that no practical step had been taken by the Board to ascertain the causes of the diseases treated.[1]

It was accordingly decided to appoint a full-time research pathologist to study the causation, infectivity, prevention and treatment of 'zymotic' diseases. In May 1913, after certain objections raised by the Local Government Board had been resolved,[2] Dr. W. Mair, MD, ChB, DPH, was appointed for one year in the first instance, with emoluments of £500 per annum. The appointment was renewed annually; and in the course of the next few years a series of reports was published on the aetiology of scarlet fever.[3] As in the past, independent studies of this and other acute infectious diseases, including diphtheria, typhoid fever and measles, continued to be made by members of the Board's medical staff.[4]

All the work of the pathological and serum production laboratories, as well as research into infectious disease, was carried on under the general supervision of Sir German Woodhead until his death in 1921. The Board then invited the assistance of a scientific advisory committee to serve in a similar capacity.[5] Following its constitution in 1923, the committee made a number of recommendations, as a result of which a degree of decentralization was carried out. The Belmont laboratories were thereafter devoted entirely to antitoxin serum production; and Dr. R. G. White, MB, ChB, formerly Director of the Serum Institute and Public Health Laboratories in Cairo, was appointed Director of Antitoxin Establishment. All routine pathological work was carried out at the hospitals. Each became self-contained and competent to deal with its own bacteriological and pathological requirements under the direction of a skilled pathologist. For work requiring special techniques, such as virulence tests, strain typing, Widal and Wassermann reactions, section-cutting, blood culture and the preparation of vaccines, two laboratories were established to serve the Board's hospitals in the northern and southern areas of London,

[1] M A B *Mins.*, vol. xlvi, 1912, p. 349.

[2] Commenting on the M A B recommendation that a full-time research bacteriologist should be appointed, the LGB held that the title should be 'pathologist' and that such an appointment should be part-time and on an annual basis. (LGB letters to the M A B, 29 January and 26 April 1913.)

[3] W. Mair, 'Experimental Scarlet Fever in the Monkey', *J. Path. Bact.*, 1915, vol. xix, p. 443; 'On the Aetiology of Scarlet Fever', ibid., 1916, vol. xx, p. 366; 'A Contribution to the Serological Classification of the Bile-soluble Diplococci', ibid., 1917, vol. xxi, p. 305; 'The Preparation of Desoxycholic Acid', *Biochem. J.*, 1917, vol. xi, p. 11; 'The Diplococcal Theory of Scarlet Fever', *M A B Annual Report*, 1919–20, p. 61; ibid., 1923–24, p. 99.

[4] See Medical Supplement (following the Appendices to this study), Section I.

[5] Members of the M A B scientific advisory committee are listed in Appendix I, Document V.

respectively. The Northern Group Laboratory was established at the North-Eastern Hospital, South Tottenham, while the Southern Group Laboratory was erected at the Park Hospital, Lewisham. This became the headquarters of the direction and centre of the work. In April 1925, Dr. J. E. McCartney, MD, ChB, DSc, was appointed Director of Research and Pathological Services. His tasks were to organize the work of the group laboratories, to plan research in the field of infectious disease, to supervise the instruction of resident medical officers in special pathological techniques, and to foster a wider research outlook among the personnel of the Board's institutions.

In July 1925, the Ministry of Health, alarmed at the rise in maternal mortality, suggested to the Asylums Board that an advance would be made in the treatment of puerperal fever if a greater number of cases were to receive the skilled medical and nursing attention available in the M A B hospitals. The disease had been made legally admissible to the Board's hospitals for both pauper and other patients in 1912, but a large number of notified cases still found their way to the poor law infirmaries. The M A B accordingly devoted part of its Eastern, North-Western and South-Western Hospitals to the treatment and study of puerperal fever. Mr. James Wyatt, MB, FRCS, who was appointed as obstetric consultant, carried out a number of investigations;[1] and work sponsored by the Medical Research Council, which had already been started in the poor law institutions, was continued in the Board's hospitals.[2]

Among other investigations conducted by the Board's staff during this period were those concerned with rheumatic infection in children,[3] and a number of contributions to the study of tuberculosis.[4] In 1928, at the request of the Ministry of Health, the Asylums Board agreed to establish at its North-Western Hospital at Hampstead a clinic for the study and treatment of cancer of the uterus. At this time cancer was being treated by radium, radon, X-rays or operation, or by one of these methods combined with another. According to the published records of certain continental clinics, the treatment of cancer by radium had been more successful in cases of carcinoma of the cervix uteri than in any other part of the body, but the results from these clinics, as well as findings in this country, were very unequal. The League of Nations, therefore, appointed a Radiological Sub-Commission in 1928 to report on radio-therapeutic methods used in the treatment of cancer of the uterus; and the participating countries—which included France, Germany, Great Britain and Sweden—undertook to issue reports from their centres on lines laid down by the Sub-Commission. The British centre was administered by the M A B and directed by Mr. Comyns Berkeley, MD, MC, FRCP, FRCS, who had been carrying out successful work in this field at the Middlesex Hospital, where he was consulting surgeon. On 1 November 1928, the Board's clinic opened with eight beds. In spending £4,000 on

[1] See Medical Supplement, Section I. op. cit.

[2] Sir A. E. Wright, *Lancet*, 1919, I, 489, and *idem*, 1923, I, 473; L. Colebrook and E. J. Storer, *Lancet*, 1923, II, 1341; L. Colebrook and E. J. Storer, *Brit. J. exp. Path.*, 1924, V., 47; and L. Colebrook, *Proc. Roy. Soc. Med.*, 1926, XIX, 31.

[3] See Medical Supplement, Section IV.   [4] Ibid., Section II, A & B.

the required radium, the M A B was the first public body to make such a purchase on this scale. About 150 women from poor law hospitals were admitted to the clinic during the fourteen months of its operation before the dissolution of the Board. The report on these cases was of limited interest, in view of the relatively brief period covered.[1]

At the time of the inauguration of the group laboratories for the study of infectious diseases, research laboratories were also being established at the Fountain, Caterham and Leavesden mental hospitals; and Dr. S. A. Kinnier Wilson, MD, FRCP, consulting neurologist, was appointed to the M A B mental health service. The rich field of material provided by the M A B mental institutions was drawn upon in a number of studies in psychological medicine.[2]

Meantime, special attention was being given to the children who had been admitted to the Board's encephalitis lethargica unit at the Winchmore Hill Hospital. Although sporadic encephalitis had long been known, encephalitis lethargica or epidemica was recognized as an independent entity on its first appearance in this country in 1918. In that year, an enquiry was conducted by the Local Government Board into this obscure disease, and four years later this was followed up by the Ministry of Health.[3] The disease, which attacked people of all ages and both sexes, was commoner in populous areas than in rural districts. Social conditions, however, appeared to have little connexion with liability to attack.[4] One of the most distressing features of the disease was its after-effects, especially those of a functional nature associated with deterioration in behaviour. Up to this time, little was known of these mental changes, which were usually permanent and sometimes of a vicious or criminal nature. The selected group of 125 children admitted in 1924 ranged from paretic juveniles of normal intellect and behaviour to moral imbeciles and potential criminals. During the next few years, an attempt was made—the Board claimed that it was the first of its kind in any country—to study the characteristics of the aftermath of encephalitis, the effects of treatment and the possible need for permanent institutional provision.[5] The epidemic form of the disease lasted until about 1930 and then disappeared from the records.

IV

The pathological and research activities of the Asylums Board were financed from the

[1] Report of the M A B Radium Centre, by Comyns Berkeley et al., M A B Annual Report for 1929–30, pp. 125–63. This report does not appear to have been published by the League of Nations Radiological Sub-Commission, but reports from the Radium Institute of Paris, the Gynaecological Clinic of the University of Munich and the Radiumhemmet of Stockholm were issued in League of Nations publication: Ser.L.o.N. P. III Health 1929, III 5 (C.H. 788, June 1929).

[2] See Medical Supplement, Section III.

[3] *Local Government Board Reports, New Series*, No. 121, 1918, 'Report of an enquiry into an obscure disease—Encephalitis Lethargica'; *Ministry of Health Reports on Public Health and Medical Subjects*, No. 11, 1922, 'Encephalitis Lethargica'.

[4] A. H. Gale, op. cit., Chap. 10 *passim*.

[5] See Medical Supplement, Section I and Section III.

same source as the rest of its expenditure—the poor rates of the metropolis. During the Board's last four years (1926–29), the total cost of serum production averaged about £9,000 annually. Bacteriological diphtheria cases were being received at the rate of over one thousand a year at this time. The combined expenditure of the pathological and research laboratories during this period averaged £5,500 annually. About half of this represented the cost of organized investigations.[1]

When the Asylums Board made its first research appointment, the financing of medical enquiries from public funds was something of an innovation, although it was not the first occasion on which research expenditure had been met out of the London rates. In 1895, the LCC established a central pathological laboratory at Claybury Asylum—the first mental hospital to be built by the Council—and appointed a research pathologist.[2] The foundation of research supported from Exchequer funds, however, is generally associated with the creation in 1913 of the Medical Research Council (formerly the National Research Committee) as a by-product of national insurance. The first systematic grant by the State of funds for the investigation of health problems was that provided by the penny-per-person-per-year retained for tuberculosis research out of the total contributions from insured persons, employers and the State under the 1911 National Insurance Act. This fund, of approximately £60,000 a year, was subsequently increased by government grants and devoted to a wider range of health problems. The work was co-ordinated by the Medical Research Council. Before this, the only grant from public funds specifically made for health investigations was an annual sum of £2,000, first administered by the Local Government Board on its creation in 1871.[3] By 1908 this sum had been reduced to £1,900 because the £2,000 had not been totally expended during a particular year. The Treasury time-limit for spending did not fit in with the exigencies of scientific work.[4] Apart from this relatively meagre degree of State support, medical advances had been financed almost exclusively from the charitable funds which supported the work of the voluntary hospitals.

[1] The cost of research conducted in association with the League of Nations Radiological Sub-Commission was probably recovered by the M A B from the League.

[2] When the LCC took over from the Justices the charge of the lunacy of London, it was recognized that there was room for improvement in pathological investigation and research and that the occasion was opportune for establishing a central laboratory replete with the equipment necessary for the study of psychological medicine in its widest sense. At the end of 1892, a special committee was convened to consider the appointment of a pathologist to the London County Asylums. As a result of the committee's report, the LCC approved the establishment of a laboratory at an estimated cost of £4,000, the provision of fittings and apparatus at a cost of £800, and the appointment of Dr. F. W. Mott, MD, FRS, as pathologist at £700 per annum. Research work was begun in 1895 (*Archives of Neurology from the Pathological Laboratory of the London County Asylums, Claybury, Essex*, vol. i (1900), pp. ix–x). The laboratory was later transferred from Claybury to the Maudsley Hospital and was given generous help by the Rockefeller Foundation.

[3] Although no systematic grant had been made by the State for research into health problems before 1871, Sir John Simon's appointment to the Privy Council under the Public Health Act, 1858, authorized enquiries by the Council into matters concerning the public health and required its Medical Officer to report to the Privy Council in relation to such matters.

[4] Sir A. Newsholme, op. cit., p. 121.

Since its inception, the Asylums Board had constantly striven to wean its hospitals away from their initial role of repositories for paupers from whom the wider community was to be protected. By the middle 1920s, largely through the development of teaching, pathological and research activities, it had brought its institutions much more nearly into line with the traditional pattern of the voluntary hospitals.

CHAPTER 18

Child Care

I

CHILDREN had always formed a substantial proportion of the M A B hospital population.[1] In addition to the mentally handicapped and infectious sick, some seven thousand healthy children had passed through the hands of the Board by the end of the century. These were poor law boys, between thirteen and sixteen years, who were provided for in the training ship *Exmouth*, for which the M A B had been responsible since 1875. In that year, the *Goliath*, a training craft belonging to the Whitechapel and Poplar guardians, was destroyed by fire, and the Local Government Board decided that it should be replaced by another vessel for the benefit of the whole metropolis. As the one central poor law authority in London, the M A B was called upon to manage the new ship.[2]

It was not until 1897, however, that the Asylums Board was charged with special duties as a metropolitan child care authority. This widening of its responsibilities was an outcome of the somewhat inauspicious movement which had been concerned since the poor law reform Act of 1834 with providing for pauper children. In the metropolis, the problem had presented itself in four phases. From 1834 to 1849, poor law children were accommodated for the most part in the workhouses, although as early as 1767 it had been enacted that children under six should be cared for outside London.[3] When the opportunism of private enterprise made it easier to comply with the law, some children were boarded out by the guardians in what became known as 'contractors' establishments', but these were viewed with disfavour by the Poor Law Commissioners. It was assumed, notwithstanding, that the shortcomings of these institutions stemmed solely from the conditions of private management, and that schools on similar lines would ensure success

---

[1] See Chapters 4 and 14 (mentally handicapped children) and Chapters 10 and 15 (infectious cases).

[2] The provision of a training ship for the instruction of boys for sea service was sanctioned by the LGB in 1875 under the terms of the Metropolitan Poor Law Amendment Act, 1869 (32 & 33 Vict. c. 63 s. 11). The *Exmouth*, an old wooden two-decker line-of-battleship, was lent to the M A B by the Admiralty and moored off Grays, Essex. The ship, which accommodated 600 boys, was replaced, first in 1903 and again in 1913, by larger vessels specially built and equipped. From 1876 until the end of 1929 more than 16,000 boys had been trained. An ex-naval officer served as captain-superintendent of the ship and was directly responsible to the special training ship committee of the M A B.

[3] 7 Geo. III c. 39, an Act 'for the better regulation of the parish poor children . . . within the bills of mortality'.

if placed in the hands of bodies responsible to the ratepayers. In 1844, therefore, Parliament empowered the Poor Law Commissioners to combine metropolitan unions and parishes into school districts 'for the management of any class of infant poor. . . '.[1] After certain restrictions to this power had been removed by Parliament in 1848,[2] work on the 'district schools' began, and by 1864 they were completed. These establishments for pauper children were in the nature of vast barrack boarding schools, and were managed by boards of guardians. This phase of development was followed by one of doubt concerning the value of the new institutions, and official enquiries were instituted. The recommendations of two investigators, in particular, are relevant to the role of the Asylums Board in this movement for ameliorating conditions for poor law children. Owing to the difficulty of classification in these large establishments, contagious disease—particularly of the eyes and scalp—spread rapidly. An ophthalmic surgeon, Mr. Edward Nettleship, FRCS, commissioned by the Local Government Board in 1874 to study the incidence of oph-thalmia among London schoolchildren, urged, like medical experts before him, that the only certain means of eradication was the provision of isolation schools.[3] During the same year, Mrs. Nassau Senior, who had been studying the institutions with special reference to the training of girls, advocated 'schools of a more homelike character, con-taining not more than twenty to thirty children of all ages'.[4] These reports gave rise to a number of further independent studies of pauper children.[5] All revealed the persistent failure of the central authority to give any comprehensive consideration to what was numerically one of the largest sections of the pauper population. About one-third of the whole were children under sixteen years.[6] During the next period—1875 to 1894—a few small-scale experiments with scattered homes and cottage homes in colonies were carried out, but the barrack schools, with their now patent defects, continued until the outcry against them resulted in the appointment in 1894 of the Departmental Committee on Metropolitan Poor Law Schools 'to enquire into the existing systems for the maintenance and education of poor law children in the metropolis and to advise as to any changes that might be desirable'.

[1] Poor Law Amendment Act, 1844 (7 & 8 Vict. c. 101 s. xl).

[2] Poor Law Amendment Act, 1848 (11 & 12 Vict. c. 82).

[3] Ophthalmia had long been the bane of the poor law schools but, despite sustained efforts at eradication, it remained undiminished during the nineteenth century. Mr. Nettleship's survey of 1874 revealed that at least 1,300 London children required isolation. Only one attempt was made to isolate such cases; this was in 1889, when the Central London School District Board established an institution at Hanwell. Even by 1897, nearly a thousand London schoolchildren were found to be suffering from ophthalmia. (Report by Mr. Sydney Stevenson, FRCS: Cmd. 8597 of 1897; and M A B Children's Committee Annual Report, 1898, pp. 53 and 62–63.)

[4] *Report by Mrs. Nassau Senior on the Education of Girls in Pauper Schools*, appended to LGB Annual Report, 1875.

[5] E. C. Tufnell (ex-Inspector of the Metropolitan District), *Observations on the Report of Mrs. Nassau Senior* (1875); Menella Bute Smedley, *Boarding-Out and Pauper Schools, especially for Girls* (1875); F. J. Mouet, *Report . . . on the Cost of Maintenance of the Children . . . from 1869 to 1873* (1876); Walter R. Browne, *Facts and Fallacies of Pauper Education* (1878); E. C. Tufnell, *The Training of Pauper Children* (1880).

[6] S. and B. Webb, *English Local Government: English Poor Law History—The Last Hundred Years*, p. 246.

The Committee's report, published in 1896,[1] amounted to a virtual condemnation of the poor law schools, the metropolitan guardians and the Local Government Board. It recommended the creation of a special authority to supervise all metropolitan poor law institutions for children, and the transfer of powers of inspection from the Local Government Board to the Board of Education. The report, which aroused strong resentment, was followed shortly by the introduction into Parliament of the Government Education Bill by Sir John Gorst, MP, a member of the Departmental Committee who had since become Parliamentary Secretary of the Board of Education. The Bill proposed that all poor law children, both in the metropolis and in the provinces, should be transferred to the care of the Education Department. The project met with considerable opposition and was eventually abandoned. Shortly afterwards, however, the Local Government Board announced its intention of creating a new metropolitan authority 'for the reception and relief' of certain classes of poor law children.[2] Supported by a number of boards of guardians, the Asylums Managers protested to the Local Government Board. They pointed out that, with their thirty years' experience and existing administrative machinery, they were well equipped to carry out the duties which it was proposed to assign to a new authority.[3] A few months later, the Local Government Board issued an order[4] instructing the Asylums Managers to assume responsibility for poor law school children suffering from contagious diseases of the eyes, skin and scalp; educationally subnormal children;[5] and those in need of long-term nursing and convalescence. This last category was assigned to the Board's care because sick children were still being boarded-out to contractors' establishments by the guardians, although the practice had been superseded in the case of healthy pauper children. The primary consideration of the contractors being financial gain, they willingly accepted every child sent to them, whether suffering from contagious disease or not, so that various infections were frequently congregated under one roof. There were at this time some 18,000 children in the care of the metropolitan poor law guardians, and it was estimated that about 2,000 of these were eligible for transfer to the Asylums Board. In addition, the Board was instructed to provide for all youthful offenders who were remanded to a workhouse under the 1866 Industrial Schools Act.

II

The M A B children's committee, which was convened to give effect to these instructions, based its policy on the major conclusions of the recent studies of poor law children. Accordingly, two important features of its programme concerned their education and accommodation. First, while the children were undergoing medical care and treatment,

[1] *Report and Evidence of the Departmental Committee on Metropolitan Poor Law Schools*, 1896: BPP, 1896, vol. xliii [Cmd. 8027, Cmd. 8032, Cmd. 8033].
[2] LGB circular to metropolitan guardians of January 1897.
[3] M A B letter to the LGB, 14 March 1897.
[4] LGB order to the M A B, 2 April 1897.
[5] The care of these feeble-minded children has already been discussed in Chapter 14 on mental deficiency.

their schooling was to be continued, according to their capacity, at a standard not lower than that of the schools from which they had come. Secondly, they were to be housed in cottages in groups of ten or twelve.

The projected 'hospital-schools' were the first of their kind, and time was needed for detailed planning and building. Meanwhile, many chronic sick and convalescent children required immediate care in health-giving surroundings. Hitherto, only two poor law authorities in London had attempted to make any special provision for such patients, and their seaside homes were acquired by the Asylums Board. At the end of 1897, St. Anne's Home at Herne Bay, with 134 beds, was opened; and the East Cliff Home at Margate, supplemented by additional blocks to accommodate one hundred patients, was opened the following June. This home was adapted for the treatment of tubercular disease of the joints, spine and glands, from which a large proportion of poor law children suffered. The Paris Municipal Council maintained a similar institution at Berck-sur-Mer, near Boulogne. A site for a third home was acquired at Rustington, West Sussex, and designed as a 120-bed sanatorium for early cases of pulmonary tuberculosis. This institution, known as Millfield, was opened in April 1904 and was the only poor law establishment in the country set apart for the treatment of phthisis.

III

By this time, sites had been acquired at Swanley in Kent and Brentwood in Essex, and hospital-schools had been erected for children suffering from ophthalmia. Each institution provided for 360 children distributed among thirty cottage homes in charge of house-mothers. The homes were divided into groups of three pairs, each group having its own staff block. In addition to a small infirmary and an isolation cottage, each of the two establishments included an ophthalmoscopic room and a bacteriological laboratory. A complete elementary school was also provided, with a non-resident teaching staff. Children, for whom application was made by the guardians, were examined in London by the ophthalmic surgeon in charge of the administration. If found to be in need of treatment, they were sent to the school, where they remained until cured. The general scheme was intended to allow classification on a medical basis and to provide a semblance of family life. White Oak, the Swanley institution, was opened in March 1903, and High Wood at Brentwood received its first patients in July 1904.

Despite the prevalence of ophthalmic disease among poor law children, the M A B hospital-schools were not readily used by the guardians in the early years. There was no statutory provision for the detection of trachoma—the commonest eye disease among the children—and the authorities could not be compelled to transfer any child from their own jurisdiction to that of the M A B. Concerned at the casual methods of selection adopted by the guardians, the Asylums Board arranged in 1913 with the managers of the London district schools for systematic inspections to be undertaken by the M A B ophthalmic medical staff. This procedure was also introduced by special arrangement into some of the extra-metropolitan poor law schools as well as into the LCC elementary schools. Payment was made to the M A B for patients admitted from these sources.

As more infective children were withdrawn from the ordinary schools, the outbreaks of eye disease diminished, and by 1919 it was possible to put the Brentwood establishment to other uses. In 1924, the other ophthalmic institution, at Swanley, was able to receive children suffering from interstitial keratitis, a non-contagious form of eye disease leading frequently to blindness.[1] It had been found that children suffering from phlyctenular keratitis who attended the out-patients' departments of the London voluntary hospitals derived little benefit from the treatment which they were expected to carry out at home, often in difficult conditions. The attention of the Ministry of Health was accordingly drawn to this situation by the British Council of Ophthalmologists. When these patients were admitted to the healthier surroundings of the M A B Swanley school, where corneal affections were skilfully treated, significant improvements were observed. By the conclusion of the Board's term of administration, it had been demonstrated beyond all doubt that its work in the ophthalmic field had been one of the most successful efforts in preventive medicine, in that it had eradicated trachoma from the London schools and had effectively controlled the spread of other forms of chronic conjunctivitis and blepharitis.

IV

Although ringworm was not usually accompanied by any physical or mental disability, children attacked by it had to be withdrawn from school on account of its contagious nature. Victims of this infection comprised the largest section of children suffering from skin and scalp diseases at this time. It was to ringworm cases, therefore, that the Board initially devoted its attention. Accommodation for four hundred patients was provided in two buildings acquired from the South Metropolitan School District, which was on the point of dissolution. Bridge School, at Witham in Essex, was opened in February 1901, and The Downs, Sutton, in February 1903. The principles and methods of management governing the scheme for ophthalmic cases were applied in the ringworm hospital-schools.

The introduction of X-ray treatment in 1905, following successful trials in the Paris municipal schools, aided the cure of ringworm and substantially reduced the duration of stay in hospital. By 1908, it was possible to close the Bridge School, and the work was concentrated at The Downs institution. From there it was transferred to the Goldie Leigh Homes, Abbey Wood, south-east London, rented from the Woolwich Guardians. Originally concerned solely with ringworm, this institution developed until it was treating a score of different diseases of the skin and scalp.

V

The chronic sick and handicapped children assigned to the care of the Asylums Board all formed part of the metropolitan poor law schools population, but the youthful offenders

[1] LGB order to the M A B, 1 July 1924.

were quite distinct. They were not necessarily poor law children and needed only short-term care. Before 1866, children, like adults, were remanded to prison when further enquiries were necessary. In 1866, the Industrial Schools Act decreed that children charged before a magistrate with offences punishable by committal to an industrial school should be kept during remand, not in prison, but in the workhouse.[1] The guardians hitherto had met this unwelcome addition to their duties with inadequate expedients. The Asylums Board, therefore, was charged with the responsibility of providing for these remanded children in surroundings which would shield them from prison and pauper life.

Having ascertained that in the recent past about 3,000 children were remanded annually to the metropolitan workhouses and that the maximum number received at any one time was 273, the Board planned accommodation in three separate homes for 150 children. Before completing their arrangements, however, the Asylums Managers took the precaution of enquiring of the London magistrates whether they would in fact remand children to the M A B homes. The magistrates replied that they could take no share in any scheme 'except it emanated from the Secretary of State for the Home Department'. They were still bound by the 1866 Act, and amending legislation was the only way out of the difficulty. Eventually, on 17 August 1901, the Youthful Offenders Act was passed empowering a court of summary jurisdiction to remand any child or young person 'into the custody of any fit person named in the commitment who was willing to receive him'.[2] In anticipation of this enactment, the M A B children's committee adapted the houses it had purchased in Pentonville Road, Harrow Road and Camberwell Green; and these were opened on 1 January 1902, the day the Act came into force.

Following a practice already instituted in Australia, each remand home was placed under a superintendent and a matron, and arrangements were made for the instruction and occupation of the children. Individual members of the Board took a personal interest in this work and pressed for the reform of penal methods for dealing with young delinquents. With Will Crooks[3] as its chairman, the M A B children's committee steadily advocated the adoption by the legislature of measures aimed at reclaiming the juvenile offender, such as the establishment of separate courts for children and their entire dissocia-

[1] The Industrial Schools Act of 1866 (29 & 30 Vict. c. 118) remained unchanged, but in 1893 it was supplemented by the Reformatory Schools Act (56 & 57 Vict. c. 48), which extended the powers of magistrates for dealing with remanded children.

[2] 1 Edw. 7 c. 20 s. 4 (1).

[3] William Crooks (1852–1921)—Will Crooks, as he was always known—was sent to the workhouse at the age of eight and later to the Poor Law School at Sutton, experiences which left a lasting impression on him and no doubt motivated his interest in under-privileged children. In adult life, he adopted radical ideas and taught and lectured in Poplar. In 1892, he was elected to represent Poplar on the LCC, and when a member of the Poplar Board of Guardians, he represented that body on the M A B. From 1898 to 1907, he served on the M A B children's committee as chairman and vice-chairman. In 1903, he was returned with a huge majority as Labour MP for Woolwich and retained his seat, except for a short period in 1910, until 1921, a few months before his death in June of that year. (*Dictionary of National Biography;* and George Haw, *From Workhouse to Westminster: The Life of Will Crooks, MP.*)

tion from the adult criminal. Most of the committee's recommendations were eventually embodied in the Probation of Offenders Act, 1907[1] and in the Children Act, 1908.[2] Although the separate children's courts recommended by the M A B committee were established, its suggestion that these should be set up informally in the places of detention was not accepted. Nevertheless, a striking measure of progress was achieved through the contributions of the M A B to these enactments, which brought to an end those legal processes for dealing with the young which had remained almost unchanged during the seven decades since Dickens wrote of Oliver Twist and Mr. Fang.[3]

The Asylums Board managed London's first remand homes until 1909. During that year, 2,046 children were received; of these only twenty were from poor law schools. The total number of cases for the year was 4,072, as some children were remanded more than once. Ages ranged from six months to twenty years. Offences included wandering, begging, gambling, residing in a house of ill-fame, prostitution, attempted suicide and, under the 1908 Act, 'in the charge of drunken parents'. Backgrounds were of every type. Of all the remanded children received in the eight years during which the Board managed the homes, the proportion from poor law schools was as low as 0·06 per cent. Ironically, the 1908 Act, which was promulgated largely as a result of the pioneering activities and persistence of the M A B, empowered the central authority to transfer the remand homes from the Asylums Board to the LCC;[4] and this was effected on 1 April 1910.

VI

In 1908, the Asylums Managers were asked to provide for yet another category of children.[5] These were the sick and convalescent in the infirmaries and workhouses of London. The children of this class already in the care of the Board were drawn only from the district schools. The transfer of this new group was not primarily in the children's interests, but in order to relieve pressure on accommodation for the adult sick poor of London. A census taken in April 1907 showed that in the metropolis there were 2,175 sick children under treatment in infirmaries and 205 in workhouses. Of these, 1,627, with 73 epileptics, were classed as mainly medical, and 680 as mainly surgical; 1,655 suffered from acute, and 725 from chronic, illness.[6] Pressure on the guardians' institutions continued relentlessly until, in the autumn of 1908, it was decided to transfer to the care of the Asylums Managers such

[1] 7 Edw. 7 c. 17.   [2] 8 Edw. 7 c. 67.
[3] Charles Dickens, *Oliver Twist* (1838), Chapter 11. See also F. T. Giles, *Children and the Law* (1959), Chapter 1. Before the Children Act of 1908, there were a number of statutes, as Mr. Giles points out, which allowed courts to deal with young delinquents in other ways than imprisonment, but only the more forward-looking and enlightened benches dealt with young offenders in these ways. The others preferred the simple, time-honoured, straightforward methods of the Middle Ages—no matter how immature the culprit—the prison cell and the birch.
[4] 8 Edw. 7 c. 67 s. 108 (12).
[5] LGB order to the M A B, 11 September 1908.
[6] Census of paupers under medical care in 128 unions taken by the LGB on 13 April 1907 at the request of the Royal Commission on the Poor Law: BPP, 1910, vol. liii [Cmd. 5077], p. 550.

sick children as could be removed. This was the prelude to the opening of what later became known as Queen Mary's Hospital for Children.

On the 136-acre site at Carshalton, which the Board had acquired in 1896, a convalescent fever hospital had been erected to accommodate 800 patients.[1] By the time it was completed in 1907, one of the smallpox hospitals had become available for convalescent fever cases and the Southern Hospital—as it was then known—consequently remained unused. It was eminently suitable for the new patients, and in four months it was equipped to accommodate one thousand children and renamed The Children's Infirmary. It included twenty-four double bungalow-pavilions in six groups, with one staff block to each group, two infirmary blocks and administrative buildings. In addition, it was equipped with lecture rooms and accommodation for the probationers of the first M A B training school for nurses. The earliest patients were received at the end of January 1909 and, on 15 May, the formal opening ceremony was performed by the President of the Local Government Board, the Right Hon. John Burns, MP. By the end of the first year, over 2,000 sick pauper children had been admitted, nearly 800 of whom were under three years of age.

In 1910, when King George V and Queen Mary succeeded to the throne, the Children's Infirmary was finally renamed 'Queen Mary's Hospital for Children', to commemorate the event. In 1912, school buildings were erected for ambulant patients and verandahs were added to provide open-air treatment for some three hundred bed patients suffering from non-pulmonary tuberculosis. Later, departments for electro-therapeutics, radiography, and dental and eye diseases were introduced. Other features included a remedial gymnasium, and workshops which produced most of the surgical appliances required. During the early years of Queen Mary's, most of the young patients were of the convalescent or chronic type. Whooping-cough was the only acute infectious disease admitted. On average about 40 per cent of the children were orthopaedic cases; some 30 per cent suffered from non-pulmonary tuberculosis; and the remaining 30 per cent were disabled by other diseases. While the average stay per patient was one year, a large number remained under treatment for four years or more. The hospital possessed the great advantage over most other institutions of being able to keep in-patients almost indefinitely. In time, Queen Mary's became world-renowned as a hospital for general diseases in children and, in particular, for orthopaedic surgery.

During the 1920s, the LCC, which already subsidized a number of beds for non-pauper children in the Board's ophthalmic schools, asked for accommodation at Queen Mary's for children suffering from tuberculosis and from the after-effects of anterior poliomyelitis. In 1926, confronted with the problem of 1,500 children absent from their schools with rheumatic illnesses, the Council asked for a further 350 beds for such cases. Substantial extensions to the hospital became necessary; meantime the LCC children were admitted to the Board's institution at Brentwood.

[1] On completion in 1907, the cost of building the hospital at Carshalton, including road-making, engineering works, etc., was £232,920. A tender for the actual erection of the buildings was accepted at the sum of £176,050. The site cost £13,550.

Throughout 1929, the Board's last complete year, 818 children were in continuous residence at Queen Mary's. The total cost of each child then averaged 46s. a week (of which 6s. 5d. represented the cost of food), compared with 18s. 4d. per week (including 4s. 2d. for food) in 1909, when the hospital opened. At the other M A B children's establishments, costs were slightly lower.[1] When the construction work at Queen Mary's was completed late in 1930—at a cost of some £200,000—accommodation had been increased to 1,250 beds, requiring a staff of 750, including 350 nurses. By this time, the hospital had passed into the hands of the LCC. Beds were no longer differentiated as 'poor law' or 'LCC'; Queen Mary's had become a public health hospital. The Local Government Act of 1929[2] had launched a municipal system of hospital care which was to abolish anomalies such as those evidenced in the work of the M A B.

It was at Queen Mary's that the detrimental effect of the poor law on public health and medical progress had been most apparent. Relatively few of the London voluntary hospitals had special departments for orthopaedic cases.[3] Queen Mary's offered the necessary facilities on an adequate scale in ideal conditions. But no systematic arrangement existed between the voluntary hospitals and the poor law institution, either for the transfer of orthopaedic cases or for the training of students in orthopaedic surgery. In the course of a survey carried out in 1920–22 of the forty-two LCC schools for physically defective children, it was found that there were just under 3,000 cripples on the rolls, 37 per cent of whom were deemed by the orthopaedic surgeon making the survey as being in need of in-treatment in the country.[4] LCC beds at Queen Mary's were limited, and non-pauper parents were deterred from applying for admission through the poor law authorities, as this frequently resulted in the children being retained in the local infirmaries. The lack of public hospital beds for orthopaedic patients and the absence of liaison between the poor law and the voluntary institutions before 1930 in effect deprived hundreds of disabled children in London of a chance of rehabilitation.

VII

One of the reasons why the Board had been charged with the care of sick and handicapped pauper children was the absence of facilities for their instruction whilst unable to attend school. The provision by the M A B of medical care combined with teaching was,

[1] See Appendix IV, Table G, for average numbers and patient-costs at Queen Mary's Hospital and the other M A B children's establishments at different periods.

[2] 19 Geo. 5, c. 17, Part I. For the effects of the Local Government Act on the M A B hospitals, see Chapter 22.

[3] In addition to the Royal National Orthopaedic Hospital, the only other London hospitals having an orthopaedic department in the earlier decades of this century were: St. Bartholomew's, St. Thomas', Guy's, the London Hospital, Great Ormond Street and the Queen's Hospital. Queen Mary's at Carshalton was the only large country institution for the treatment of orthopaedic cases besides the Sir William Treloar's voluntary hospital at Alton.

[4] Report on LCC Schools for Physically Defective Children by Mr. Elmslie, orthopaedic surgeon to St. Bartholomew's Hospital, of 5 December 1922, cited by Dr. W. T. Gordon Pugh in M A B Annual Report for 1922, p. 201, *et seq.*

therefore, in the nature of an experiment. While the medical services for children were the responsibility of the M A B children's committee, schooling in the homes and hospitals was supervised by a special M A B education committee. The medical superintendent of each institution was responsible to the children's committee through the Board's chief medical officer in charge of children's services, while a head teacher, with assistant teachers, was responsible to the education committee. The curriculum was kept as wide as possible and included many varieties of handwork. For children not fit enough to attend classes in the school buildings, teaching was carried on in the wards. Progress in general subjects was tested and reported on periodically, and records kept for the whole period of the patient's stay. Recreation, outings and physical instruction were provided outside teaching hours under the supervision of nurses and instructors. The young patients were encouraged to organize their own entertainments and even the chronically disabled participated in the boy scout and girl guide movements. To further outside interest in the children, the Board sanctioned the appointment of local residents as visitors. As far as possible, an institutional atmosphere was deliberately eliminated from the children's homes and hospitals.[1]

In 1900, the Asylums Managers associated themselves with a representative committee of managers of metropolitan poor law schools in order to press their view that pauper school children should be placed under the jurisdiction of the Board of Education for educational purposes. In so doing, they reasserted the intention of the aborted Government Education Bill of 1896 and anticipated a similar recommendation of the Poor Law Minority Commissioners.[2] In 1905, this objective was achieved and in that year, for the first time, M A B teaching arrangements were inspected by officials of the central education authority. The Board of Education applied to the hospital-schools the regulations and curricula designed for the teaching of children in day schools for the physically disabled. While these were followed reasonably closely in essentials, the M A B children's committee adapted them to suit the different conditions in its own residential establishments. For some twenty years, the Asylums Board restricted expenditure on children's education to 6s. per head per annum, but in 1929 this capitation limit was raised to 7s. By this time, 121 teachers were being employed to give tuition to nearly 2,300 handicapped children.[3] A special committee appointed by the Board of Education in 1908 to enquire into the instruction of pauper children, described the M A B schools as 'remarkably good', 'generously equipped', 'suitably staffed and conducted on the most approved lines', while it assessed the standard of education as 'entirely satisfactory'.[4]

[1] The educational work of the M A B is described in detail in a report on hospital-schools by Dr. W. T. Gordon Pugh appended to M A B Annual Report for 1925–26, pp. 355–59.

[2] *Report of Royal Commission on the Poor Law, 1905–9* (Minority), BPP, 1910, vol. xxxvii, p. 501.

[3] In 1909, head teachers (non-resident) in M A B hospital-schools received up to £120 p.a., while assistant teachers, some of them certificated, received from £50 to £90 p.a. By 1929, the maximum for head teachers was increased to £225, while that for assistants ranged from £108 to £211 p.a.

[4] *Board of Education Report on an Enquiry into the Educational Work in Poor Law Schools* (HMSO), 1 July 1908, p. 8; and *M A B Annual Report*, 1908, pp. 19–20.

VIII

During the greater part of the nineteenth century, preoccupation with industrial progress engendered indifference towards the welfare of the individual in society, particularly of the child. Despite this unprogressive ethos, the M A B directed its efforts towards providing equally for the medical, educational and social needs of the under-privileged children in its care. 'Taking only a sub-division of their work', wrote Local Government Board Inspector Sir Arthur Downes in 1911, 'the Asylums Managers now have under admirable care and with infinite classification approximately four thousand poor law children. . . .'[1] For those of low mental calibre, efforts were directed to developing such potential as they possessed. For the chronic sick and handicapped, medical care[2] and equipment of a high order were provided, while treatment was combined with tuition of a standard not previously accorded to rate-aided children. And with the same forward-looking policy, the Asylums Managers pioneered the reclamation of youthful offenders from the depravation of workhouse, prison and criminal proceedings. In short, the history of child care under the aegis of the M A B illustrates the emergence of the new concern for the welfare of the young, which fructified in both voluntary and statutory action during the first quarter of the twentieth century. As Professor Titmuss has pointed out, 'society was beginning to count and reassess the health costs of industrial progress in terms of the life chances of its next generation. . . .'[3]

[1] Note by Sir Arthur Downes in *Comments on the Proposals for the Reform of the Poor Law* by Charles Booth (1911), p. 16.

[2] The Medical Supplement to this study includes (section IV) references to articles by paediatricians based on their work in the M A B children's institutions.

[3] Richard M. Titmuss, 'Health', in M. Ginsberg (ed.) *Law and Opinion in England in the Twentieth Century*, (1959), p. 304.

CHAPTER 19

Tuberculosis[1]

I

ALTHOUGH phthisis was known in the nineteenth century as the 'morbus pauperum', no special provision was made for the tuberculous poor. Apart from the care of sick children, many of whom were consumptive, the M A B had no statutory concern with the disease until the second decade of the twentieth century, when residential treatment for tuberculosis was included among the benefits provided by this country's first measure of national insurance. From 1912, the Board played an active part in the State anti-tuberculosis crusade.

In Victorian England, 'consumption' was one of the outstanding diseases responsible for high mortality. Through the researches of Villemin[2] and Koch,[3] its infectious nature was established in 1865 and the tubercle bacillus was isolated and identified in 1882. By the turn of the century, public opinion was aroused to the necessity for preventive action. The National Association for the Prevention of Tuberculosis had been formed in 1898, and in the following year appeared one of the most valuable contributions to the subject— *The Prevention of Consumption* by Robert Philip, pioneer of the social approach to the problem.[4] In 1901, the British Congress on Tuberculosis met in London, and in the same year a Royal Commission was appointed to study the relationship of the disease in animals and man.[5]

---

[1] Background material for this chapter has been drawn from: C. Fraser Brockington, *Short History of Public Health*, Chapter XIV; J. H. Harley Williams, *A Century of Public Health in Britain*, Part III; and Sir Arthur Newsholme, *Fifty Years in Public Health*, Chapters XXVIII and XXX; and, *idem*, *The Last Thirty Years in Public Health*, Chapters XIV and XV.

[2] Jean Villemin, a French Army surgeon, clearly demonstrated the communicability of tuberculosis in 1865.

[3] Robert Koch, a German Jewish physician, discovered the *bacillus tuberculosis* in 1882 as the essential cause of phthisis, destroying the old theory of constitutional peculiarities and establishing the possibility that tuberculosis was preventible.

[4] See Sir Robert W. Philip, *Collected Papers on Tuberculosis* (OUP, 1937). Robert Philip, the Edinburgh physician, in promoting the social aspects of tuberculosis prevention, launched the first dispensary, the Victoria Dispensary for Consumption, in 1887. This focus of all preventive and curative agencies was the model upon which dispensaries were later founded in the national organization against tuberculosis.

[5] Reports of the Royal Commission on Tuberculosis for 1904, 1907, 1909 and 1911: BPP, 1904, vol. xxxix, 129 [Cmd. 2092]; 1907, vol. xxxviii, 1 [Cmd. 3322]; 1909, vol. xlix, 365 [Cmd. 4483]; and 1911, vol. xlii, 173 [Cmd. 5761].

The concern of the metropolis was voiced by a conference of parochial authorities convened in July 1900 'to consider the advisability of special accommodation being provided under the management and control of a metropolitan authority for the treatment by "open-air methods" of phthisical patients chargeable to the metropolis'. When it was put to the M A B that it should provide the necessary sanatoria, the guardians were informed that the Board would be ready to consider the matter if there should be a general request from the metropolitan local authorities.

In April 1905, the M A B received a deputation representative of a number of interested bodies, including the Society of Medical Officers of Health and the Royal Institute of Public Health. The Board was urged to make provision for isolating and treating the consumptives of London, of whom seven to eight thousand died every year, primarily because they found difficulty in securing admission to hospital. It was suggested that the Metropolitan Poor Act of 1867[1] and the Public Health (London) Act of 1891[2] should be made applicable to pulmonary phthisis and thereby empower the Asylums Board to take the necessary action.[3] After consulting sixty-nine metropolitan local authorities and the governors of hospitals for consumptives, the Asylums Board requested the central authority to offer its judgment on the deputation's suggestion. In March 1906, the Local Government Board replied that the matter had been given careful consideration but that the information submitted did 'not appear to afford sufficient justification for the very heavy outlay which would be involved in the proposal'.[4]

Even at this date, tuberculosis was not a notifiable disease in London,[5] so that it would have been difficult to assess the number or class of patients likely to require treatment. Further, in these pre-national insurance days, it was unlikely that breadwinners suffering from incipient phthisis would have been willing to submit to prolonged hospital treatment. Another objection to unilateral action in the metropolis was the risk of consumptives flocking to the capital from other parts of the country to obtain treatment at the expense of London ratepayers. Apart from these considerations, the reluctance of the Asylums Board to press the matter further stemmed from its conviction that tuberculosis presented a problem of such magnitude that it demanded government intervention on a national scale.

II

Five years later, Lloyd George's National Insurance Act of 1911 set in motion the State anti-tuberculosis campaign. 'Sanatorium benefit' was a particular feature of the

---

[1] 30 & 31 Vict. c. 6 s. 5.   [2] 54 & 55 Vict. c. 76 s. 80.
[3] M A B Mins., vol. xxxix, 1905, p. 95.   [4] LGB letter to the M A B, 22 March 1906.
[5] Certain towns in England had a scheme of voluntary notification of tuberculosis as early as 1899, but it was not until 1903 that notification was first made compulsory in Sheffield by means of a private bill. In 1908, the LGB, using its powers under the Public Health Acts, issued regulations requiring compulsory notification of all cases which came under the poor law medical officers. Public Health (Tuberculosis) Regulations of 1912, which consolidated earlier regulations, required universal compulsory notification of all forms of tuberculosis.

workers' insurance scheme inaugurated by this enactment.[1] Provision was also made under the Act for the domiciliary treatment of insured consumptives by their panel doctors; for the building of tuberculosis institutions; and for research into the disease. The Insurance Committees—a new series of local authority which administered the medical provisions of the Act—were empowered to make arrangements for the treatment of workpeople insured under the Act and also, if they thought fit, of their dependants. This was to be done by negotiation with 'persons or local authorities (other than poor law authorities)' who managed approved sanatoria.[2] The qualification 'other than poor law authorities' was a last-minute addition to section 16 (1) of the Act, doubtless intended to emphasize the fact that the new insurance principle was completely dissociated from public assistance. The special position in London of the M A B hospitals for infectious diseases seems to have been overlooked. For the past twenty years, the Board had controlled some 8,500 isolation beds, which had been available to the whole metropolitan community without distinction and without reference to poor law procedure. Furthermore, the Board was already providing for nearly 2,000 sick children, 48 per cent of whom were tuberculous.

Before the 1911 Act became operative in July 1912, it had become increasingly clear throughout the country that any effective scheme for the eradication of tuberculosis must be comprehensive. Only about one-third of the population would be covered by the 1911 Act. In February 1912, a Departmental Committee—The Astor Committee—was appointed to report on a general policy for dealing with tuberculosis; and two months later it presented an interim report.[3] The need for comprehensive schemes to be worked out by the major local authorities was the essence of its recommendations. As regards London, it was suggested that consideration might be given to the possibility of the M A B providing some of the required accommodation. The Committee estimated that the number of beds needed under a national prevention scheme would be about one to every five thousand of the population. On this basis it appeared that nine hundred to one thousand beds would be required for London. The Local Government Board agreed generally with the Committee's findings, and in May 1912 sent out a circular urging the county and county borough councils to formulate schemes for the treatment of tuberculosis. Whether by design or oversight, the London County Council was the only major local authority in the country which failed to receive the circular. The whole matter was thus left in the separate hands of the metropolitan borough councils, with no provision for co-ordination.

On the eve of the appointed day, provision in London for sanatorium benefit was not impressive. The LCC—of a political complexion different from that of the Government—felt slighted. The M A B, assuming that it was the proper authority to make sanatorium

---

[1] 1 & 2 Geo. 5 c. 55 s. 8 (i).

[2] Ibid., ss. 16 (1) and 17.

[3] *Departmental Committee on Tuberculosis* (Chairman, Mr. W. Astor) *Interim Report, 1912*, BPP, 1912–13, vol. xlviii, 1 [Cmd. 6164]; *Final Report*, 1913, ibid., 29 [Cmd. 6641].

provision in London, was incensed by its exclusion from the scheme and the implication of section 16 (1) of the 1911 Act that its hospitals were 'tainted with pauperism'. In July 1912, the Asylums Board presented a memorandum to the Local Government Board emphasizing the fact that, if effect were to be given to the provisions for sanatorium benefit in London on a large scale in any reasonable time, it could only be done by utilizing existing machinery and institutions. The Asylums Board was willing to find the accommodation required.[1] During the same month, a conference of metropolitan borough councils resolved that the provision of sanatoria should be entrusted to the M A B. Owing to the paucity of alternative accommodation in London—as in the country generally[2]—this seemed the obvious arrangement. The Local Government Board was in a quandary. In October 1912, it informed the Asylums Board and the LCC that legislation to enable the M A B to participate in a London scheme for sanatorium provision could not at that time be obtained. Nevertheless, 'it was hoped that by some friendly arrangement the community would have the benefit of the proved experience and organized administration of the Board'.[3]

In December 1912, the Local Government Board made its peace with the LCC. A nominal grant of £10 was made to the Council in order to bring it within the scope of the financial arrangements applicable to sanatorium authorities under the 1911 Act.[4] The Council was then asked to submit a plan for the whole metropolis, which would weld into one co-ordinated and harmonious scheme the existing authorities—the Council itself, the Insurance Committee, the M A B and the borough councils, together with the voluntary hospitals and dispensaries. In the course of further discussions between the Council and the Local Government Board, it was confirmed that the LCC was the metropolitan tuberculosis authority, with responsibility for ensuring that the necessary accommodation was available. 'Much of this', the Local Government Board suggested, 'could, no doubt, be economically and efficiently provided by the M A B. . . .'

Meantime, in order to circumvent the statutory exclusion of the M A B from the prevention scheme, a tripartite agreement was concluded in November 1912 whereby the London Insurance Committee arranged for the provision of accommodation with the LCC, which in turn negotiated with the Asylums Board. Five hundred tuberculosis beds were thus made available at the M A B Downs Sanatorium, Sutton, and the Northern Hospital, Winchmore Hill. There is little doubt that the prompt participation of the Asylums Board in this circumlocutory procedure minimized the confusion which existed in London at the outset of the anti-tuberculosis campaign, a state of affairs which the Charity Organization Society sought to unravel by instituting an enquiry on its own

[1] M A B communication to the LGB, 14 July 1912.
[2] On the eve of the passing of the 1911 National Insurance Act, there were only about 1,300 beds available for tuberculosis cases in local authority institutions in the country and 4,200 in 84 voluntary sanatoria. (Sir Arthur Newsholme, *International Studies on the Relation between the Private and Official Practice of Medicine* (1931), Vol. III, p. 226.) The Astor Committee estimated that about twice that number would be required.
[3] LGB letter to the M A B, 19 October 1912, a copy of which was sent to the LCC.
[4] LGB letter to the LCC, 11 December 1912.

account.[1] Some time later, Mr. John Burns, President of the Local Government Board, endeavoured to lubricate the creaking machinery by declaring in the House of Commons that, 'thanks to the public spirit of the M A B, tuberculous insured patients in the London sanatoria have been provided with treatment . . . to which no criticism can be wisely or fairly directed.'[2]

Within a year, the Board's institutions had treated some 2,000 insured patients, but in so doing they had been acting *ultra vires*, as they had done during the smallpox epidemics of their early days. From the outset, the Asylums Board had persistently impressed upon the Government the need for promoting legislation to regularize its participation in the London 'sanatorium benefit' scheme. With the support of the LCC parliamentary committee, it succeeded in securing an amendment to the 1913 National Insurance Act. This empowered the Board to make provision for insured tuberculous patients and their dependants through agreements with any county or county borough council. Further, the Act specifically decreed that, for this purpose, the Asylums Board was not to be deemed a poor law authority.[3] Not for the first time had the status of the M A B been hybridized by statute.[4]

It still remained, however, for the Board's position to be clarified so far as provision for uninsured patients was concerned. In July 1912, as a result of representations by the County Councils' Association, the Government had agreed to bear half the cost of treating both the uninsured and the dependants of insured workers for whom it was already liable under the 1911 Act. Any comprehensive scheme for residential treatment of tuberculosis in the County of London would have to include these classes. The M A B was not yet legally in a position to receive uninsured persons, and, apart from sick children who happened to be tuberculous, it had no specific authority to provide for the numerous patients suffering from tuberculosis in the poor law infirmaries of London. Of these there were, at this time, some 2,300 chronic and advanced cases, 86 per cent of whom were uninsured persons.

In 1913, the Public Health (Prevention and Treatment of Diseases) Act was passed. This statute, which saw the beginnings of the country's tuberculosis services, empowered local authorities—in accordance with the Astor Committee recommendations—to formulate tuberculosis schemes and to put into operation such plans as were authorized by the central authority.[5] This provision, coupled with the sanction accorded to the

---

[1] *The Prevention and Treatment of Tuberculosis in London.* Report by the Charity Organization Society (1913).

[2] *Hansard*, 1913, vol. liii (5th series) col. 1916 (Mr. Burns).

[3] 3 & 4 Geo. 5 c. 37 s. 39.

[4] Under enactments 46 & 47 Vict. c. 35; 52 & 53 Vict. c. 56; 54 & 55 Vict. c. 76; 3 & 4 Geo. 5 c. 28; and 3 & 4 Geo. 5 c. 37, the poor law status of the M A B had been waived in respect of particular functions.

[5] 3 & 4 Geo. 5 c. 23 s. 3. Concerning public health, county councils hitherto had been merely federations of existing local sanitary authorities. By the Public Health (Prevention and Treatment of Disease) Act, 1913, the county council was created an authority for executing the orders of the LGB with regard to the prevention of 'cholera or any other . . . infectious disease'. The Act also empowered county councils, or any sanitary authority, to make arrangements, approved by the LGB, for the treatment of tuberculosis.

Asylums Board by the Public Health (London) Act of 1891 to admit non-pauper patients into its isolation hospitals,[1] enabled the M A B to make arrangements for the institutional care of uninsured tuberculous persons.[2] In 1914, in the exercise of its new powers, the LCC delegated to the M A B its responsibility for making arrangements with the County Insurance Committee for sanatorium treatment for insured persons and their dependants. The Council also obtained Local Government Board approval of its comprehensive scheme for the whole County. This provided that M A B tuberculosis beds, already eligible for insured patients, should be used also for the uninsured. Thus, at the outbreak of World War I, the Asylums Board had been brought into the national tuberculosis scheme as a fully-fledged public health authority.

III

During the first part of the war, the M A B was providing some six hundred tuberculosis beds—about five hundred in hurriedly converted and unsuitable buildings and one hundred in the London fever hospitals. In order to double this number, the Board purchased sites at Godalming, East Grinstead and Ellisfield, near Basingstoke, on which to erect three modern sanatoria. For the building of new tuberculosis institutions throughout the country, £1,500,000 had been made available under the National Insurance and Finance Acts of 1911.[3] Subject to certain limitations, the Local Government Board provided three-fifths of the capital outlay on sanatoria. Owing to higher wartime priorities, however, the building of the new M A B institutions had to be shelved. Nevertheless, in accordance with its powers under the 1913 National Insurance Act, the Asylums Board concluded agreements with local authorities outside London to receive tuberculosis patients, including ex-service men. On average, some 2,500 cases were admitted annually to the M A B sanatoria and hospitals during the war years.

After the war, the LCC and the County Insurance Committee negotiated concerning the assumption of responsibility by the Council for the provision of residential accommodation for insured persons. The Council's pre-war comprehensive scheme had provided that such an arrangement might be concluded, if desired by the Insurance Committee. In 1919, this transfer was effected, together with the handing over of responsibility for ex-service patients. The agreements concluded between the M A B and the Insurance Committee also came to an end. In this way, the LCC became responsible for the residential treatment of all persons suffering from tuberculosis in the County—insured and uninsured, adults and children, civilians and ex-service men; and it made this provision by

---

The local authority schemes formulated under this enactment included the appointment of tuberculosis officers and of nurses for home visiting; dispensaries for early diagnosis; after-care committees on a voluntary basis; and sanatoria in increasing numbers.

[1] 54 & 55 Vict. c. 76 s. 80.   [2] LGB letter to the M A B, 24 September 1913.

[3] Financial provision for capital outlay in connexion with the acquisition by local authorities of tuberculosis sanatoria was made by the National Insurance Act, 1911, section 64 (1) and by the Finance Act, 1911, section 16 (1) (b).

arrangement with the M A B and other authorities willing to provide the accommodation. Most of the other local authorities in England and Wales had been similarly engaged in taking over from the Insurance Committees responsibility for tuberculosis provision. This was the prelude to the cessation of sanatorium benefit under the national insurance scheme.

During the years in which sanatorium benefit was provided, the cost of treating patients was defrayed from Insurance Committee funds so far as insured persons and their dependants were concerned, and by government and insurance funds so far as ex-service men were concerned. The maintenance of all other patients was aided by an Exchequer grant amounting to half the net deficiency between the total cost of carrying on the sanatoria and the amounts received from Insurance Committees and any other sources. In London, the outstanding deficiency was met by the Asylums Board in the same way as its other commitments—by precepts upon the metropolitan poor law authorities. No grants were received in respect of tuberculous poor law patients, who remained a separate category in health administration until the dissolution of the destitution authorities in 1930.

Under the National Insurance Act of 1920, sanatorium benefit ceased to be included among the benefits conferred by Part I of the 1911 Act.[1] From 1 May 1921, Insurance Committees no longer had the duty of providing in-patient care for tuberculosis cases, which now became the responsibility of county and county borough councils. From the same date, contributions payable under the Acts no longer included payment towards the cost of institutional treatment. Insured patients retained the right to domiciliary attendance as a medical benefit, but shared the entitlement of the rest of the community to sanatorium treatment as a social service under the local authorities. And so ended the brief but significant association of tuberculosis sanatorium provision with the national insurance principle.

In order that the transfer of responsibility should be as smooth as possible, the Public Health (Tuberculosis) Act of 1921 conferred statutory sanction upon the administrative arrangements already agreed between the Local Government Board and the major local authorities.[2] The financial arrangements of the administering authorities were not significantly changed save that the Exchequer grants were extended to cover the additional responsibility incurred by the authorities in the absence of insurance funds. Since the publication of the Astor Committee Reports in 1912 and 1913, most of the local authorities had been putting its recommendations into practice. In addition to adequate sanatoria and hospitals, these included the provision of dispensaries for diagnosis and treatment, and the organization of educational work and after-care. Under the 1921 Act, their implementation became a statutory duty, so that in each local authority area there developed a unified system for the prevention and treatment of tuberculosis.

[1] 10 & 11 Geo. 5 c. 10 s. 4. This provision (cessation of sanatorium benefit) did not apply to Ireland.
[2] 11 & 12 Geo. 5 c. 12. Of the 145 major local authorities in England and Wales, 124, including the LCC, had already made their arrangements before the passing of the 1921 Act.

IV

In London, the system was not as unified in practice as elsewhere. Lacking institutions of its own, the LCC was obliged to rely largely on the M A B for the residential care of tuberculosis patients. The Asylums Board made available such beds as it was called upon to provide, and retained the administrative and financial control of the sanatoria entirely in its own hands. This was resented by the Council, which feared an encroachment on its public health preserves. Shortly after the co-ordination of central health services, following the Ministry of Health Act, 1919, the LCC formulated a scheme for centralizing all the London health services under its own control as part of a 'Greater London' plan. To justify taking over all the functions of the M A B, the Council cited the institutional arrangements for tuberculosis and complained of the potential inconvenience of its having to rely on the goodwill of another authority over which it had no direct control. The LCC conceded that 'this important body has certainly performed its duties very efficiently', but emphasized that the constitution of the Board had 'long been considered anomalous' and that it had become 'increasingly difficult to determine where the domain of the Council should end and that of the M A B should begin'.[1] The imperialistic designs of the LCC had no immediate effect on the M A B, and events set in motion by post-war reconstruction, including the Ullswater Commission on the Government of Greater London (1921–23),[2] saved the Board for another decade from annexation by the LCC.

Meantime, the tuberculosis branch of the M A B hospital empire steadily developed. The first addition after the war was the Pinewood Sanatorium at Wokingham, which was taken over fully equipped and staffed in June 1919. This institution, standing in 82 acres of wooded grounds on the Upper Bagshot Sands, had been established originally by voluntary effort. In 1898, it had been acquired by the National Association for the Prevention of Tuberculosis shortly after its formation, at a meeting convened at Marlborough House by the Prince of Wales (later King Edward VII). Pinewood, first used for eighty male patients, was subsequently enlarged to accommodate twice that number. Later in 1919, the Board purchased the Hendon Infirmary from the City of Westminster guardians. This institution, standing on a site of some 27 acres, was renamed the Colindale Hospital and opened in January 1920. Eventually, it was extended to accommodate some 350 patients. For surgical cases, the Board purchased and adapted the Empire Hotel at Lowestoft, which was renamed St. Luke's Hospital and opened in 1922 for about 200 cases. This was followed shortly by the opening of the King George V Sanatorium, which had been erected to accommodate some 230 patients on the Godalming site purchased during the war.[3] In addition to medical treatment, the patients at King George's—

[1] *Report of the LCC Committee on Health Administration in London*, dated 31 October 1919 (adopted by the Council on 19 December 1919).

[2] See Chapter 22.

[3] The King George V Sanatorium was the Board's only purpose-built tuberculosis institution. The other M A B establishments for tuberculous patients had been acquired and adapted. Following the War, as a result of the findings in 1919 of an inter-departmental committee, the Treasury made grants to stimulate

nearly all male pulmonary cases—were provided with light manual work and suitable industrial training. Later, a treatment and training centre was experimentally established at the Sanatorium for convalescent female patients from other M A B tuberculosis institutions. After a period of from six to twelve months' treatment and probationary nursing or domestic work, the 'trainees' were appointed as ordinary members of the Board's sanatorium staff. In 1926, an institution in Lee, south-east London, was acquired from the Greenwich guardians and adapted for about 320 male patients. This became known as the Grove Park Hospital. For ex-service men suffering from advanced pulmonary tuberculosis some 150 beds were set aside in four of the Board's London fever hospitals. For children, the Princess Mary's Hospital had been built during the war on the site of East Cliff, Margate, the former children's home. In addition to this accommodation for 270 surgical patients, more than 500 beds were devoted to similar cases at Queen Mary's Hospital, Carshalton, while the children's institutions at Rustington and Brentwood were reserved for pulmonary cases.

By 1929, there were nearly 22,500 tuberculosis beds in the whole of England and Wales. One-third of these were provided by voluntary organizations, while the remainder were in local authority institutions.[1] These included 2,700 M A B beds, most of them in nine special establishments.[2] During the last quinquennium of the Board's administration (1924–29), approximately 4,500 tuberculosis patients were admitted each year. In 1929, some £254,000 was spent on maintaining a daily average of nearly 2,000 sanatorium patients. Based on a net expenditure, the weekly cost per patient in 1929 averaged 43s. 10d., compared with 28s. during the early part of the war (1915).[3]

The national anti-tuberculosis scheme had worked relatively smoothly in London once the initial difficulties had been resolved. In large measure, this had been due to the enthusiastic co-operation of the M A B. Nevertheless, the disadvantages of separating the social and clinical aspects of control had been brought into relief. The involvement of the Asylums Board in the prevention campaign had further demonstrated that a 'two-nations' system of health administration was an anomalous impediment to any scheme of socialized medical care.

---

the immediate construction of new sanatoria at the rate of £180 per bed, subject to a maximum of three-fifths of the total cost. (See *Hospital Gazette*, November 1919, p. 24.)

[1] Sir Arthur Newsholme, *International Studies* . . ., op. cit., Vol. III, p. 226. The total of 22,500 tuberculosis beds excludes those in voluntary *general* hospitals.

[2] For details of M A B tuberculosis institutions, see Appendix I, Table VI, section C.

[3] See Appendix IV, Table H, for tuberculosis patient-costs in selected years. (Rates, taxes and semi-capital expenditure are excluded from these calculations.) For an analysis of revenue expenditure in M A B sanatoria, see Appendix IV, Table D.

CHAPTER 20

The Homeless Poor

I

ALTHOUGH the M A B was primarily a hospital authority, it was by origin a central poor law authority for London. The 1867 Metropolitan Poor Act had decreed that 'asylums' might be provided under the Act, not only for the infectious sick and the insane, but also for 'other classes' of the rate-aided poor.[1] The Asylums Board was thus liable to be called upon to administer relief outside the spheres of curative and preventive medicine. Shortly before World War I, the need for a centralized relief agency was nowhere more apparent than in connexion with those social castaways collectively known to the poor law as 'casual paupers'. On one night in February 1910, a census disclosed that there were some 6,600 homeless persons in London's parks and streets. Together with the occupants of licensed common lodging houses and casual wards the total exceeded 25,000.[2]

In 1912, the Asylums Board was therefore entrusted with the administration of all the casual wards of London, hitherto the responsibility of some thirty separate boards of guardians. While a 'casual pauper' was defined in law as 'any destitute wayfarer or wanderer applying for or receiving relief . . .',[3] the genuine wayfarer was found in very small numbers amongst the itinerant poor seeking relief. The problem presented by London's hordes of homeless persons, and the systematic attempts of the M A B to resolve it, were inseparably bound up with the history of vagrancy as a whole.

II

The early statutes of labourers, enacted in the times when serfdom was collapsing, show the attempts to deal with vagrants as runaway slaves breaking the law which fixed their wages, place of residence and work; and it was not long before they came to be looked upon as potential criminals. The modern history of the subject begins with an Act of 1495,[4] under which local authorities were bidden to search for all 'vagaboundes idell and suspecte

[1] 30 & 31 Vict. c. 6 s. 5.
[2] M A B Annual Report for 1912, Appendix IX (Casual Wards Committee Report), quoting statistics of the census of homeless persons in London, taken by the MOH to the LCC on the night of 14 February 1910.
[3] 34 & 35 Vict. c. 108.   [4] 11 Hen. VII c. 2.

223

persones lyvying suspeciously', to put them in the stocks for three days, giving them bread and water only, and then to turn them out of the township. From time to time during the next three hundred years, legislation aimed to combat vagrancy by sternly punitive measures. According to the preambles of some statutes, these were necessitated by 'the increase of vagrancy and the consequent increase of crime and disorder' (1530),[1] or by previous legislation not having had 'that success which hath byn wisshed' (1547).[2] This Act of 1547 provided the punishments of branding and slavery for those who would neither work nor 'offer themselves to labour with anny that will take them according to their facultie'. Such penalties, however, may not have been regarded as unduly severe in an age when larcenies exceeding one shilling in value were punishable by death and when repeated attempts had already been made to establish a system for the correction and re-formation of the vagrant, on the one hand, and for the relief of the aged and infirm, on the other. An Act of 1597 required the Justices to build and equip houses of correction, to be used in addition to the county goals for vagrants, while transportation was devised as a means of ridding the country of 'sturdy beggars and idle and disorderly persons'.[3] New definitions of the vagrant are found early in the eighteenth century, when the offence was no longer merely the vagrant mode of life but his chargeability to the poor rate, particu-larly of a parish in which he had no settlement.[4]

By the nineteenth century, the vagrancy law had become extraordinarily complicated; twenty-seven of the forty-nine Acts of the preceding three hundred years were still in operation. An Act consolidating this legislation lasted little more than one year,[5] and was replaced by the Vagrancy Act of 1824 'for the punishment of idle and disorderly persons and rogues and vagabonds'.[6] This enactment, which was almost entirely a measure of repression, had the effect of raising the number of vagrants committed to prison from about 7,000 in 1825 to nearly 16,000 in 1832. The period after 1824 was notable for the steady recognition of the principles first formally stated by the 1832–34 Poor Law Com-mission, which made it clear that the growing burden of vagrancy would only be reduced if the relief given to vagrants was such as only the really necessitous would accept; that no diminution could be effected unless the system were general; and that no enactments to be executed by parochial officers would be rigidly adhered to in all parishes unless under strict control. The Poor Law Act of 1834, nevertheless, made no special reference to vagrants, since the primary duty of the guardians was regarded as the provision of relief for the destitute within their district. But the necessity for dealing with the poor who came in from other localities soon established itself. The Poor Law Commissioners accordingly instructed guardians to keep vagrants in a separate ward of the workhouse, and to set

[1] 22 Hen. VIII c. 12.   [2] 1 Edw. VI c. 3.   [3] 39 Eliz. c. 4.

[4] 17 Geo. II c. 5. This enactment, which prescribed punishment for vagrants who became chargeable to a parish in which they had no settlement, empowered quarter sessions to order a public whipping and im-prisonment for six months for any woman wandering and begging who was delivered of a child in a parish to which she did not belong (section 25). The whipping of women was abolished by 32 Geo. III c. 45 s. 3.

[5] 3 Geo. IV c. 40.   [6] 5 Geo. IV c. 83.

them to work on prescribed tasks.[1] When the Poor Law Board succeeded the Commissioners in 1848, reports were received from the inspectors concerning the consequences of the lack of uniformity and the laxity in the treatment of vagrants. Thereupon, the attention of guardians was drawn to the necessity for repressing the growing evil of vagrancy and the importance of exercising greater discrimination in administering relief to the itinerant poor.[2] In 1871, the Pauper Inmates Discharge and Regulation Act[3] sought to clarify the duties of the destitution authorities concerning the detention and dietary of casual paupers, while in 1882 the Casual Poor Act[4] amended these provisions and imposed more deterrent conditions for persistent applicants. This was followed by General Orders issued by the Local Government Board in 1882, 1887 and 1897.[5] Both men and women vagrants were required by these orders to work three hours for one night's lodging and nine hours for each entire day of detention. Tasks for men included oakum-picking, stone-breaking, digging, wood-cutting and corn-grinding; quantities were specified according to the period of detention. Women also picked oakum or were given tasks of washing, scrubbing or needlework. As regards diet, the regulations provided that 'persons over 7 years of age' detained for one night should be given supper and breakfast, each consisting of 6 ozs. of bread with 1 pint of hot gruel containing not less than 2 ozs. oatmeal, or of hot broth. The midday meal of those detained for more than one night consisted of 8 ozs. of bread and $1\frac{1}{2}$ozs. of cheese or 6 ozs. of bread and 1 pint of soup. Children under 7 years were given $\frac{1}{2}$ pint of milk for each period of 8 hours. Those under 2 years were allowed an additional $\frac{1}{2}$ oz. of sugar, and those between 2 and 7 were given 4 ozs. of bread and $\frac{1}{2}$ oz. of cheese.[6]

These legislative and administrative measures for controlling the relief of the homeless poor applied throughout the country. But in London supplementary schemes for establishing vagrant asylums had been formulated by the central poor law authority in 1845 and 1857, although they were never carried into effect.[7] Another, and more successful,

---

[1] General Order to Poor Law Guardians, 1842, and 5 & 6 Vict. c. 57 s. 5.

[2] PLB Minute to Poor Law Guardians, 4 August 1848.

[3] 34 & 35 Vict. c. 108.   [4] 45 & 46 Vict. c. 36.

[5] LGB General Orders to Boards of Guardians, 18 December 1882, 3 November 1887 and 4 May 1897.

[6] In 1866, a dietary for vagrants was prescribed for the first time by the central authority, but the order had reference only to London. In that regulation, the pint of gruel for supper for all persons above 9 years of age was withdrawn from March to September in each year. (Poor Law Board Annual Report, 1866–67, p. 37.)

[7] Poor Law Amendment Act, 1844 (7 & 8 Vict. c. 101 s. 41) authorized the formation of districts in London and certain other large towns for the provision of 'asylums' for the temporary relief and setting to work of the destitute homeless poor. Accordingly, in 1845 the Poor Law Commissioners prepared a scheme of districts in the metropolis for this purpose but it met with considerable opposition. In 1846 a Select Committee of the House of Commons was appointed to enquire into the manner in which the Poor Law Commissioners had exercised their powers under this enactment. The Committee took a mass of evidence but expressed no opinion on the question submitted to it. The evidence attributed the increase in vagrancy largely to the action of the Commissioners in issuing instructions in 1837–39 which resulted in workhouse masters relieving *all* applicants, whether destitute or not. Evidence pointed strongly to the harmful effects and the increase of vagrancy which might be expected from the building of asylums for the homeless.

attempt to deal with vagrancy in London was made in 1864 by the Houseless Poor Act. Following a recommendation of the 1861–64 House of Commons Select Committee on Poor Relief,[1] this enactment required that metropolitan guardians should provide casual wards for vagrants in the capital and that the cost of maintaining these refuges should be a common charge on the whole of the metropolis.[2]

In 1904, the President of the Local Government Board, Mr. John Burns, appointed a departmental committee to study the whole question of vagrancy. This included representatives of the Local Government Board, the Home Office and the Prisons Commission. Reporting in 1906, the committee emphasized the need for central control and uniform administration, and proposed that casual wards throughout the country should be placed under the police authorities. This was no new idea. It had been suggested first in 1848, and revived in 1871 on the introduction of the Pauper Inmates Discharge and Regulation Act. But it was discarded on the grounds that it might divert the police from their other duties and that it would involve considerable expense. The departmental committee made other important recommendations concerning diet, detention, offences, labour colonies and assistance to work-seekers.[3]

Concerning the metropolis, the committee commented on the relatively high cost of some casual wards. During 1903, daily expenditure per inmate had averaged 1s. 8½d., and in one ward it had reached 4s. 9d. So far as concerned detention and tasks, there existed no uniformity whatever. Twenty-eight wards were administered by so many boards, each with a different opinion on some point or another. In consequence, vagrants flocked to certain London wards where detention and work were not enforced. In 1904, of the 21,000 refusals to admit on account of want of room at various wards in London, two-thirds occurred in five wards.

No action was taken on the committee's recommendations pending the deliberations of the 1905–9 Royal Commission on the Poor Law. Meanwhile, the numbers of the homeless poor continued to rise, particularly in London. The first major innovation resulting from the committee's report was the issue on 10 November 1911 by the Local Government Board of the Metropolitan Casual Paupers Order. This constituted the Asylums Board the sole authority in London for the relief of the itinerant destitute. In effect, the control and management of all the casual wards of London were centralized under the hospital authority.

III

On 1 April 1912, the twenty-eight metropolitan wards ceased to be administered by the guardians. All except four, which were integral parts of workhouse structures, were transferred to the M A B. The main principle of the Board's policy was that, for the relief of

[1] *Report of the Select Committee on Poor Relief*, 31 May 1864: BPP, 1864, vol. ix (349), 187.
[2] 27 & 28 Vict. c. 116. See Chapter 2, p. 22, note 2.
[3] *Report of the Departmental Committee on Vagrancy*, 1906: BPP, 1906, vol. ciii, p. 1.

vagrants, London should be administered as a homogeneous whole, in strict conformity with existing statutory regulations. At the same time, no effort was to be spared to assist helpable cases to become self-supporting. The system of unification produced immediate results. The annual census of homeless people in London, which for some years had been conducted by the LCC Medical Officer of Health during one night in February, showed that on 14 February 1913—nine months after the centralization of the metropolitan wards—these centres admitted only 546 applicants, a reduction of 50 per cent on the nightly average of the past two years. On the same census night, those found sleeping out and loitering in the streets numbered 1,200, again 50 per cent of the average of census-night figures since 1904. This was accompanied by no increase in casual pauperism in adjacent areas, nor in the numbers of those sleeping in London's licensed common lodging houses, which, at about 21,000, remained approximately the same as for the two previous census-nights.[1]

In the history of vagrancy, with each new measure of control, numbers had fallen, only to rise again until the next repressive enactment. The initial decrease following centralization under the Asylums Board, however, was maintained up to and during World War I. In 1914, daily admissions to the metropolitan casual wards—which had been reduced to nine—fluctuated between 160 and 300, according to season, while the homeless found in the streets and shelters on the census-night of February 1914 numbered less than 550. During the war, casual ward admissions rarely exceeded 100 a day and in July 1919 they declined to a record low daily average of 24. Later, with the economic depression, numbers rose again to as high as 800 a day at the end of 1927.

When the Asylums Board was first entrusted with the administration of the casual wards, vagrancy in London had long been a growing and notorious evil, largely attributed to indiscriminate charity and maladministration by the poor law authorities. The complexity of the problem stemmed from the heterogeneous character of the casual pauper population. In effect, the itinerant destitute comprised four broad categories, the ratio of each to the whole varying according to social conditions. First, there were the *bona fide* working men in search of employment. The 1904–6 departmental committee estimated that this type then represented less than 3 per cent of the whole. Secondly, there were those who undertook casual labour for a short time but were incapable of sustained work and tended to degenerate into habitual vagrants. Thirdly, there were the elderly and infirm who clung to their liberty, preferring a sequence of casual wards to the workhouse. Fourthly, there were the hardened 'professional' beggars, systematically avoiding work in an endeavour to live parasitically on the community. Detection of the habitual vagrant was aided by the M A B central register of casual ward admissions and the rigid enforcement of the statutory regulations prescribing detention and work for persistent applicants to the wards. Superintendents telephoned their admission lists each morning to the Board's head office, and, after these had been compared with the central register, they were told which vagrants to detain. During the Board's first eight months, some 22,000 identifications were made in this way, compared with 20,000, the annual average of previous years during which

[1] M A B Casual Wards Committee Report, op. cit.

Local Government Board visiting officers haphazardly called at the wards in search of occupants whom they recognized.

Towards the end of 1912 a discriminatory method of granting relief and temporary shelter was evolved by the M A B setting up a central 'clearing house' for casuals, known as the 'Night Office'. The scheme was devised by the metropolitan poor law inspectors' advisory committee on the homeless poor, which had formerly assisted the President of the Local Government Board. Following the transfer of the wards, the committee co-opted the chairman and one other senior member of the Asylums Board and continued as an advisory body. The Night Office was intended to secure that every person loitering or sleeping out in London should have the offer of lodging and food for the night. Police on duty between 10 p.m. and 2 a.m. carried tickets which they handed to persons found without shelter. These contained directions to apply to the Night Office, which was situated on the disused steamboat pier near Waterloo Bridge. (At the end of 1921 this centre was transferred to the Charing Cross Railway Bridge.) Here the case of each applicant was considered. The Board's staff were in telephonic communication with all the metropolitan casual wards and with the Salvation Army, the Church Army and other voluntary organizations which had agreed to participate in the scheme. According to the discretion of the director of the Night Office (a former casual ward superintendent who knew many of the *habitués*), applicants were directed either to a charitable institution or to a casual ward and furnished with an admission ticket specifying the destination. During the first month of operation (November 1912), when the system was something of a novelty, some 3,500 tickets were issued by the police, and 3,000 recipients applied to the Night Office. About 2,000 of these were directed to casual wards, but more than half did not use their admission tickets. Of the 900 or so applicants who were offered beds in voluntary institutions, more than 100 failed to reach their destinations. During the ensuing months, the numbers receiving tickets from the police fell significantly but the pattern of refusals remained very much the same. Following World War I, the monthly average of applicants to the Night Office ranged between 1,200 and 1,600, and these were distributed fairly evenly between the casual wards and the voluntary institutions. The elderly and infirm were assisted to accommodation in guardians' institutions, and women, alone or with children, were nearly always directed to voluntary organizations. Only one ward (Southwark) offered beds for women, but most wards provided beds for couples. Before the war, from 10 to 20 per cent of wayfarers were women, only a few being accompanied by children. In 1929, of 73,250 admitted to the casual wards of London during the year, upwards of 2,500 were women and 100 were children.[1]

Extending its practice of classification and discriminatory treatment, the Board opened a hostel in 1923 where helpable cases genuinely seeking employment might reside in conditions less restricted than in the wards. Between 1924 and 1929, 1,000 to 2,500 such cases were admitted annually. Those discharged to situations obtained by the Board, direct or through labour exchanges, rose from 300 in 1924 to nearly 1,000 in 1929.[2]

[1] M A B Annual Report, 1929–30, p. 59.   [2] Ibid., p. 39.

During its eighteen years' administration of London's casual wards, the Asylums Board approached the age-old problem of vagrancy by procedures hitherto untried. Classification and discrimination, tempered by humanity and reason, were the basic principles of the system. Structurally and administratively, the casual wards were improved; the dietary was revised; newspapers were provided; and the old tasks of a deterrent character, such as stone-breaking, were almost entirely abandoned. The occasional were differentiated from the habitual vagrants; the irreclaimable were deterred, while the resources of voluntary and statutory services were co-ordinated to assist such as could be helped to a better way of life.

Both the Majority and Minority Reports of the 1905–9 Royal Commission on the Poor Law had recommended that the functions of boards of guardians should be exercised by authorities having jurisdiction over wider administrative areas. The centralization of London's casual wards under the M A B was the sole attempt in twenty years to implement that recommendation. When, in 1929, the Local Government Act fundamentally altered the administration of the poor law in this direction all over the country,[1] the centralization of casual pauper relief in London reached its second milestone. After 1930, the system initiated by the Asylums Board was continued with little change under the LCC. In 1935, a consultative committee was added under the chairmanship of the Council's chief officer of public assistance, Sir Allan Powell, formerly Clerk to the M A B. In the same year a new welfare office was opened and administered on the lines of the former 'Night Office'.

The administration of London's casual wards by the M A B from 1912 to 1930 marked the end of the six-century-old policy of repression and its replacement by the practice of rehabilitation. It also represented a significant step towards the national system of relief for the homeless. The 'casual ward' and the 'vagrant' have been replaced by the 'reception centre' and the 'wanderer without a settled way of living'.[2] The problem of the vagrant has been reduced but not resolved: an intractable core survives to defy the 'Welfare State'.

[1] 19 Geo. 5 c. 17, Part I.
[2] 11 & 12 Geo. 6 c. 29 s. 17 (1).

CHAPTER 21

War-Work, 1914–1919

A STUDY of the Asylums Board would be incomplete without a reference to its contribution to the war effort between 1914 and 1919. During this period, a number of M A B institutions were requisitioned by the War Office for military purposes. Chief among these were the fever hospitals at Woolwich and Tooting—the Brook and the Grove. The Brook War Hospital—as it was called—was enlarged to accommodate 1,000 service patients; and, with eight auxiliary institutions for convalescent cases, it treated over 30,000 sick and wounded between September 1915 and November 1919. The Grove Military Hospital, with some 550 beds, admitted another 21,000 patients from every field force and theatre of war between February 1917 and September 1919. Special sections of the hospital were earmarked for infectious diseases, tubercle of the lung, skin, scabies and venereal cases.[1] Both the Brook and the Grove remained under the direction of the Board's senior staff. The Southern (Lower) Hospital—formerly part of the convalescent smallpox hospital at Darenth—was lent to the War Office in 1915 for the use of enemy sick and wounded. Later in the war, the Southern (Upper) Hospital and the M A B North-Eastern Hospital at South Tottenham were placed at the disposal of the United States military authorities, who retained the M A B medical superintendents as representatives of the American Red Cross.

By the middle of 1915, some 90,000 civilian hospital beds throughout the United Kingdom had been made available for sick and wounded service men.[2] About one-third of these were in carefully selected poor law infirmaries,[3] and another 6,500 were in M A B fever hospitals and sanatoria.[4] This depletion of the Board's isolation hospitals service, however, led to no serious inconvenience for sick civilians. Except in the autumn and winter of 1915–16, the incidence of acute infectious diseases in the metropolis—as in the country generally—was comparatively low throughout the war period.[5] As Professor Richard

---

[1] Particulars of the diseases treated in the M A B war hospitals may be found in M A B Annual Report, 1919–20, pp. 49–50.

[2] For details concerning the mobilization of civilian hospital beds in the U.K. during World War I, see B. Abel-Smith, *The Hospitals, 1800–1948*, Chapters 16 and 17, *passim*.

[3] *Poor Law Officers' Journal*, 2 July 1915, p. 783.

[4] M A B Annual Report, 1919–20, op. cit.

[5] *Ministry of Health First Annual Report*, 1919–20 [Cmd. 923], pp. 30–31.

Titmuss has pointed out, 'the privations and calamities attendant upon war' have been 'held at bay' on more than one occasion when this country has been engaged in hostilities.[1]

In addition to lending beds for service men, the M A B was called upon to accommodate and organize destitute enemy aliens. A workhouse belonging to the Holborn guardians was taken over for this purpose and opened in August 1914. In all, nearly 400 internees, mostly Germans and Austrians, were admitted and cared for until this work was transferred to the military authorities before the end of the year.

The principal war-work undertaken by the M A B, however, was the provision and management of institutions for war refugees. When Belgium was invaded by Germany, it was expected that those seeking asylum would arrive in such large numbers that the task of providing for them would be beyond the powers of any voluntary organization. Early in September 1914, therefore, the Asylums Board was invited to undertake the work. This was organized by a committee consisting of the Chairman, Vice-Chairman and Clerk to the M A B,[2] and administered by officials of the Board. The nucleus of the staff was drawn from its regular service and supplemented by voluntary helpers.

All preliminary arrangements were made to receive the first influx of refugees at the Crystal Palace on the evening of 4 September 1914. When they arrived, however, it was found that it had been commandeered by the Admiralty, unknown to the Local Government Board, who had placed it at the disposal of the M A B. Immediately, the search for alternative accommodation began. A number of buildings, most of them former workhouses and casual wards, were requisitioned. Some had been unoccupied for a considerable time and lacked equipment and essential services. However, by the evening of the following day, they had been made habitable. The exiles were all registered on arrival; an employment exchange was set up to deal with those for whom work could be found; a military bureau under the Belgian military authorities enrolled those suitable for army service; and representatives of the War Refugees Committee arranged for those requiring hospitality in the country.

In mid-September 1914, the Alexandra Palace was taken over, equipped to receive 4,000 refugees, and placed under the direction of the Board's principal medical officer, Dr. H. E. Cuff. From its opening until after the fall of Ostend a month later, a great stream of refugees passed through the Palace at an average rate of 500 a day. When the refugee ship *Amiral Ganteaume* was lost in the Channel on 26 October 1914, nearly 2,000 survivors were admitted after midnight. By the time the Palace closed in March 1915, it had dealt with 32,000 refugees in all.

The Earl's Court exhibition buildings were also placed at the Board's disposal. These premises, covering thirty acres intersected by two railways, were taken over on 15 October 1914 immediately following the close of the summer exhibition, when they were still cluttered with the general paraphernalia of booths and show cases. These were removed,

[1] Richard M. Titmuss, *Problems of Social Policy* (1950), pp. 529–31 and note 4, p. 531.
[2] Mr. (later Sir) Woolley Walden, chairman of the M A B; the Very Rev. Canon Sprankling, vice-chairman; and Mr. (later Sir) Duncombe Mann, Clerk to the Board.

staff and equipment brought in, and by the evening of the same day upward of 1,500 refugees were received, fed and housed. The strain of the first few days caused the medical officer in charge to suffer a breakdown in health, and Mr. (later Sir) Allan Powell, who was then Assistant Clerk to the Board, took over and managed the refugee centre for the duration. Eventually, accommodation for some 4,000 persons was provided at Earl's Court. The Empress Theatre alone, under a single-span roof, supplied dining accommodation for over 3,000 in the arena, as well as beds for 1,400 in the dismantled seating galleries.

By the end of October 1914—less than three months after the declaration of war—the M A B was maintaining over 12,000 refugee beds.[1] It was at first assumed that only temporary housing would be required pending the distribution of the exiles throughout the country, but it soon became apparent that a more permanent settlement would be needed for large numbers who could not be placed elsewhere. For the remainder of the war, the Earl's Court 'Refugees' Camp' fulfilled the double function of receiving arrivals requiring temporary accommodation and of providing for 'settlers'. In addition to Belgian and French civilians, the first category included army recruits and allied soldiers en route for the front or on leave from the army. Later, when the Russian débâcle began, provision was made for large numbers of soldiers and civilians who had been in Russia and were being repatriated through England. These included people of almost every allied race, particularly French, Italians, Serbians and Poles.

The medical, spiritual and recreative needs of the refugees were provided for; suitable buildings were adapted as places of worship, schools, nurseries, hospitals, laundries and workshops. Schooling for 600 resident children was organized in the Earl's Court Camp, as well as evening classes for the adults. Munitions and other works were installed in which large war contracts were undertaken, while women's workshops produced army clothing. The resident workers received wages which, allowing for the cost of maintenance,

[1] The following institutions were used by the M A B for the accommodation of refugees during World War I:

Institution	Number of Beds	Opening Date	Closing Date
Poland Street Workhouse, Oxford Circus, London, W.	800	5 Sept. 1914	16 Sept. 1914
Hackney Wick Casual Ward	200	6 Sept. 1914	30 May 1916
Silver Street Workhouse, Edmonton	1,200	7 Sept. 1914	2 May 1918
St. Giles' Home, Endell Street, London, W.C.	1,000	9 Sept. 1914	3 Dec. 1914
Alexandra Palace	4,000	14 Sept. 1914	29 March 1915
St. Anne's Home, Streatham Hill, London, S.W.	500	12 Oct. 1914	31 March 1916
Millfield House, Edmonton	450	14 Oct. 1914	28 Sept. 1916
Earl's Court Exhibition	4,000	15 Oct. 1914	7 July 1919
M A B Park Fever Hospital, Lewisham	800	16 Oct. 1914	27 Oct. 1914
St. Marylebone Casual Ward	95	22 Oct. 1914	16 Oct. 1915
War Refugees' Hospital and Dispensary, Sheffield Street, London, W.C.	40	3 Feb. 1915	7 June 1919
Surrey House, Wandsworth	20	1 July 1916	7 June 1919

equalled outside rates. Many thousands were placed in outside work, after training; and over 5,000 were recruited from the Camp for the Belgian Army.

A measure of classification was attempted. Cases requiring more supervision and control than was possible in the general refuges were accommodated in institutions in Edmonton which had been acquired for the M A B mental health service. Of this 'difficult' class, 12,000 refugees passed through the hands of Dr. D. L. Gordon, medical superintendent of the Fountain Hospital, who administered the Edmonton institutions. For refugees of the professional class, a separate hostel was maintained in association with the Earl's Court Camp.

Towards the end of the war, 1,200 refugees from Russia arrived in England. They had been in contact with smallpox, so were isolated at the Board's Joyce Green Hospital, where only two cases eventually developed. After a few weeks they joined the other refugees at Earl's Court. Following the armistice, the Earl's Court Camp served as a depot in connexion with the repatriation of some 100,000 refugees from England.

On the whole, singularly little difficulty was experienced concerning the health of the refugees. Serious cases were sent to the nearest infirmary, while infectious cases were admitted to the Board's fever hospitals. For those who were billeted in the London area, a 40-bed hospital and a dispensary were opened in Sheffield Street, off Kingsway, London. In all, about 70,000 visits of out-patients were recorded.

Among the unsung victories of World War I must be included the successful resolution of the countless difficulties involved in providing asylum for the allied exiles. Apart from the sheer weight of numbers, obvious problems were inherent in the composition of the refugee population: civilians and soldiers of various nationalities; a continuously changing sector on the one hand, and a restless, resident sector on the other. Staff shortages, food rationing, and a dearth of labour and materials to maintain the acres of decaying temporary structures added to the stress.

Numerous visitations were received from eminent personages, who bestowed encouraging commendations upon the work. The Duchess of Vendôme, sister of the, then, King of the Belgians, described the Earl's Court Camp as 'une vraie cité de charité'. To the task of governing this 'city of charity', the Asylums Board had brought its accumulated experience and expertise in the service of the sick and needy. For nearly half a century, as its coat-of-arms appropriately proclaimed, the motto of the M A B had been: *Miseris succurrere disco.*

CHAPTER 22

Dissolution

D ESPITE its unique position in the metropolis and its extensive public health functions the M A B was jettisoned with the rest of the country's destitution authorities, as a result of the Local Government Act of 1929. Although the Board's fate might appear, at first sight, like death by misadventure, a closer look at general social trends and contemporary local events suggests that liquidation was almost unavoidable.

The creation of new social services since the early years of the century[1] had expanded the province of public health and reduced the scope of the poor law. The 1834 relief administration had become increasingly inappropriate, and demands for the dispensation of public assistance in fresh forms had grown out of a clearer understanding of the aetiology of poverty. In London, especially, administrative reform was long overdue. By 1929, the poor law was being administered in the capital by twenty-five boards of guardians, four school boards and the Asylums Board—more than nine hundred members, in all, operating a system based on the illusion that 'the poor' were a separate, homogeneous sector of the community. At the same time, advance by the M A B into the public health field had provoked an imperialist LCC to prepare for annexation. On the one flank, therefore, the Asylums Board was threatened by the general trend towards a radical reform of the poor law, and, on the other, by the growing demand for the unification of London's local government.

During its first thirty years, the Board's development had depended to a large extent on the outcome of its conflicts with the central authority, but, during the second half of its lifetime, its struggle for survival was influenced mainly by its relationship with the LCC and by the deliberations of the various royal commissions and departmental committees appointed to investigate poor law or local government reform.

As early as 1908, the Royal Commission on the Care of the Feeble-Minded had sounded the death-knell of the M A B by specifically recommending the transfer of its mental institutions to the LCC.[2] This was in no way a reflection on the Board's management of

---

[1] The social services of the early twentieth century included old age pensions; national insurance against unemployment, sickness and invalidity; and gratuitous domiciliary and institutional treatment for tuberculosis.

[2] *Report of the Royal Commission on the Care and Control of the Feeble-Minded*, 1908: BPP, 1908, vol. xxxix [Cmd. 4202], Recommendation xcvi, p. 360.

the mentally afflicted. The Commissioners commended the M A B as 'a progressive and efficient local lunacy authority' with 'a very clear and enlightened policy'. Nevertheless, they applied indiscriminately to London the scheme which they had formulated for the rest of the country, namely, that the existing lunacy authorities—the county and county borough councils—should be responsible also for the care of the mentally deficient.[1] The fact that the M A B had provided effectively for the harmless chronic insane of London for the past four decades appears to have carried less weight with the Commissioners than the appeal of administrative tidiness.

A few months later, in February 1909, the M A B was made aware again of the uncertainty of its future by the conclusions of the Royal Commission on the Poor Law.[2] The general denunciation of parochial administration in both the Majority and Minority Reports spelt doom to all existing destitution authorities. After decrying the incapacity of boards of guardians to provide adequately for the young, the sick, the mentally defective and the aged, the Minority Commissioners declared that 'no alteration in the membership, no change in the constitution, no enlargement in the area would remedy the defects that now stand revealed'. The Asylums Board had supplied the Commission with detailed information concerning its forty years of specialized work on behalf of these deprived groups.[3] Nevertheless, it was obliged to share in this sweeping condemnation. The Minority Commissioners were wholly at variance with their colleagues on the fundamental issue as to whether the dispensation of relief should be divided between various semi-independent committees or entrusted to one separate body; and, in furtherance of their objective to 'break up' the poor law, they urged the former plan.

The Majority Commissioners were more favourably disposed towards the M A B. They affirmed that 'the Metropolitan Asylums Managers have efficiently discharged as a central body for London the task entrusted to them'. What was needed, they suggested, was 'a disinterested authority practised in looking at all sides of a question, especially when it is a family rather than one individual that requires rehabilitation'. They even discussed the possibility of a transformed M A B becoming the future poor law authority for London, but eventually decided in favour of a statutory committee of the LCC. Neither of the reports, therefore, provided the Asylums Board with much assurance.

The greatest measure of support for the survival of the M A B was contributed by one of the Majority Commissioners, Dr. (later Sir) Arthur Downes. As senior medical inspector of the Local Government Board for poor law purposes, Dr. Downes had materially assisted in improving relations between the Asylums Board and the central authority, and had familiarized himself with the detailed working of the Board's institutions. In a separate memorandum, Dr. Downes declared that the defects in poor law administration which

---

[1] See Chapter 14.

[2] *Reports of the Royal Commission on the Poor Law*, 1905–9: BPP, 1909, vol. xxxviii: Majority Report, p. 1 *et seq.*; Minority Report, p. 719 *et seq.* [Cmd. 4499].

[3] *Minutes of Evidence of the Royal Commission on the Poor Law*, BPP, 1909, vol. xl [Cmd. 4684], pp. 334–66.

had been indicated could be remedied by a strengthening and an extension of existing powers, on lines already established. For London, which presented an exceptional problem, he accordingly advocated one central and independent authority. He was convinced that the organization of relief could be combined effectively with the administration of asylums and hospitals, as both these were essentially instruments of public relief. Fever hospitals and ambulance services in London, he pointed out, had been administered admirably by such an authority, and the arrangement admitted of many advantages which otherwise could not be secured, such as the scientific application of principles of administration, the development of a trained and organized service, the control of finance, contracts and supplies, and the adaptation of accommodation according to the needs of the time.[1]

Following the publication of the Poor Law Commission's reports, divided counsels persisted. One school of thought was led by Charles Booth, the Liverpool shipowner who had conducted a scientific study of London's poverty.[2] In a series of pamphlets, he elaborated the principles which he had submitted to the Poor Law Commission during the period in which he was a member.[3] Instead of dividing the classes to be provided for between different committees, he advocated independent authorities administering various types of relief in enlarged areas, which would be formed by the adequate grouping of existing unions. These enlarged districts would be extended still further by combination, according to the subject treated. His plan for the whole country involved nineteen 'combinations', or regions, and fifty-four groups. He cited the M A B as having prepared the way for such a plan. In a preface to one of Charles Booth's pamphlets, Sir Arthur Downes pointed out that this regional principle had been the keynote of the 1867 Metropolitan Poor Act, and urged that no final decision concerning future legislation should be arrived at 'without a careful examination of the more than forty years' experience of the departure then taken by Mr. Gathorne Hardy'.[4]

As history has shown, poor law reform was neither rapid nor revolutionary. After twenty years, it was the Minority Report of the Poor Law Commsision which made the greater impact upon the Statute Book. Meantime, the Board's fears of immediate annihilation were dispelled as the area of its responsibility was widened to include the care of sick children, tuberculous patients and the homeless poor.[5] With its recruitment into the war effort,[6] its continued existence seemed assured, at least for the duration.

---

[1] Memorandum by Dr. A. Downes, BPP, 1909, vol. xxxvii, p. 674 *et seq.*

[2] Charles Booth, *Life and Labour of the People in London* (17 vols.: 3rd edn. 1902–3).

[3] Charles Booth, *Poor Law Reform* (1910); *Reform of the Poor Law by the Adaptation of the existing Poor Law Areas and their Administration,* 'being a further consideration of the proposals contained in a memorandum included in the *Report of the Royal Commission on the Poor Law* (Appendix vol. xix)' (1910), BPP, 1910, vol. li, 217 [Cmd. 4983]; and *Comments on Proposals for the Reform of the Poor Law,* with Note by Sir Arthur Downes (1911). Charles Booth had been a member of the 1905–9 Royal Commission on the Poor Law but had resigned for health reasons before it completed its work.

[4] Charles Booth, *Comments on Proposals . . .* op. cit., p. 16.

[5] Chapters 18, 19 and 20.

[6] Chapter 21.

At the height of the war, however, the threat to the Board's survival was unexpectedly revived. In 1917, with the problems of the post-war period in view, a committee of the Ministry of Reconstruction was appointed to study the better co-ordination of public assistance in England and Wales and other matters affecting the system of local government. With Sir Donald Maclean as chairman, its members included Lord George Hamilton, chairman of the 1905–9 Commission on the Poor Law, with Sir Samuel Provis and Mrs. Sydney Webb representing its Majority and Minority, respectively. The Committee took no evidence and based its conclusions generally on the recommendations common to the Commission's two main reports. These were adopted unanimously and published in 1918.[1] So far as the Asylums Board was concerned, the Committee dismissed it in a line, proposing that its work should be transferred to the LCC. All poor law guardians were to be abolished without delay and their functions merged with those of the major local authorities. Seven years later—in 1925—the Committee's recommendations were accorded a resolution of approval by the House of Commons.[2] At this time implementation was inopportune.

Meanwhile, such uncertainty as the Board might have entertained for its future was allayed by proposals of various reconstruction committees, supported by the House of Commons, for the creation of subordinate legislatures within the United Kingdom.[3] A parliament for federal London would have involved the formation of one or more central organizations for the administration of relief and public health matters. In this event, the M A B confidently assumed that it would be invited to perform either or both of these functions.

In 1919, the LCC—possibly also with a metropolitan parliament in view—pressed for an urgent enquiry by the Government for the purpose of determining the services which should be brought under a single Greater London administration. The memorandum, which was drawn up by the Council as a basis for discussion by an independent tribunal, outlined a future province of London which would include the five home counties. For this area, all local government matters, including health, were to be controlled by one authority.[4] This document was followed closely by another setting out a scheme of health administration and management of residential institutions in the new London province. The LCC was to be the statutory authority for health services throughout the enlarged County, with power to organize and supervise the services for which the borough councils

[1] Ministry of Reconstruction, Local Government Committee. *Report on the Transfer of Functions of Poor Law Authorities in England and Wales*, 1918; BPP, 1917–18, vol. xviii, p. 529 [Cmd. 8917].

[2] *Hansard*, vol. 184, 5th series, col. 1532 (Mr. Neville Chamberlain, 27 May 1925).

[3] The proposed creation of subordinate legislatures within the United Kingdom was the subject of (a) a resolution of the House of Commons in 1919 (*Hansard*, 4 June 1919, 5th series, col. 2126); (b) the Conference on Devolution presided over by the Speaker in 1919 (BPP, 1920, vol. xiii, 1151 [Cmd. 692]); (c) the Report of the Consultative Committee of the Ministry of Health on the post-war provision of medical and allied services, presided over by Lord Dawson of Penn (Ministry of Health, Cmd. 6937, 1920); and (d) the Interim Report of the Departmental Committee on Unhealthy Areas (Ministry of Health, June 1920, p. 4).

[4] Report of the LCC Local Government, Records and Museums Committee on *A 'Greater London' Administration*, adopted by the Council on 21 October 1919 (LCC Publication 2024).

were to remain responsible. The recommendations included the transfer *en bloc* to the Council of all the M A B institutions and their 'highly competent staff'. The report conceded that 'it would probably be desirable that the Council should have the benefit of the experience in hospital management of some of the members of the M A B'.[1]

The Asylums Board, on the contrary, considered that this would not be at all desirable. It pointed to the impracticability of the administrative work of the fifty M A B residential institutions, with their 16,000 patients and 9,000 staff, being undertaken by the Council, particularly as it planned, in addition, to take over from the metropolitan guardians twenty-four infirmaries containing some 15,000 patients; thirty-one homes and schools, with a population of about 12,000; and thirty-eight workhouses, accommodating nearly 38,000 inmates. The experience of the M A B had proved that it was by the personal interest of a large body of representatives, who were prepared to give the greater part of their time to this special work, that the welfare of the patients was secured and the efficient management of the institutions maintained. The Board could only view with apprehension and uncertainty the inclusion of this work with that of the general municipal duties of the Council. As an alternative to the LCC proposals, the Asylums Managers suggested that the metropolitan borough councils and the LCC should be represented on the M A B, and that its name should be changed to one more clearly indicating the nature of its work.[2]

In 1921, as a result of the representations of the LCC, a Royal Commission, with Lord Ullswater as its chairman, was appointed to study the need for alterations in the local government of London. Despite its distinguished membership, the Ullswater Commission has been described as 'an unmitigated fiasco', largely on account of the feebleness with which the LCC presented its case.[3] All the Council could offer as evidence in support of the proposed appropriation of the functions of the M A B was 'the obvious advantage . . . in getting rid of another authority'.[4] In the absence of any claims that greater efficiency or economy would be secured or that the public would be better served, the advantage was not obvious, and the M A B representatives made this plain when giving evidence. Deprecating the LCC's plan to assume additional functions, they suggested that the M A B should be entrusted with any further institutional work which it might be decided to centralize. The LCC mental hospitals, for instance, might appropriately be transferred to the M A B mental health sevice. In the Board's opinion, the only way of governing the proposed province of London would be by an overall legislative body, with district councils to deal with purely local government affairs, and central administrative authorities to control public utility services, education, health and public assistance. These authorities would be composed of directly-elected, co-opted and centrally-nominated members. Such a plan, the Board's representatives submitted, would bring new methods to the solution

[1] LCC *Report on Health Administration in London*, 31 October 1919, adopted by the Council on 19 December 1919.

[2] M A B Annual Report, 1920–21, Appendix B, pp. xl–xlvii.

[3] W. A. Robson, *The Government and Misgovernment of London*, Chap. XIV (1939).

[4] *Minutes of Evidence of the Royal Commission on the Local Government of Greater London* (1923), Part I, QQ.334–39.

of a unique problem.[1] The implication was, of course, that the M A B should be the central administrative authority for health and, or, poor relief. The Commission appeared impressed by the Board's evidence, which was described as 'particularly helpful'. In rejecting the LCC proposals for a Greater London authority, the Majority Commissioners, reporting in 1923, recommended no change so far as the work of the M A B was concerned.[2] Once more the Board's chances of survival were in the ascendant.

No further cause for concern occurred until the beginning of 1926, when Mr. Neville Chamberlain, Minister of Health, invited the M A B to comment on a draft circular which he proposed to address to boards of guardians in England and Wales, apprising them of provisional plans which entailed their liquidation.[3] In London, it was proposed that the powers and duties of the M A B and of the parochial authorities should be transferred to the LCC, which was to assume responsibility for all London health services, including those of the borough councils. By deputation and written communication, the Board played every card it held in a desperate attempt to persuade the Minister of Health that London's public health institutions were of sufficient importance and extent to justify their control by a fully representative central body endowed with statutory powers.[4] The views of the Board were duly acknowledged, and no more was heard concerning its destiny for another two years.

In February 1928, however, the M A B was granted what purported to be a four-year reprieve. The Minister of Health invited the Board to undertake for this period the administration of the Metropolitan Common Poor Fund.[5] The following month, it was empowered to perform this function by the Local Government (Emergency Provisions) Act.[6] The position of the M A B was buttressed once again.

Hopes were sustained for but a few weeks. An unexpected announcement was made by the Chancellor of the Exchequer, the Rt. Hon. Winston Churchill, when he introduced his 1928 budget. The government had decided to legislate for the de-rating of industrial premises in order to help industry and reduce the heavy unemployment from which the country was suffering. This was to be combined with a measure for the revision of local government, which would involve the abolition of poor law guardians and the transfer of their duties to county and county borough councils.[7]

Within a year, these proposals had become law. So far as the Asylums Board was concerned, the Local Government Act of 1929 decreed that its functions should be transferred

[1] Ibid. Evidence of the Chairman and Clerk to the M A B, Part VI, p. 917 *et seq.* and M A B Annual Report, 1921–22, pp. 48–49.

[2] *Report (Majority) of the (Ullswater) Royal Commission on the Local Government of Greater London*, 1921–23: BPP, 1923, vol. xii, Part I, p. 567 [Cmd. 1830].

[3] Letter from the Ministry of Health to the M A B, 4 January 1926.

[4] Letter from the M A B to the Ministry of Health, 2 May 1926; M A B *Mins.*, vol. lx, 1926, pp. 107–8.

[5] For details of the circumstances leading to this arrangement, see Note on the Metropolitan Common Poor Fund, Appendix IV.

[6] 18 & 19 Geo. 5 c. 9.

[7] *Hansard*, vol. 216 (5th series), cols. 843–53 (Mr. Winston Churchill, 24 April 1928).

to the LCC on 1 April 1930.[1] When the Bill was being debated in the House of Commons. the operation of the 'guillotine' precluded any discussion of the provisions relating to London, as the whole of this section was passed *en bloc* in a few minutes. Consequently, no reference whatever could be made to the work of the M A B. Members of the Board had to content themselves with Mr. Neville Chamberlain's explanation of the reasons for their dissolution. The M A B, he pointed out, derived its membership from the poor law guardians; as these were being abolished, the need consequently arose for a change in the Board's constitution. But Parliament could not be asked to set up another authority in London since the LCC had expressed its willingness to undertake the Board's work.[2]

It would have been difficult to convince the dedicated members of the M A B that London's public hospitals would be managed better by an LCC committee than by an *ad hoc* hospital authority with six decades of experience behind it. In separating health policy from the poor law, the 1929 Local Government Act empowered major local authorities throughout the country to provide 'curative hospitals for the general public', appropriating poor law beds for that purpose. Despite its unique public hospital provision, London was made no exception to the new national pattern. The M A B was liquidated, not because it no longer served its purpose efficiently, but because it was constitutionally anachronistic. By origin, it was a poor law authority and was thus part of the parochial system which was creaking under the economic stresses of the time. Further, the Asylums Board was an *ad hoc*, undemocratically constituted body. For about a century, the complexities of London local government had encouraged the creation of *ad hoc* bodies as an easy solution to administrative problems. But, as the efficiency of local government came to depend more upon the closer co-ordination of public and social services, there were definite drawbacks in having such bodies functioning in isolation. Furthermore, the M A B was composed of members who were nominated either by the central authority or by local boards of guardians. Since 1888, when the LCC was created in succession to the undemocratically elected Metropolitan Board of Works, it had developed an elaborate system of democratic government which had worked demonstrably well for four decades. An indirectly elected, *ad hoc* body, which did not fit into this pattern, was unlikely to be tolerated indefinitely. The economic foundering of the centuries-old poor law thus enabled the LCC to annex a vast, ready-made network of hospital and allied services, and permitted the central government to divest itself of the direct responsibilities it had assumed by its initial incursion into the field of institutional medical care.

The 'take-over' was effected relatively smoothly owing to previous collaboration between the M A B and the Council. There were no complications concerning areas of jurisdiction, since the administrative County of London was almost identical with the Metropolitan Asylum District.[3] The expertise of the Asylums Board in hospital manage-

---

[1] 19 Geo. 5 c. 17, Part I, s. 18 (e).   [2] M A B Annual Report, 1928–29, p. 29.

[3] The area of the administrative County of London was almost the same as that which was given to the Metropolitan Board of Works under the Metropolitan Management Act, 1855 (see Robson, op. cit., p. 164 and Chapter VI). The Metropolitan Asylum District, created in 1867, comprised the unions and parishes

ment and relief was not entirely lost; the Council co-opted a number of the Board's leading members on to the committes concerned with public assistance and public health, and recruited some of the senior M A B officials to administrative appointments.

On Saturday, 29 March 1930, the sixty-third anniversary of the Royal Assent to the 1867 Metropolitan Poor Act, the M A B held its final meeting, presided over by its last chairman, the Viscount Doneraile.[1] Described by the Minister of Health, the Rt. Hon. Arthur Greenwood, as 'in many ways the most remarkable local government body in the world',[2] the M A B passed into history on 1 April 1930, with its unfortunate name still unchanged. On that day the LCC commanded over 76,000 beds.[3] Some 24,000 of these were inherited from the Asylums Board. In all, the M A B empire comprised fifteen infectious disease hospitals, with nearly 9,000 beds; ten tuberculosis sanatoria, with over 2,000 beds; an epileptic colony and five mental institutions providing for over 9,000 patients; and five hospital-schools for nearly 2,000 sick children; as well as two pathological laboratories, an antitoxin establishment, and two ambulance systems—for road and river.[4] By 1 April 1932, the five M A B institutions for the mentally ill and subnormal became part of the LCC mental health service. The other M A B remedial institutions, together with most of the London poor law infirmaries, were brought under the control of the Council's Public Health Department,[5] while the M A B hospital-schools were absorbed into the LCC school medical service.[6]

'The effects of the Act upon the organization of public medical and institutional services', affirmed the Ministry of Health in its sixteenth annual report, 'have been nowhere more strikingly illustrated than in London, and nowhere upon so great a scale'.[7] The response of London to the 1929 Act was, in effect, the direct outcome of that landmark in its social history, the Metropolitan Poor Act of 1867, which initiated the erosion of the poor law and the founding of this country's first State hospitals.

---

within the metropolis as defined by the 1855 Act (Poor Law Board Order of 15 May 1867). This statute took as its area the metropolis as defined by the Registrar-General for the purposes of the Bills of Mortality (see Robson, op. cit., p. 57).

[1] Chairmen and other senior members and officers of the M A B are listed in Appendix I, Document V.

[2] Speech by the Minister of Health on the occasion of a farewell dinner for members of the M A B, held at the Hotel Victoria on 20 March 1930.

[3] LCC publication No. 3657, *The LCC Hospitals: a Retrospect* (1949), Appendix II. The *actual* number of beds under the control of the LCC on 1 April 1930 was 71,771 (op. cit., p. 12). The total number of beds 'certified' in each institution by the Ministry of Health and approved by the Board of Control (mental beds) totalled 76,539.

[4] See Appendix I, Document VI, following, for details of the M A B institutions at the time of their transfer to the LCC. The total number of beds *transferred* totalled 22,572. The total bed complement for which the M A B institutions were 'certified' at the time of the transfer was 24,137.

[5] Concerning the LCC's handling of the transfer of poor law hospitals and institutions under the 1929 Local Government Act, see LCC Annual Reports for 1930 and 1931, Vol. IV, Part I. Later developments are fully described in Ministry of Health Annual Report for 1934-35, [Cmd. 4978] and LCC publication No. 3657, *The LCC Hospitals: a Retrospect*.

[6] Established under the Education (Administrative Provisions) Act, 1907 (7 Edw. 7 c. 43 s. 13 (b)).

[7] Ministry of Health Annual Report, 1934-35, p. 95.

CHAPTER 23

Conclusion

I

ALTHOUGH the M A B services were only a regional innovation, their origins and development provided signposts which pointed to the emergence of State responsibility for personal health and welfare in this country. Once the State had assumed direct control of institutions for the sick poor, it came to touch the lives of more and more people. In making specialized provision for the infectious sick and chronic insane, the M A B system anticipated the recommendations of the 1905–9 Minority Poor Law Commissioners, who urged that the needy should be dealt with according to the cause and character of their distress rather than by virtue of their poverty, and that they should be removed from the ambit of the poor law to specialized local authority care.[1] This is precisely what had happened to the dependants of the M A B since its creation. By 1891, the Asylums Board had become virtually a public health authority in so far as concerned the isolation, treatment and transport of the infectious sick; and by 1913 its poor law status was similarly superseded in respect of the institutional care of the mentally deficient and the tuberculous.

The Board's work from 1897 on behalf of sick and handicapped children also represented a break with the principles and practice of the poor law in that, for the first time, pauper children were treated specifically in relation to their disability and not primarily because they were destitute. The fields of public health, orthopaedics, education, and even penal reform, were all affected by this pioneer work, which resulted in the establishment of the first State hospital-schools. One important outcome of the Board's activity in this sphere was the dramatic diminution of skin and eye diseases in London schools and the consequent rescue from pauperism of countless children who might otherwise have been dependent on the State for life. No less far-reaching was the improvement in conditions for youthful offenders. By the time the Board handed over its functions in this field to the LCC in 1910, it had established the first remand homes and been instrumental in the provision of separate juvenile courts. Here again, the Board's intervention served to reduce the scope of the poor law and to bring one more category of the needy a stage nearer to the wider area of general collective provision.

The financial arrangements of the M A B served no less as a link between the 'paternal' and the 'welfare' State, inasmuch as the Metropolitan Common Poor Fund—successfully

[1] S. and B. Webb, *The Break-Up of the Poor Law*, pp. 306–7 and 497–98.

242

applied throughout the metropolis for over sixty years to meet the upkeep of the M A B institutional and ancillary services—represented the widest application in this country of the collectivist principle before its adoption on a national scale.

II

The transitional roles of the M A B before the welfare revolution become more meaning-ful when considered in relation to the development of other sectors of contemporary hospital provision in London and the provinces,[1] and to the impact made upon them during this evolutionary period by the 1867 intervention of the State in the field of remedial care.

The separate infirmaries established in London for the general sick poor following the Metropolitan Poor Act were financed, like the M A B hospitals, from the Metropolitan Common Poor Fund. Thus encouraged, they increased. By 1891, they numbered twenty-four, with some 12,500 beds, but even then not every London poor law district had a separate infirmary, and about 4,000 patients still occupied beds in the general workhouses.[2] By this time, however, the poor, including those above the pauper class, had come to regard the infirmaries as State-supported hospitals where they could be treated without the taint of pauperism.

In the provinces, public hospital provision for the sick poor followed about a generation after the founding in London of the M A B 'asylums' and the first separate poor law in-firmaries. Its growth was slower since it lacked the incentive of the Common Poor Fund, but certain events gave it a stimulus. The rate-aided sick, formerly disenfranchised, ob-tained the vote under the Medical Relief Disqualification Act of 1885. The growing selectivity of the voluntary hospitals, induced by the increasing departmentalization of medicine, forced chronic and less 'interesting' cases into the infirmaries. Where no volun-tary institution existed, greater demands were made on the poor law hospitals. Patients who were not strictly destitute came to be more freely admitted as a result of the acceptance of a wider definition of the term 'destitution', as recommended by the 1905–9 Poor Law Commission. A more enlightened central policy led to improved standards and amenities in infirmaries throughout the country. Such were the influences which popularized and expanded poor law hospital provision.

Institutional medical care was less advanced under the sanitary authorities. They had been generally lethargic in implementing their powers to provide for the sick under the public health statutes of 1866 and 1875. In the provincial towns and rural areas where the voluntary hospitals admitted infectious cases,[3] the local authorities found no more reason

---

[1] The evolution of all sectors of hospital provision in the country from 1800 is discussed in detail by Brian Abel-Smith in *The Hospitals, 1800–1948*.

[2] *Third Report of the Select Committee of the House of Lords on Metropolitan Hospitals*, 1892: BPP, 1892, vol. xiii, p. clviii.

[3] Of the voluntary hospitals visited by Dr. J. S. Bristowe and Mr. T. Holmes in 1863, the following provincial and rural hospitals admitted fever cases, usually in separate 'fever houses': Newcastle Fever,

to accept their responsibilities than did the metropolitan sanitary authorities whose negligence led to the illegal use by the general public of the early M A B smallpox hospitals. During the last years of the nineteenth century, however, a demand for isolation accommodation followed the emergence of new theories of infection and the compulsory notification of infectious disease. Further, the Isolation Hospitals Acts of 1893 and 1901[1] tended to limit the provision of hospitals by the local authorities to those for infectious diseases, whereas the Public Health Act of 1875 had empowered them to provide generally for the 'treatment of the sick'.[2] The Isolation Hospitals Acts aimed to centralize under the county councils the numerous small fever hospitals which had grown up throughout the country, and to stimulate the building of large county institutions on the lines of the M A B system. They failed in these objectives. By 1911, some 32,000 fever beds existed in hundreds of small units; and when the 1929 Local Government Act came into force, upwards of 40,000 local authority beds, mainly for infectious diseases, were distributed among 1,800 localities. Standards varied but, following the example of the M A B isolation hospitals, most of them provided free treatment on public health grounds.

While the poor law and sanitary authority hospital services had been reacting to State intervention, expansion had been taking place in the general voluntary system, especially in London. Reform would have been demanded sooner or later, but the timing, content and direction of the steps taken to resolve the problems arising from the unco-ordinated proliferation of voluntary hospitals suggest that they, too, were influenced by the 1867 entry of the State into the field of medical care. Everywhere else, except America, hospitals were subsidized in some way, or controlled, by the State. In England before 1867, the central government had never been involved in the management of civil institutional services for the sick. But within a few years of the founding of the M A B hospitals, there were constant demands for some kind of State action in the voluntary sector.[3] Most of these took the form of requests for an official investigation into the administration of hospitals. Parliamentary grants, State inspection, State control of finances, central co-ordination of management—these were among the remedies suggested for resolving the grievances with which the voluntary sector abounded. Between 1875 and 1881, at least

---

Birmingham General, Royal Manchester, United Bath, Bedford, Brighton, Cambridge, Chester, Chichester, Derby, Lancaster, Leicester, Nottingham, Oxford, Reading, Stafford, Whitehaven, Wolverhampton. All the Scottish hospitals and about half of the Irish hospitals admitted fever cases (Sixth Report of the MO to the Privy Council, 1863, Appendix 15, Table on pp. 569–70).

[1] 56 & 57 Vict. c. 68 and 1 Edw. 7 c. 8.   [2] 38 & 39 Vict. c. 55 s. 131.

[3] The following are typical statements of authoritative concern in regard to the state of voluntary hospital management at this time. In a letter to *The Times* (2 May 1878), Sir T. Fowell Buxton, one-time treasurer of the London Hospital, wrote: 'From a long acquaintance with hospital management, I am convinced that its principal defects both in London and the country arise from want of organization and co-operation and from the absence of all central control and of government inspection.' In an article in the *Lancet* (16 July 1881, p. 82), Dr. F. J. Mouat, MD, FRCS, retired Deputy Inspector-General of Hospitals, affirmed that 'the state of London hospitals is so anomalous . . . that it would be almost better for the State to take charge of them all than to leave them in their present unsatisfactory position. What London really wants is a central authority to harmonize the action of the various hospitals . . .'

four influential deputations petitioned the Home Secretary for a Royal Commission. The British Medical Association and the National Association for the Promotion of Social Science were among the pressure groups demanding an official investigation.

When the Royal Commission of 1881–82 was studying the metropolitan fever hospitals, requests were made for its terms of reference to be extended to cover all London hospitals. Hopes were disappointed, and demands for an official enquiry persisted throughout the ensuing decade. Although some form of government control was advocated by extreme reformers, it was generally agreed that State intervention should be limited to an enquiry, and that centralization should replace unitary independence. It was regarded as logical by some that institutional co-ordination should include the poor law sector,[1] as in Sweden, where charitable and public institutions were closely linked.[2] Centralized purchasing of hospital supplies was advocated. London, it was suggested, should emulate Paris and establish 'a central store at which all hospitals could purchase at a little over cost price every article of consumption from an egg to a wooden leg'.[3] A central board of control, acting in harmony with the Local Government Board, might also regulate admissions of the acute sick; administer 'a metropolitan ambulance brigade'; deal with all outbreaks of infectious disease; establish joint convalescent homes and institutions for the chronic sick and the incurable; provide dispensaries; inaugurate a register 'for the employment of damaged lives'; and in these various ways 'render hospital accommodation more useful and lighten the burden of the State'. Such were the visions of a number of hospital reformers who banded together in the early 1880s under the auspices of the National Association for the Promotion of Social Science.[4] In 1882, encouraged by the improved prospects which the findings of the 1881–82 Royal Commission promised for the infectious disease hospitals of London, they appealed to the Home Secretary for State intervention.[5]

Representations continued until July 1889, when the case for an enquiry was presented to the House of Lords by Lord Sandhurst. It fell to the promoter of the M A B hospitals, Gathorne Hardy (now Viscount Cranbrook), to reply on behalf of the Government. The following year, a sixteen-member Select Committee of the Upper House was appointed. Its detailed study of all the charitable and rate-aided hospitals of London[6] lasted until

[1] *Third Report of the Select Committee of the House of Lords on Metropolitan Hospitals*, 1892, op. cit. Evidence of Sir E. Hay Currie, one-time vice-chairman of the M A B (para. 276), and of Sir H. Burdett (para. 284).

[2] In Sweden, the hospitals, though managed by separate governing bodies, had been brought into close association by the government by means of a three-level scale of charges: grade I patients paid a substantial sum and obtained anything they cared to have, subject to medical control; grade II patients paid much less but a remunerative rate for all they received at the hospital; grade III patients (paupers) were paid for on an agreed scale by the poor law authorities. (*Trans. NAPSS*, 1881, H. C. Burdett, 'Is it desirable that hospitals should be placed under State supervision?' pp. 508–9.)

[3] H. C. Burdett, *Trans. NAPSS*, 1881, p. 509.

[4] T. Gilbart-Smith, MA, MD, 'What Reforms are desirable in the Administration of Hospitals?' *Trans. NAPSS*, 1882, pp. 390–448.

[5] Petition addressed to the Home Secretary by the NAPSS, *Trans. NAPSS*, 1882, pp. 427–30.

[6] Lord Sandhurst's motion recommending an enquiry into the voluntary hospitals of London emphasized that general opinion in the provincial towns was in favour of a similar enquiry into their hospitals. (*Hansard* (H of L), 29 July 1889.)

1892.[1] Moved by the great weight of evidence in favour of a central board, the Committee urged the establishment of such a body.[2] Prophetically, it warned that, in default of such action, a time might come when it would be necessary for the voluntary hospitals 'to have recourse either to government aid or municipal subvention'. One of the chief causes of the voluntary hospitals' predicament, the Committee believed, was 'the intervention of the State in 1867', which, 'by bringing into being the M A B hospitals and poor law infirmaries, had radically altered the relationship between the sick poor and the voluntary hospitals. . . '.[3] The founding of this country's earliest State hospitals had thus affected all existing sectors of institutional provision for the acute sick, while at the same time it had given rise to the movement which, as we have seen, culminated in 1913 in public care for the mentally handicapped.

III

While certain aspects of present-day hospital development may be traced to nineteenth-century influences, some instances of 'history repeating itself' are discernible in the absence of any direct causal link. For instance, a number of similarities may be found if a comparison is made between the principles and practice of the M A B and of hospital management today.[4] The constitution of the M A B, like that of Regional Hospital Boards, was based on the administrative principles of agency and legal independence. It was an incorporated body with perpetual succession which acted for, and was directly responsible to, the Minister accountable for local government affairs. All members of Regional Hospital Boards are nominated by the head of the 'parent' authority on the advice of interested bodies. The M A B, with one-quarter of its members appointed in this way and the rest selected by the metropolitan guardians, was no less undemocratically constituted. While, on paper, the acts of the Asylums Board were circumscribed by the will of the central authority, Regional Hospital Boards have been accorded scope to develop and organize along their own lines. The M A B, nevertheless, evolved organically, largely as a result of ineffective central authority control during its formative decades. Another aspect of similarity concerns structure. The organizational pattern of a central 'command' for

[1] See *Third Report of the Select Committee of the House of Lords on Metropolitan Hospitals*, op. cit.

[2] Ibid., pp. cv–cvi. No immediate action was taken on this recommendation of the Lords Committee.

[3] Ibid., p. cvii, para. 624.

[4] The present-day system of hospital regionalization and grouping was mainly the outcome of such studies as the Dawson Report (*Interim Report on the Future Provision of Medical and Allied Services*, Cmd. 693, 1920); the Cave Committee Report (*Voluntary Hospitals Committee, Final Report*, Cmd. 1335, 1921); the Onslow Commission Report (Ministry of Health: *Voluntary Hospitals Commission, Interim Report*, 1923); the BMA Report, *A General Medical Service for the Nation*, 1928; the report of the Sankey Commission (*Report of the Voluntary Hospitals Commission*, British Hospitals Association, 1937); the *Draft Interim Report of the Medical Planning Commission*, 1942; and the Beveridge Report (*Social Insurance and Allied Services*, Cmd. 6404, 1942). The present-day system also owes much to particular influences such as the work of the Nuffield Provincial Hospitals Trust, formed in 1939, and also to the experience of the operation of the Emergency Medical Service under the Ministry of Health in preparation for World War II.

planning, with sub-divisions for operational purposes, was adopted by both the pioneer board and its twentieth-century successors. While in the case of the former it evolved spontaneously, for the latter it was specifically devised. The grouping system of today was imposed *ab initio* for the purpose of welding into a national whole the traditionally differing systems of the constituent 'streams'. In the earlier system, however, grouping of units by function was the logical outcome of its extension into new branches of institutional care.

One of the fundamental differences between the two systems concerns finance. Whereas present-day Regional Hospital Boards derive their income from exchequer funds, that of the M A B was raised from the London poor rates. Although the central authority had powers to limit certain items of M A B expenditure, financial sanctions were a less effective lever of compulsion in the days of the M A B than they are today. On rare occasions, when thwarted to extremes, the M A B threatened to resign in a body—a course still conceivably open to Regional Hospital Boards. The most notable difference, however, is one of operation. The Asylums Board with over seventy members—two to three times the size of a modern hospital board—was an 'all-purposes' body, with both directive and managerial functions, and from its own members appointed all management and other committees.[1] In operation, the more comprehensive system pointed to the advantages of a policy-making body putting its theories into practice and directly experiencing the results of its planning.

Postscript: As this study goes to press, the Labour Government's proposals for the future of the National Health Service suggest that the Regional Hospital Boards referred to in this section are unlikely to endure for more than a few more years.[2]

IV

Most of the lessons resulting from the M A B experiment in large-scale hospital management have since been re-learned and re-applied except, possibly, the need in health administration for adequate statistical tools. Inaugurating its work when public health was administered almost in a statistical vacuum, the M A B began by furnishing the local sanitary authorities with a regular pestilential picture of the metropolis drawn from its hospital admissions records. Later, when the M A B became the statutory 'clearing house' for returns received under the notification laws, statistics played a vital role in the development of the Board's own services. An organized arsenal of statistical data was built up for aiding

[1] Members of Hospital Management Committees may also be members of a Regional Hospital Board, but most of them are not.

[2] Government proposals include the creation of about ninety area health boards (corresponding with the projected new local authority areas) to unify the three separate branches of the health service—the hospitals, GPs, and local community services, with some two hundred subordinate district committees. The planning of hospitals and specialist services would be in the hands of about fourteen regional councils, whose functions were intended to be largely advisory. The scheme, as set out in *The Future of the National Health Service* (HMSO, February 1970), foreshadows a broad extension of central direction and control.

every aspect of work—administration, prevention, vaccination, propaganda, finance, planning, pathological services and medical research.

Besides improving the techniques of hospital management, the M A B recognized and attended to the social and psychological aspects of institutional care. A brief glance at trends in social thought while the M A B was emerging may throw some light on the forces which influenced its policies. Although Benthamism and the notion of the free play of enlightened self-interest were dominant for much of the nineteenth century, philosophies in certain oases of social reform already were germinating the basic principles of the 'welfare state'—the inherent worth of the individual and his entitlement to social security and opportunity for personal development. The sanitary idea—the assumption by government of preventive responsibility for personal health—had been promoted by Chadwick on the basis of 'the greatest happiness of the greatest number'. Later sanitarians and reformers came to expose the fallacies of Benthamism. In the 1860s, John Stuart Mill re-assessed the utilitarian concept of happiness in terms of spiritual condition, as opposed to material acquisition.[1] This presupposed a breach with the notion of a 'natural harmony of interests' and its replacement by legislation aimed at the removal of impediments to individual development. The mid-1860s also saw the publication of *Ecce Homo* by Sir John Seeley. This moving work included a re-assessment of 'the law of philanthropy' as affected by 'the progress of science and civilization'. The tasks of the nineteenth-century Christian, it was asserted, were

> to investigate the causes of all physical evil, to master the science of health, to consider the question of education . . . of labour . . . and . . . of trade with a view to health, and while all these investigations are made, with free expense of energy, time and means, to work out the re-arrangement of human life in accordance with the results they give.[2]

While such influences as these were beginning to place social emphasis on the individual, as distinct from society in general, the workhouse 'scandals' of the middle 'sixties were bringing to light the plight of the helpless poor. During the year in which *Ecce Homo* first appeared, Mr. Gathorne Hardy was in fact making investigations into the metropolitan workhouses 'with free expense of energy, time and means'. His belief that the world was governed by a personal God was with him a guiding and living influence.[3] He aimed to inject a new, humane element into the bleak paternalistic function of the State, not by demolishing or breaching the poor law system of 1834, but by building on to it, in the knowledge that it contained the seeds of its own reform. This extension in 1867 represented a major landmark on the road to the welfare revolution of the twentieth century. But the State at this time was concerned less with the well-being of the individual than with that of the community—'the greatest number'. Public hospital provision was

---

[1] J. S. Mill, *Utilitarianism* (1863), Chapter III; and *Autobiography* (pub. posth. 1873), *passim*.
[2] Sir John Seeley, *Ecce Homo* (1866), Chapter XVII, 'The Law of Philanthropy', p. 190, *et seq.*
[3] A. E. Gathorne-Hardy (ed.), *Gathorne-Hardy, First Earl of Cranbrook—a Memoir* (1910), vol. I, p. 5.

acceptable to the legislature mainly insofar as it protected society from infectious and insane paupers.

Dr. William Brewer, who led the Asylums Board through the almost insuperable difficulties of its first fourteen years, was also a deeply religious man, in tune with the need to wed the new science of health to practical philanthropy. He was a close associate of John Stuart Mill, and, judging from his utterances and actions, there is little doubt that he was influenced by the reformer's undoctrinaire, essential socialism. After Dr. Brewer's death in 1881, his policy, based on a reverence for human beings, was perpetuated by Sir Edwin Galsworthy, M A B chairman for the next twenty years, and by his successors. To the influences which inspired these leaders, as well as their like-minded colleagues on the Board, their medical superintendents, and their associates, Dr. Bridges[1] and Sir Arthur Downes of the Local Government Board, must be attributed in large measure the fundamental difference between the intentions of the M A B's original terms of reference and the socially-orientated policies by which they were implemented and expanded.

From the outset, the Board accepted its charges not as paupers but as patients and members of a social unit. The M A B infectious disease hospitals, unlike the London voluntary hospitals, were deliberately located to serve the convenience of patients. Mothers were encouraged during epidemics to accompany and nurse their young children in hospital. Medical considerations being equal, the standard of amenities in the home served as the criterion for admission when accommodation was limited. Compensation for the breadwinner when submitting to isolation was continually urged by the Board, although without success.

The far-sighted concern of the M A B and its medical staff for the child is evidenced by such innovations as the hospital-schools for the physically handicapped, special training for subnormal children, small-group foster-parent homes for ESN children, remand homes for juvenile delinquents, and research into the after-effects of encephalitis lethargica in the young. In short, the child was regarded in the M A B institutions as a person and a member of the coming generation—a viewpoint with which the State had scant concern in the nineteenth century.

The complex administrative network of an organization dealing with thousands of patients in vast institutions might well have tended towards depersonalization, but there is ample evidence to testify to the Board's concern for the integrity of the individual. In the vast, isolated mental institutions, for example, occupation was a prominent feature. For the sick and aged who were unable to participate, a special infirmary was provided in an urban environment within reach of relatives. At Colindale and Grove Park—two large sanatoria devoted to the hopeless and dying—efforts were made to maintain the morale of

[1] Of Dr. John H. Bridges, Professor L. T. Hobhouse wrote: '. . . One or two historians have recognized him as prominent among the little band of civil servants whose names are written for the few who care to decipher them in the record of that social recovery from the chaos of the Industrial Revolution which was the great though incomplete work of the second half of the nineteenth century.' (Preface, p. xv, to S. Liveing, *A Nineteenth-Century Teacher, John Henry Bridges, MB, FRCP.*)

long-stay patients by the constant movement in and out of observation cases. On the whole, the experience of the M A B does not suggest that vast buildings should be avoided but that, if economies and technological advances necessitate large institutions, their short-comings should be acknowledged and minimized, in particular by special consideration for the heightened proneness of patients to fears of personal submergence in a limitless, clinical universe.

In its later years, the M A B system, with its ambulance services, medical education, nursing training, pathological laboratories, antitoxin production and research units, was far removed from the pauper 'asylums' over which the Board waged battles in its early days with an obscurantist central authority. Most of these developments had resulted from the close collaboration of the Asylums Managers with their medical staff. As a public authority, the M A B was probably unique in the extent to which it sought and accepted medical counsel. The greater part of public health legislation relating to London between 1873 and 1891 was influenced by the repeated representations of the Asylums Managers based on medical evidence.

V

While the M A B founded and developed this country's earliest public fever hospitals, 'imbecile asylums' and hospital-schools, its success in these undertakings can be attributed in no way to its relationship with the central authority as prescribed by the 1867 inaugural statute. During the greater part of the Board's first three decades, the head of the 'parent' department assumed direct and detailed authority over all its activities and retained undivided responsibility and accountability to Parliament. By the end of the century, however, reorganization and the infusion of new blood into the Local Government Board brought about a more enlightened regime.[1] While retaining accountability for the M A B, Presidents from the mid-nineties gradually relaxed the detailed supervision of earlier years and communicated only major lines of policy to the Asylums Managers, allowing them wide decision-making powers and freedom to plan within approved financial limits. With its eminent central authority nominees and other expert members, its comprehensive committee system, and its own financial and medical inspectorates, the Asylums Board obviously was not in need of guidance from the lay civil servants of the central department. The change in the relationship first became manifest when the M A B was instructed in 1897 to act as the metropolitan authority for the care of handicapped and delinquent children. Following the initial notification, the M A B was left entirely free to plan,

---

[1] During the presidency of Sir Charles Dilke (1882–85), a committee under Sir John Lambert was appointed to consider staff reorganization at the LGB. As a result, eight clerkships of the Higher Division were thrown open to public competition, a reform which eventually increased the efficiency of the LGB. (H. Preston-Thomas, *Work and Play of a Government Inspector*, p. 195; and Stephen Gwynn and Gertrude Tuckwell, *The Life of Sir Charles Dilke*, vol. i, p. 505). A committee appointed by the Treasury in 1897 resulted in further reforms (*Report of Committee . . . to enquire into the sufficiency of the clerical staff of the LGB . . .* (Cmd. 8731 and 8999 of 1898).

inaugurate and develop this new branch of its work. This proved to be one of its most imaginative and far-reaching ventures. There is no doubt whatever that, compared with its first three decades, the second thirty-year period of the Board's administration was by far the more fruitful and harmonious, and that the greatest contributory cause was its operational freedom.

Most of the difficulties of the Board's earlier years stemmed from the experimental nature of the policy which brought it into being and of the functions it was called upon to perform. The overriding powers which the 1867 legislation bestowed upon the Poor Law Board—and its successors—were more a function of the poor law principles of 1834 than of a specifically formulated policy for public hospital management. On the one hand, was a government department administered by 'poor law-minded' laymen, unconcerned with medical counsel and armed with the new executive weapon of delegated legislation. On the other hand, was a regional hospital board which far exceeded the calibre and size of the local management committees envisaged in the 1867 Act. To the department were assigned the functions of 'top management', while the hospital board was accorded a subsidiary role. In the early days it looked for a lead in matters of moment and found only a system of petty control. In times of crisis its sense of urgency was met by passivity and prevarication. Precipitating causes of disharmony were inherent in the relationship itself. The antithesis was constituted by the very nature of central executive functions, on the one hand, and by pressing demands calling for qualities of leadership, on the other. The functions of a government department are essentially impersonal and permit of little scope for enlightened compassion. The demands of a hospital authority concern the arrest of suffering, sickness and death. Administration in a central department is conducted in accordance with the policy of government and in obedience to the expressed will of Parliament. Its acts are circumscribed by the requirements of the democratic process and consequently are subject to all the delays and dilemmas which that entails. In Bagehot's words, 'a skilled bureaucracy . . ., though it boasts of an appearance of science, is quite inconsistent with the true principles of the art of business.'[1] When the legislature endows a central department with great powers of compulsion and prohibition, it confers upon it, *ipso facto*, the role of leadership. But, even if possessed by officials as individuals, the qualities implied in this role—including the capacity for reasoned and, where necessary, instant, decision-making— are likely to be stultified by the bureaucratic machine. If the controlling levels of administration of a public service demand flexibility and immediate response, these are not to be sought in a central government department, by virtue of the very nature of its frame of reference. Co-operation there may be, but where a subservient role exists on one side, decisive leadership is expected on the other. Concerning the nature of executive responsibility, it has been said: 'Co-operation, not leadership, is the creative process; but leadership is the indispensable fulminator of its forces'.[2] Throughout the history of the M A B, its activities were subject to the conflicting demands of public accountability on the one

[1] W. Bagehot, *The English Constitution* (1872), p. 280 (Nelson edn.).
[2] C. T. Barnard, *The Functions of the Executive* (Harvard University Press, 1956), p. 259.

hand, and of managerial flexibility on the other; but the greater harmony and unfettered advances of its later years were the direct outcome of a tacit understanding of these demands and of an effort to reconcile them.

In the last analysis, one basic conclusion which may be drawn from this study is that a State-directed social service can be an instrument of dynamic progress, always provided that the central controls are imaginatively devised and applied in the best interests of those for whom the service is created, and foster unthwarted the human qualities of those who minister to their needs.

APPENDIX I

Constitution and Structure of the M A B

DOCUMENT I

STATUTES AND PRINCIPAL ORDERS GOVERNING THE CONSTITUTION, DUTIES
AND DISSOLUTION OF THE METROPOLITAN ASYLUMS BOARD, 1867–1930

CONSTITUTION

The Metropolitan Asylums Board was established by an *Order of the Poor Law Board*,[1] dated
15 May 1867, which also combined the London unions and parishes into the 'Metropolitan Asylum
District', pursuant to the provisions of the *Metropolitan Poor Act of 29 March 1867* (30 & 31 Vict.
c. 6).[2]

The *Metropolitan Poor Act, 1867*, provided for 'the establishment in the metropolis of asylums
for the sick, insane and other classes of the poor, and of dispensaries; for the distribution over the
metropolis of portions of the charge for poor relief; and for other purposes relating to poor
relief in the metropolis.'

The Act empowered the Poor Law Board to combine into districts the unions and parishes
of the metropolis for the purpose of establishing the 'asylums' and also to issue orders to the
managers of any such asylum districts.

DUTIES

(i) *Infectious Disease Patients*

The *Order of the Poor Law Board of 15 May 1867*, constituted the Metropolitan Asylums Board

> 'for the reception and relief of the classes of poor persons chargeable to some union or parish
> in the [metropolitan asylum] district . . . who may be infected with, or suffering from, fever,
> or the disease of smallpox, or may be insane'.

'Fever' (scarlet fever, enteric fever, typhus) and smallpox

Central authority admission regulations of *10 February 1875* prescribed that an infected person
should have a relieving officer's order and a poor law medical certificate before being admitted
to the M A B 'asylums'. Only if non-admission 'might be attended with dangerous results' was
a patient allowed entry without the required documentation.

The *Divided Parishes and Poor Law Amendment Act of 1876* (39 & 40 Vict. c. 61 s. 42) provided
for the recovery of maintenance charges in respect of *non-pauper patients* admitted in these
exceptional conditions and thereby, for the first time, implicitly legalized the reception of non-
paupers into poor law institutions.

The *Poor Law Act of 1879* (42 & 43 Vict. c. 54 s. 15) empowered, but did not compel, the
metropolitan local sanitary authorities to enter into agreements with the M A B for the reception
of *non-pauper patients* suffering from the above diseases (but this was not implemented by the
authorities).

The *Diseases Prevention (Metropolis) Act, 1883* (46 & 47 Vict. c. 35) removed the civil disabilities which until that date had been sustained by patients admitted into the M A B hospitals.
(This was renewed annually until 1891.)

---

[1] The distinction of names of the central authority is one of date: Poor Law Board up to June 1871;
Local Government Board, July 1871 to June 1919; Ministry of Health, from 1 July 1919.

[2] The Metropolitan Poor Act, 1867, is summarized in Document II, following.

Diphtheria

The admission of pauper diphtheria cases to the Board's hospitals was provisionally sanctioned by the *Local Government Board* on *17 October 1888*; and the *Poor Law Act of 1889* (52 & 53 Vict. c. 56) gave statutory authorization for the reception of *all* diphtheria cases (section 3 (1)).

Socialization of M A B Infectious Disease Hospitals

The *Poor Law Act, 1889*, empowered the Metropolitan Asylums Board to admit metropolitan *non-pauper* cases of fever, diphtheria and smallpox (section 3 (1)). Boards of guardians were directed to pay the maintenance costs of such non-pauper patients and to recover these expenses from the patient or any person legally liable to maintain him (section 3 (2)). 'The said expenses, so far as the same are not recoverable by the guardians,' the Act continued, 'shall be repaid to them out of the Metropolitan Common Poor Fund'[1] (section 3 (3)).

The *Public Health (London) Act, 1891* (54 & 55 Vict. c. 76), which consolidated earlier poor law legislation relating to the metropolis, re-enacted in section 80 (paras. (1) and (2)) the terms of section 3 (paras. (1) and (2)) of the 1889 Act, op. cit., but omitted all reference to the recovery of the maintenance costs by the guardians. The third paragraph of section 3 of the 1889 Act was reduced to: 'The said expenses shall be repaid to the board of guardians out of the Metropolitan Common Poor Fund.' (section 80 (3) of the 1891 Act). As from *1 January 1892*, therefore, the M A B infectious disease hospitals became free to every patient in London suffering from fever, diphtheria or smallpox, irrespective of ability to pay.

Other diseases treated in the M A B hospitals

By *Order dated 18 February 1911*, the *Local Government Board* sanctioned the admission to any of the M A B infectious disease hospitals of 'poor persons suffering from such infectious or contagious diseases other than those above-mentioned as they might thereafter determine.' The following diseases subsequently became the subject of LGB orders.

Measles and Whooping-Cough

On *18 February 1911*, the *Local Government Board* sanctioned the admission of poor children suffering from measles or whooping-cough received through the metropolitan authorities, while by further *Orders, dated 30 May 1911*, and *9 August 1912*, issued pursuant to the provisions of the *Public Health (London) Act, 1891* (Sec. 80), the *Local Government Board* sanctioned the admission, subject to certain restrictions, of non-pauper cases of measles and whooping-cough respectively.

Puerperal Fever

On *2 July 1912*, the *Local Government Board* (under its *Order of 18 February 1911*) authorized the M A B to receive into its fever hospitals, through the poor law authorities, poor persons suffering from puerperal fever; and by *Order dated 20 August 1912* prescribed that, subject to certain restrictions, non-pauper cases should also be admitted.

Venereal Disease

Under *Local Government Board Orders of 12 September 1916*, and *13 October 1919*, the Board made provision for the treatment of parturient women and other women and girls suffering from venereal disease.

[1] For further details concerning the Metropolitan Common Poor Fund, see Appendix IV.

Under *Local Government Board Order of 29 September 1917*, the Board provided for the treatment of *children suffering from ophthalmia neonatorum.*

Zymotic Enteritis

Under *Ministry of Health* authority of *27 August 1924*, certain cases of zymotic enteritis were also received into the Board's infectious disease hospitals.

Carcinoma of the Uterus

By *Ministry of Health Order dated 26 September 1928* the Board made provision in their isolation hospitals for the treatment by radium of certain women suffering from cancer of the uterus.

Tuberculosis

The Board entered into arrangements with the London County Council for the provision of residential treatment of tuberculous patients in the County of London under *National Insurance Acts, 1911 to 1920* (1 & 2 Geo. 5 c. 55; 3 & 4 Geo. 5 c. 37; 7 & 8 Geo. 5 c. 62; and 10 & 11 Geo. 5 c. 10); *Public Health (Prevention and Treatment of Diseases) Act, 1913* (3 & 4 Geo. 5 c. 23); and *Public Health (Tuberculosis) Act, 1921* (11 & 12 Geo. 5 c. 12).

(ii) *Ambulance Services*

By the *Poor Law Act, 1879* (42 & 43 Vict. c. 54 s. 16), superseded by *Section 79 of the Public Health (London) Act, 1891*, the Board was empowered to provide ambulance services for the removal of pauper infectious patients from their homes to the hospitals. Under the *Poor Law Act, 1889*, the Board was authorized to remove infectious patients (poor law and non-pauper cases) to the M A B hospitals and to any other destination.

(iii) *Medical Instruction and Research*

Under the *Poor Law Act, 1889* (52 & 53 Vict. c. 56 s. 4), provision was made at the Board's infectious disease hospitals for the instruction of medical students and of candidates for the diploma in public health. Provision was also made in separate establishments for pathological and bacteriological work, and for the manufacture of diphtheria antitoxin, while research was conducted in the Board's isolation, mental and children's hospitals (see Medical Supplement following).

(iv) *Compulsory Notification of Infectious Disease*

Under the *Infectious Disease (Notification) Act, 1889* (52 & 53 Vict. c. 72), and the *Public Health (London) Act, 1891* (54 & 55 Vict. c. 76 s. 55 (4)), the Board received from the metropolitan Medical Officers of Health details of infectious disease occurring in the metropolis, notified by medical practitioners attending infectious patients. The returns were collated and published by the Asylums Board.

(v) *Mental Patients*

Poor Law Board Order, dated 15 May 1867, included the 'insane' amongst the classes of poor for whose reception and relief the Board was constituted.

Local Government Board Order, dated 10 February 1875, defined the persons to be admitted into the Board's mental hospitals as 'such harmless persons of the chronic or imbecile class as could be lawfully retained in a workhouse; but no dangerous or curable persons, such as would, under the statutes . . . require to be sent to a lunatic asylum, shall be admitted' (section II (2)).

Local Government Board Order, dated 2 April 1897, included *feeble-minded children* amongst the classes of poor persons to be received by the Board, and authority was subsequently given for the retention of these cases after 16 years of age. These provisions were subsequently incorporated in the *Metropolitan Asylums (Mentally Defective Persons) Order, dated 29 December 1911*, which defined the subnormal young persons to be received as

'persons not certified as lunatics, who by reason of mental defect are incapable of receiving proper benefit from ordinary instruction, or cannot be properly trained in association with other persons in ordinary schools or institutions, or are incapable of using ordinary means or precautions for protecting themselves from injury or improper usage or treatment, or are incapable of maintaining themselves by work, provided that any such poor person on admission into an asylum belonging to the Metropolitan Asylums Managers shall not exceed 21 years of age.'

On *1 January 1918*, the Local Government Board consented, for a period of five years, to the reception into certain of the Board's mental hospitals and industrial colonies of cases certified under the *Mental Deficiency Act, 1913* (3 & 4 Geo. 5 c. 28). On *3 March 1923*, the period was extended for a further five years, and on the *9 May 1928*, for a third period of five years.

On *20 August 1924*, the *Ministry of Health* issued an instrument authorizing the Board to receive *poor persons over the age of 70 years* who had not at any time been certified as 'lunatics' and who by reason of mental infirmity required institutional care and treatment.

(vi) *Sane Epileptics*

In *1916* the Board undertook to receive *sane epileptic children*. By the *Metropolitan Asylums (Epileptics) Order, dated 26 March 1917*, the Board was empowered by the Local Government Board to provide for the treatment of sane epileptic poor law adults.

(vii) *Children*

Boys training for sea service

The provision of a training ship for the training of boys for sea service was sanctioned by the *Local Government Board in 1875*, under the terms of the *Metropolitan Poor Amendment Act, 1869* (32 & 33 Vict. c. 63 s. 11).

Sick and disabled poor law children

By *Orders of the Local Government Board dated 2 April 1897* and *11 September 1908*, and an *Order of the Ministry of Health dated 1 July 1924*, the Asylums Board was constituted as a central metropolitan authority for dealing with various classes of poor law children, viz., *the sick and convalescent* and those suffering from *ophthalmia*, *ringworm* and *interstitial keratitis*.

Juvenile Offenders

Under *Local Government Board Order of 2 April 1897*, the Asylums Board was charged with the care and accommodation of children who were ordered by two justices or a magistrate to be taken, under the *Industrial Schools Act, 1866*, to a workhouse or an asylum of the district. The Board began this work in 1902, following the *Youthful Offenders Act, 1901* (1 Edw. 7 c. 20).

The M A B thereafter steadily advocated the adoption by the legislature of measures tending towards the reclamation of the juvenile offender, the establishment of separate courts for children, and their entire dissociation from the adult criminal. Its recommendations were eventually embodied in the *Probation of Offenders Act, 1907* (7 Edw. 7 c. 17), and the *Children Act, 1908* (8 Edw. 7 c. 67), the former coming into force on *1 January 1908* and the latter on *1 April 1909*. Although the M A B was the pioneer of special treatment for juvenile offenders and had instituted the first remand homes, the Local Government Board was empowered, under the *Children Act of 1908*, to transfer the M A B remand homes to the London County Council, and this was effected in 1910.

(viii) *Casual Poor*

On *10 November 1911, the Local Government Board* issued the *Metropolitan Casual Paupers Order* forming a district, co-terminus with the existing Metropolitan Asylum District, for the relief of the casual poor of the Metropolis. The Order also provided, under the *Pauper Inmates Discharge and Regulation Act, 1871* (34 & 35 Vict. c. 108 s. 10), that the Metropolitan Asylums Board should be the Board for the new district. Before the issue of this Order, every metropolitan board of guardians was required by the *Metropolitan Houseless Poor Act, 1864* (27 & 28 Vict. c. 116), to provide casual wards, and the expenses in connexion with vagrants were repayable to the guardians by the Metropolitan Board of Works until 1867, when they were made a charge on the Metropolitan Common Poor Fund under section 69 (9) of the *Metropolitan Poor Act of 1867*.

As contemplated in the *Casual Paupers Order*, the Local Government Board issued on *28 March 1912* the *Metropolitan Casual Wards (Transfer) Order*, transferring to the Board those of the casual wards provided under the 1864 Act which it was proposed to continue.

The effect of these two Orders was to centralize the control under the Board, from *1 April 1912*, of most of the casual wards administered before that date by the separate boards of guardians.

In connexion with the casual wards, the Board undertook the management of a scheme for dealing, in co-operation with the police and voluntary agencies, with the homeless poor at night.

On *18 May 1923*, the *Ministry of Health* sanctioned a scheme for assisting helpable cases, selected from the casual wards or applying to the M A B night office, to regain employment, and agreed to the reservation for this purpose of one of the casual wards as a hostel for men.

(ix) *War Work, 1914–19*

Destitute Enemy Aliens

Local Government Board letters of *10* and *27 August 1914*, and *3 September 1914*, requested the Asylums Board to make provision for the care and accommodation of destitute persons of German, Austrian and Hungarian nationality.

War Refugees

Local Government Board letter of *3 September 1914* also requested the M A B to provide for housing a large number of Belgian refugees expected to arrive in Britain, placing at its disposal the Crystal Palace on *9 September 1914*. On *13 October 1914*, the *Local Government Board* placed the Earl's Court Exhibition premises at the disposal of the M A B for the duration (the Admiralty having requisitioned the Crystal Palace unknown to the Local Government Board).

On *28 June 1918*, the M A B was charged with the care of 1,140 Russian refugees who had been in contact with smallpox.

(x) *Metropolitan Common Poor Fund*

In pursuance of the *Local Authorities (Emergency Provisions) Act, 1928* (18 & 19 Geo. 5 c. 9), the M A B undertook for a period of four years the control of the Metropolitan Common Poor Fund, which had been administered since its inception in 1867 by the Poor Law Board, the Local Government Board and the Ministry of Health. (For details of the Fund see Appendix IV.)

DISSOLUTION

Under the *Local Government Act, 1929* (Part I) (19 Geo. 5 c. 17), boards of guardians were abolished as from *1 April 1930*. The Metropolitan Asylums Board—a *de jure* poor law authority—also ceased to exist from that date, the functions of the Board being transferred to the London County Council, which thereafter became responsible for the services hitherto maintained by the M A B.

DOCUMENT II

SUMMARY OF THE METROPOLITAN POOR ACT, 1867,[1] UNDER WHICH THE M A B WAS ESTABLISHED

'An Act for the Establishment in the Metropolis of Asylums for the Sick, Insane, and other Classes of the Poor, and of Dispensaries; and for the Distribution over the Metropolis of Portions of the Charge for Poor Relief; and for Other Purposes relating to Poor Relief in the Metropolis. [29 March 1867.]'

Short Title

1. This Act may be cited as 'The Metropolitan Poor Act, 1867'.

Interpretation of Terms

2. The term 'the Poor Law Acts' means the Poor Law Amendment Act of 1834 and the Acts extending or amending it. The 'Poor Law Amendment Act of 1844' is the 7 & 8 Vict. c. 101 relating to district schools.

Limitation of Act to the Metropolis

3. This Act extends only to unions and parishes which are wholly or for the greater part included in the Metropolis as defined by the Metropolis Management Act, 1855, and in this Act the term 'Metropolis' means the Metropolis as so defined.

Poor Law Board Orders

4. Any order of the Poor Law Board under this Act shall not be deemed a General Order within the operation of the Poor Law Acts.

---

[1] This *condensed* version of the Act is appended for convenience of reference in the context of the foregoing study. The full text may be consulted in *Public General Statutes*, 1867 (30 & 31 Vict. c. 6) and *British Parliamentary Papers, 1867*, vol. iv, p. 261 et seq. Statutes extending or amending this Act, so far as they relate to the M A B, are cited in the preceding document (pp. 254–9).

District Asylums

Asylums to be provided

5. Asylums to be supported and managed under the Act may be provided for the reception and relief of the sick, insane, or infirm, or other class or classes of the poor chargeable in unions and parishes in the Metropolis.

Formation of Districts

6. For the purpose of these asylums the Poor Law Board may by order combine into districts parishes and/or unions in the Metropolis as it thinks fit.

Number of Asylums

7. For each district there shall be an asylum or asylums as the Poor Law Board directs.

Managers of the Asylums

8. For the asylum(s) of each district there shall be a body of managers constituted as provided by this Act. These managers and their successors shall be an incorporated body with perpetual succession, with power, subject to the orders of the Poor Law Board, to take, hold and dispose of lands and other property for purposes of the asylum district.

Constitution of Managers

9. The managers shall be partly elective and partly nominated.

Election of Managers

10. Elective managers shall be elected from time to time by the guardians of the unions and parishes forming the district from among themselves or from ratepayers qualified to be guardians or partly from one and partly from the other.

Nomination of Managers

11. Nominated managers shall be nominated from time to time by the Poor Law Board from among Justices of the Peace or from among ratepayers resident in the district and assessed to the poor rate therein on an annual rateable value of not less than £40, or partly from one and partly from the other.

Number, qualifications, etc.

12. The Poor Law Board shall prescribe:

The total number of managers and the proportion of the elective and nominated managers so that the prescribed number of the nominated managers does not ever exceed one-third of the prescribed number of elective managers;
the number of elective managers to be elected for each union or parish in the district;
the qualifications of the managers;
their tenure of office;
the mode and times of election; and
the quorum for their meetings.

Validity of acts of Managers

13. Any act or proceeding of the Managers shall not be invalid by reason only of any vacancy in their body or by reason of any failure, defect, irregularity, or disqualification occurring in connexion with elections or nominations.

Prohibition against Managers being concerned in contracts

14. All penalties laid down in the Poor Law Acts on guardians and their officers for being concerned, for their own profit, in contracts etc. connected with the maintenance of workhouses shall apply to the Managers and their officers.

Building for asylum

15. The Poor Law Board may direct the Managers to purchase, hire or build and to fit up a building (or buildings) for the asylum of such nature and size and according to such plan and in such manner as the Poor Law Board may think fit; and the Managers shall carry out such directions.

Purchase or hiring of lands, etc. by the Managers

16. The Managers shall have powers in this connexion similar to those vested in guardians; but the consent of ratepayers or owners of property in a union or parish shall not be necessary with respect to any sale, lease etc. of any workhouse, building or land by guardians or overseers to the Managers.

Power to borrow money

17. The Managers may borrow money for purchasing lands or buildings and for building, equipping and furnishing buildings erected or hired for the asylum and may charge the poor rates of the district with the money so borrowed and interest, subject to the following provisions:

    1. The amount borrowed shall not exceed one-third of the aggregate annual expenditure on the relief of the poor within the whole district (exclusive of reimbursements) for the period of three years ending on the 25 March preceding the borrowing of the money;

    2. The amount borrowed shall be charged on the poor rates of the unions forming the district in the proportions in which they contribute to the maintenance of the asylums;

    3. The amount borrowed shall be paid off with interest by equal annual instalments not exceeding twenty.

Adaptation of existing workhouses for asylums

18. The Poor Law Board may direct that any workhouse may be used for an asylum and thenceforth the building shall be for the common use of the district: and an annual sum determined by the Poor Law Board shall be paid to the guardians of the union to which the workhouse belongs.

Reimbursement to Managers of expenditure

19. The Poor Law Board may make an adjustment between the owners and the Managers in respect of any substantial improvement made by the latter in respect of buildings acquired as under section 18 above.

Furniture etc. for asylum

20. The Managers shall provide for the asylum necessary fixtures, furniture and conveniences, and such as the Poor Law Board directs.

Mode of admission into asylum

21. The mode of admission into the asylum shall be such as the Poor Law Board directs.

Powers and duties of Managers in respect of inmates

22. The Managers shall have the same powers as guardians for the relief, maintenance and management of the inmates of the asylum; and shall provide such medicines, appliances and requisites for the medical and surgical care and treatment of the inmates and cause these to be furnished and used as directed by the Poor Law Board.

Application of parts of the Poor Law Amendment Act of 1844 (7 & 8 Vict. c. 101)

23. The following provisions of the Poor Law Amendment Act of 1844 shall extend to the asylum as if it were an asylum under that Act or a workhouse, and as if the Managers were a District Board under that Act:

Section 43 (so far as it relates to the rules of the Poor Law Board for the government of the asylum or its inmates, and to religious assistance and instruction) and also Sections 50, 54, 57 and 59.

Chargeability, etc. of inmates

24. With reference to chargeability, burial and other incidents, the asylum shall in relation to each inmate thereof be deemed to be in the union or parish from which such inmate is sent; but births and deaths in the asylum shall be registered by the Registrar in whose district the asylum is situated.

Appointment, etc. of paid officers

25. The Managers shall have the same powers as guardians for the appointment, control and payment of paid officers of the asylum and the grant of superannuation allowances to them.

The duties, number, salaries etc. of the paid officers shall be such as the Poor Law Board may approve or direct.

Enforcement of orders of Managers

26. Legal and reasonable orders of the Managers shall be obeyed.

Committees of Managers

27. The Managers may appoint committees of members of their body—subject to Poor Law Board regulations—and delegate to them any of the powers of the Managers.

Orders of the Poor Law Board as to Managers

28. The Managers shall be subject to orders of the Poor Law Board in the same way as guardians.

Use of asylums as medical schools

29. Where the asylum is provided for the reception and relief of the sick or insane it may be used for purposes of medical instruction[1] and for the training of nurses, subject to Poor Law Board regulations.

Representative of Commissioners in Lunacy

30. Where the asylum is provided for the reception and relief of the insane, the Commissioners in Lunacy may, if they think fit, depute one of their body or a special commissioner to attend meetings but not to vote; every such asylum shall be considered as a workhouse within the meaning of the Lunacy Acts.

Expenses of providing asylum and salaries

31. The following shall be defrayed by contributions from the unions and parishes forming the district:

expenses incurred in connexion with the purchasing, hiring, repairing and equipping of asylum buildings;
rent, or compensation payable to guardians in respect of a workhouse;
cost of furniture, conveniences, medicines, medical and surgical appliances and other necessaries required for keeping the asylum in proper order for daily use; and the salaries and maintenance of the officers.

Charges for maintenance etc.

32. Expenses incurred in connexion with food, clothing, maintenance, care, treatment and relief, or for burials, of inmates of the asylum, shall be separately charged to the respective unions or parishes from which the inmates of the asylums are sent.

Audit of accounts

33. The Poor Law Board shall appoint an Auditor of the district. The accounts shall be prepared and submitted to the Auditor in the same way as the accounts of guardians.

Powers of Auditors

34. The Auditor shall have the same powers as the Auditor of unions in regard to disallowances, reductions, etc. Appeal shall be to the Queen's Bench Division or the Poor Law Board.

Circulation of abstracts of accounts

35. Abstracts of accounts shall be sent to the boards of guardians within one month of each audit.

Remuneration of Auditor

36. The remuneration of the Auditor shall be fixed by the Poor Law Board.

[1] The provision in Section 29 concerning medical instruction was repealed by the Metropolitan Poor Amendment Act, 1869 (32 & 33 Vict. c. 63 s. 20), and re-enacted by Poor Law Act, 1889 (52 & 53 Vict. c. 56 s. 4).

Appointment of new Auditor

37. The Poor Law Board may remove an Auditor and appoint his successor.

Medical Outdoor Relief [Dispensaries]

Building for dispensary

38. The Poor Law Board may direct the guardians of a union or parish to provide a dispensary or dispensaries and to build and equip etc. such building(s) as the Poor Law Board thinks fit.

Dispensary Committee

39. There shall be a committee of management for the dispensary, to be called the Dispensary Committee.

Election of Committee

40. The Dispensary Committee may be elected from the guardians themselves and/or from ratepayers assessed at not less than £40 annual poor rate.

Number etc. of Committee

41. The Poor Law Board shall prescribe the number of members, tenure of office, mode and times of election etc. of the Dispensary Committee.

Places for seeing sick poor etc.

42. The guardians of each union providing a dispensary must provide proper places where medical officers of the union may attend such sick poor as attend for advice, and where meetings of the Dispensary Committee may be held.

Appointment of dispensers etc.

43. The Dispensary Committee shall appoint proper persons to be dispensers of medicine at the dispensary and such other officers and servants as they think fit.

Provision and dispensing of medicines

44. The guardians shall, on the requisition of the Dispensary Committee, provide proper medicines, appliances and requisites for the care and surgical treatment of the sick poor relieved out of the workhouse and the same shall be dispensed and furnished to such of the poor entitled to relief as require the same, on the prescription or written direction of the District Medical Officer, subject to such regulations as the Poor Law Board may direct.

Modification of districts, salaries etc.

45. For giving effect to the provisions of this Act relating to medical relief outside the work-house, the Poor Law Board may vary, as it thinks fit, medical districts, salaries and contracts with District Medical Officers existing at the passing of this Act or hereafter.

District and Separate Schools

District School Boards: application of Common Poor Fund[1] to expenditure; addition of nominated members to Boards

[Sections 46 to 49 provide for District School Boards' expenditure on buildings, officers' salaries etc. to be met from the Common Poor Fund and for the addition of nominated members to the District School Boards.]

[1] See Sections 61–72, following.

Workhouses for Classes of Poor

Reception in workhouses of poor belonging to other unions or parishes

[Section 50 provides for the transfer of particular classes of the poor from one workhouse in the Metropolis to another with a view to separate houses being used for special classes.]

Lands

Acquisition of land for extending institutions

[Sections 51–54 lay down conditions for the acquisition of sites for the building of workhouses, hospitals and schools under this Act and provide for the incorporation in this Act of the Lands Clauses Consolidation Act, 1845, and amending legislation. Compulsory purchase shall apply only to land required for extending a workhouse, hospital or school existing at the passing of this Act and then not without a previous order of the Poor Law Board preceded by public announcement of intention to acquire such land.]

Contributions of Unions and Parishes

Basis of contribution

55. Unions' contributions shall be assessed in proportion to the annual rateable value of the property in the union, according to valuation lists or the latest poor rate or other basis as the Poor Law Board determines.

Calls for contributions

56. The Managers of the asylums and the District School Boards may call on the guardians for such contributions as they consider necessary for the asylums or schools.

[Sections 57 and 58 provide for the collection of contributions from the unions and for remedies in the case of non-payment of contributions.]

Medical Indoor Relief

Contracts with workhouse medical officers

59. In order to facilitate provision for the appointment, where requisite, of resident workhouse medical officers, and for better classification and management of the sick poor in a separate hospital or building, or in an infirmary kept distinct from the rest of the workhouse, the Poor Law Board may vary any contract with any medical or other workhouse officer and direct that he be paid compensation by way of increased salary, annuity, or lump sum, as the Poor Law Board thinks fit.

Houseless Poor

Repeal of reimbursement by Metropolitan Board of Works

60. As from 29 September 1867, Sections 1 and 2 of the Metropolitan Houseless Poor Act, 1864, are repealed except with respect to any claims outstanding at that date.

Metropolitan Common Poor Fund[1]

Establishment of the Metropolitan Common Poor Fund

61. There is to be a fund, raised by contributions from the unions and parishes of the Metropolis, to be known as the Common Poor Fund.

[1] See Note on the Metropolitan Common Poor Fund, Appendix IV.

Assessment of contributions to the Common Fund

62. There shall be a Receiver of the Common Poor Fund to be appointed, paid, and be removeable, by the Poor Law Board.

Receiver to open account at Bank of England

63. The Receiver shall open an account with the Bank of England, known as the Account of the Receiver of the Metropolitan Common Poor Fund.

Assessment of contributions to the Common Fund

64. The Poor Law Board shall periodically assess on the unions and parishes of the Metropolis the amount of their respective contributions to the Common Poor Fund in proportion to the annual rateable value of the property therein comprised, to be determined according to the valuation lists or, where there are none, according to the latest poor rate for the time being for the union or parish, or on such other basis as the Poor Law Board directs.

Collection of the Common Fund

The 65. Poor Law Board shall periodically issue to the guardians of each union or parish a precept requiring them to pay the amount of their contribution; the guardians shall raise the amount of their contribution out of the poor rates of the union or parish and pay the contribution to the credit of the account of the Receiver; no such precept shall be liable to be taken into any court of law; nor shall any order of the guardians or any rate made after the passing of this Act be liable to question in any such court, provided always that the guardians shall be entitled to have credit in part-payment of their contribution for the amount which may be repayable to them out of the Common Poor Fund in respect of expenditure during the preceding half year.

Collection of contributions by local authority where there is no poor rate

66. In any place where there is no poor rate the Poor Law Board may issue the precept for contributions to the Common Poor Fund to the Masters of the Bench, Treasurer, Governors or any other body or persons having control or authority there.

Levying of rate by local authority

67. Such local authority may levy a rate in the nature of a poor rate for the purpose of the contribution on persons occupying rateable property in such a place.

Remedies for recovery of contributions

68. In the case of non-payment of contributions, the Receiver shall have the same remedies in law as the guardians have for recovery from overseers of contributions from parishes.

Application of the Common Fund

69. Expenses incurred for the following purposes after 29 September 1867, shall be repaid out of the Common Poor Fund:

    1. Maintenance of lunatics in asylums, registered hospitals, and licensed houses, and of insane poor in asylums under this Act, except such expenses as are chargeable on the county rate;
    2. Maintenance of patients in any asylums specially provided under this Act for patients suffering from fever or smallpox;

3. All medicines and medical and surgical appliances supplied to the poor in receipt of relief by guardians under this Act or any of the Poor Law Acts;

4. Salaries of all officers employed by the guardians in respect of poor relief, by the Managers of district schools under the Poor Law Amendment Act, 1844, and by the Managers of asylums under this Act, and also the salaries of the dispensers and other persons employed in dispensaries under this Act provided the appointments have been sanctioned by the Poor Law Board;

5. Compensation to medical officers of workhouses and other officers of a union whose contract or office may be affected by this Act;

6. Fees for registration of births and deaths;

7. Fees and other expenses of vaccination;

8. Maintenance of pauper children in district, separate, certificated, and licensed schools;

9. Relief of destitute persons certified by the Auditor, and provision of temporary wards or other places of reception approved by the Poor Law Board under the Metropolitan Houseless Poor Acts of 1864 and 1865.

Mode of repayment out of the Common Fund

70. After each half-yearly audit the Auditors must certify to the Poor Law Board the amounts expended by the unions and parishes in respect of the above expenses and the Poor Law Board shall direct the Receiver to repay the amounts out of the Common Fund.

Receiver's salary etc.

71. Salaries of the Receiver and his assistant shall be paid out of the Common Poor Fund.

Drawing on Receiver's Account

72. The Account of the Receiver at the Bank of England shall be drawn upon in accordance with the regulations of the Poor Law Board.

Poor Relief under Local Acts

Constitution of guardians for parishes under Local Acts

73. The relief of the poor in every union or parish in the Metropolis governed by a Local Act shall be administered, after a day to be stated in an order by the Poor Law Board, by a board of guardians elected according to the Poor Law Acts, notwithstanding anything in such Local Act.

Powers of new board of guardians

74. The guardians so constituted under this Act, notwithstanding anything in any Local Act, shall have the same powers and authority and be subject to the same orders and regulations as guardians elected under the Poor Law Acts.

Transfer of property to new guardians

75. The property of a union or parish governed by a Local Act and held for purposes of poor relief shall be transferred to the guardians constituted under this Act and they shall use it for poor relief as would formerly have been the case and they shall pay all debts lawfully incurred by the previous guardians.

Continuance of existing officers

76. Officers appointed under any such Local Act shall be entitled to continue in office after the constitution of the new board of guardians. If they are deprived of their office by reason of the operation of this Act the Poor Law Board may award them compensation.

Retention of rating powers by existing bodies

77. Nothing in this Act shall deprive any body constituted under a Local Act of any power thereby vested in it of making and levying poor rates, and every such body shall be deemed overseers within the Poor Law Acts.

Parts of sections 64 and 65 of 7 & 8 Vict. c. 101 repealed

78. So much of Section 64 of the Poor Law Amendment Act of 1844 as prevents the union of parishes governed by Local Acts, without consent of the guardians, and Section 65 of that Act, are repealed as far as they relate to the Metropolis.

Boards of Guardians

Power of Poor Law Board to nominate additional guardians

79. The Poor Law Board may nominate, to be members of a board of guardians of a union or parish in the Metropolis, Justices of the Peace, or ratepayers resident in the union or parish assessed to the poor rate therein on an annual rateable value of not less than £40, but so that the number of guardians so nominated does not, together with the ex-officio guardians, ever exceed one-third of the full number of the elected guardians.

Officers

Appointment of officers on failure of Managers etc.

80. If the Managers of an asylum or Dispensary Committee under this Act, or any board of guardians in the Metropolis, fail to appoint any officer whom by law they are required to appoint following a period of fourteen days after the receipt of a Poor Law Board requisition to make such an appointment, the Poor Law Board may appoint a fit person to be such officer.

Borrowing

Extension of borrowing powers

81. Where the guardians of a union or parish in the Metropolis require to borrow money for the purposes of the Poor Law Acts, the principal sum borrowed may be any sum not exceeding one-half of the aggregate amount of the rates raised for the relief of the poor in that union or parish within three years ending on the 25 March preceding the borrowing of the money.

Provision for orders of removal and of maintenance

82. Nothing in this Act shall prevent any local poor law authority from obtaining any order of removal or any order of maintenance in respect of any pauper by reason of the expenses of such pauper being repaid out of the Common Fund.

DOCUMENT III:

CLASSES OF PERSONS PROVIDED FOR BY THE M A B AND THE YEAR
IN WHICH THE RESPONSIBILITY WAS DELEGATED TO THE BOARD

(A) PHYSICALLY AFFLICTED PATIENTS

(i) *Cases of Infectious and Contagious Diseases*

1867   Scarlet fever; Typhoid fever; Typhus; Smallpox. Poor law cases only before 1883.

1888   Diphtheria. Poor law and non-pauper cases admitted from 1888. Free treatment after 1891.

1883; 1893; 1894   Asiatic cholera. Accommodation available in case of need.

1905   Plague. Accommodation available in case of need.

1907   Cerebro-spinal meningitis.

1911 (Feb.)   (Poor law).

1911 (May)   Measles (Non-Pauper).

1911   Whooping-cough (Poor law).

1912   Whooping-cough (Non-Pauper).

1912; 1926   Puerperal fever and Puerperal pyrexia.

1919   Trench fever; Malaria; Dysentery.

1924   Certain contagious conditions of the eye (children received through the LCC).

1924   Zymotic enteritis.

(ii) *Tuberculosis and other diseases*

Tuberculosis:

1897   Poor Law children.

1911   Insured persons under the 1911 National Insurance Act.

1913–1921   Non-insured persons.

Venereal Disease:

1916   Parturient women.

1919   Other women and girls.

1917   Infants suffering from ophthalmia neonatorum.

Children's Diseases:

1897   Ophthalmia and Ringworm (children).

1924   Interstitial keratitis and Infantile paralysis.

1925   Marasmus.

1925–1929   Encephalitis lethargica (cases suffering from after-effects).

1926   Rheumatic fever, acute Endocarditis, Chorea.

Carcinoma:

1928   Women suffering from carcinoma of the uterus.

(B) MENTALLY DISORDERED PATIENTS AND EPILEPTICS

1867   Harmless poor law 'imbeciles' (adults and children—capable of improvement and non-improvable).

1891 Suitable cases certified under the Lunacy Acts transferred from the London County 'lunatic asylums'.

1897 Feeble-minded poor law children (uncertified).

1916–1917 Sane epileptics (Poor Law).

1918 Cases certified under the 1913 Mental Deficiency Act (poor law and non-pauper).

1924 Mentally infirm persons over 70 years of age (poor law) who had not previously been certified.

(C) HEALTHY CLASSES

1875 Poor law boys training for sea service.
      (Non-poor law boys were later received through the LCC and by private agreement.)

1902–10 Juvenile offenders (M A B Remand Homes were transferred to the LCC in 1910).

1912 Homeless poor.

1914–1919 Destitute enemy aliens and War refugees.

DOCUMENT IV

COMMITTEE STRUCTURE OF THE M A B DURING THE LAST DECADE OF ITS ADMINISTRATION
(11 Main Committees and 53 Sub-Committees)

Committee	Main Functions
The Board in plenary session (73 members)	Determination of questions of policy and principles; the sanctioning of all new schemes affecting accommodation, of working conditions, hours, salaries and wages; the actual appointment and promotion of the chief office staff, the chief institution officers, i.e. Medical Superintendent, Matron, Steward, Chaplain, and the consulting medical staff; the settlement of contracts for all works exceeding £100, and in general the approval of expenditure over £100 in one sum.
1. *General Purposes Committee* (all members of the Board) *Sub-Committees:*	Consideration of all questions of policy and all questions affecting the Board's work as a whole.
(i) Accommodation	General questions of accommodation, especially changes of use between different departments; and acquisition and disposal of properties.
(ii) Education	All matters concerning the education of children.
(iii) Establishment	Central Office and clerical staff.
(iv) Institution Staff	All general questions relative to conditions of employment, hours and wages, uniforms, dietary, insurance, compensation, negotiations with trades unions, appeals.
(v) Laundry	Consideration of administration and technical practices in the Board's laundries; expenditure on laundries, output, etc.
(vi) Legislation	Questions of legislation affecting the Board's work.

(vii) Medical and Nursing	Professional matters relating to the medical and nursing services of concern to all the Board's departments; and supervision of work of chief medical officers.
(viii) Statistical	Supervision of collating, processing and publication of statistical data; revision of methods of keeping records, etc.

2. *Finance Committee* (12 members)

Regulation of finances: estimates of income and expenditure; loans and repayments; financial proposals of spending committees; supervision of administration of superannuation acts, insurances, banking, assessments, work of accounting officers, etc.

One Sub-Committee

Consideration of questions relating to stocks and inventories; detailed examination of accounts, passbooks, statements of balances, etc.

3. *Works Committee* (16 members)

Supervision of all matters relating to building works, and control of professional and technical staff.

Two Sub-Committees
(i) Detailed consideration of plans, specifications and estimates.
(ii) Central professional and technical staff.

4. *Contract Committee* (24 members)

Provision of all articles required at institutions, with a few minor exceptions; control of description and quality of supplies; recruitment of technical advisers; management of central stores for the reception, warehousing, examination and distribution of goods.

One Sub-Committee

Printing and stationery.

5. *Isolation Hospitals Committee* (36 members)

Control of isolation hospitals, river ambulance service and laboratories; arrangements for medical instruction, training of fever nurses, bacteriological and research work; accommodation and distribution of nurses.

Sub-Committees:
Two central

Consideration of arrangements affecting all hospitals.
(i) Special medical and nursing questions.
(ii) General.

Fourteen visiting

Control and management of separate isolation hospitals.

6. *Tuberculosis Committee* (27 members)

Control of institutions for tuberculosis; arrangements for training nurses.

Sub-Committees:
One central

Consideration of questions affecting all institutions for tuberculosis.

Eight visiting	Control and management of separate tuberculosis institutions.
7. *Children's Committee* (25 members) *Sub-committees:*	Control of institutions for children; arrangements for training nurses, etc.
One central	Consideration of questions affecting all children's institutions.
Five visiting	Control and management of separate children's institutions.
8. *Mental Hospitals Committee* (30 members) *Sub-committees:*	Control of mental hospitals, training colony and epileptic colony.
One central	Consideration of questions affecting all mental institutions.
Six visiting	Control and management of separate mental institutions.
9. *Training Ship Committee* (12 members) *One Sub-Committee:*	Management of training ship. Finances of training ship.
10. *Casual Wards Committee* (12 members) *Two Sub-Committees:*	Control and management of casual wards and of schemes for dealing with the homeless poor. (i) Control of the Hostel and the 'Night Office' (Welfare Office). (ii) Questions arising from tasks, dietary, etc. in the casual wards.
11. *Ambulance Committee* (12 members)	Control and management of ambulance and transport services.

DOCUMENT V:

CHAIRMEN, VICE-CHAIRMEN AND CLERKS TO THE M A B (1867–1930) AND
MEDICAL OFFICERS AND CONSULTING STAFF (1930)

Chairmen of the Board		*Vice-Chairmen of the Board*	
William Brewer, MP, JP, MD	1867	Alfred Suter	1867
Sir Edwin Galsworthy, JP, DL	1881	B. H. Adams, JP	1875
Sir Robert Hensley, JP	1901	Sir Edwin Galsworthy, JP, DL	1877
Sir Augustus Scovell, JP	1904	Sir Edmund Hay Currie	1881
J. T. Helby	1907	The Rt. Hon. J. G. Talbot, MP, JP	1888
Walter Dennis, JP	1910	P. M. Martineau, JP, DL, LLB	1904
Sir Robert Walden, CBE, JP, DL	1913	Colonel Sir William Smith, DL, MD	1910
The Very Rev. Canon Sprankling, CBE	1919	The Very Rev. Canon Sprankling, CBE	1913

Chairmen (cont.)

Walter Eickhoff, JP	1922
Sir Francis Morris, JP	1924
The Rt. Hon. the Viscount Doneraile	1928

Vice-Chairman (cont.)

Thomas Cornell	1919
Sir Francis Morris, JP	1922
The Rt. Hon. the Viscount Doneraile	1924
George Brittain, JP	1928

Clerks to the Board

W. F. Jebb	1867
Sir Duncombe Mann	1891
Sir Allan Powell, CBE	1922

Chief Medical Officers (1930)

Infectious Disease Hospitals Service	F. H. Thomson, MB, CM, DPH
Children's Institutions and Surgical Tuberculosis Services	W. T. Gordon Pugh, MD, BS
Medical Tuberculosis Service	James Watt, MA, MD, ChB, DPH
Mental Hospitals Service	E. B. Sherlock, MD, BSc, DPH, Barrister-at-Law
Director of Research and Pathological Services	J. E. McCartney, MD, ChB, DSc

Consulting Medical and Surgical Staff (1930)

Miss Margaret M. Basden, MD, BS, FRCS
Comyns Berkeley, MA, MD, MC, FRCP, FRCS
H. Charles Cameron, MA, MD, BCh, FRCP
R. Davies-Colley, CMG, FRCS
Miss Phyllis D. Dixon, MB, BS, MRCS, LRCP
Charles J. Heath, FRCS
T. B. Layton, DSO, MS, FRCS
J. M. H. MacLeod, MA, MD, FRCP
M. S. Mayou, FRCS

F. F. Muecke, CBE, FRCS
George Perkins, MC, MA, MB, BCh, FRCS
J. E. H. Roberts, OBE, FRCS
W. G. Sutcliffe, OBE, FRCS
W. H. Trethowan, FRCS
F. A. C. Tyrrell, FRCS
A. G. Wells, MB, BS
S. A. Kinnier Wilson, MD, FRCP
C. Worster-Drought, MA, MD, MRCP, MRCS
James M. Wyatt, MB, BS, FRCS

Scientific Advisory Committee (1930)

F. H. Thomson, MB, CM, DPH	Chief Medical Officer of the M A B Infectious Disease Hospitals Service (Chairman)
Sir G. S. Buchanan, CB, MD, BSc	Senior Medical Officer, Ministry of Health
Prof. H. R. Dean, MD	Professor of Pathology in the University of Cambridge (Bacteriology)
C. Morley Wenyon, CMG, CBE, MB	Wellcome Bureau of Scientific Research (Protozoology)
Prof. J. C. G. Ledingham, CMG, DSc, FRS, FRCP	Lister Institute of Preventive Medicine (General Pathology and Immunology)
Prof. Hugh MacLean, MD, DSc	Director of the Medical Unit in St. Thomas' Hospital (Biochemistry)
Prof. M. Greenwood, DSc, FRCP, FRS	Professor of Epidemiology and Vital Statistics in the University of London

DOCUMENT VI:

M A B INSTITUTIONS AT THE TIME OF THEIR TRANSFER TO THE LONDON COUNTY COUNCIL (1930).

Institution	Location	Date of Opening	Number of Beds[1]
A. ISOLATION HOSPITALS			
Fever			
Brook	Shooter's Hill, SE.18	31 Aug. 1896	552
Eastern	Homerton Grove, E.9	1 Feb. 1871	561
Grove	Tooting Grove, Tooting Graveney, SW.17	17 Aug. 1899	556
North-Eastern	St. Ann's Road, South Tottenham, N.15	8 Oct. 1892	661
North-Western	Lawn Road, Hampstead, NW.3	25 Jan. 1870	410
Park	Hither Green, Lewisham, SE.13	8 Nov. 1897	612
South-Eastern	Avonley Road, New Cross, SE.14	17 March 1877	511
South-Western	Landor Road, Stockwell, SW.9	31 Jan. 1871	323
Western	Seagrave Road, Fulham, SW.6	10 March 1877	479
Convalescent (Fever)			
Northern	Winchmore Hill, N.21	25 Sept. 1887	562[2]
Southern (Upper)	Dartford, Kent	October 1890	777
Southern (Lower) (formerly Gore Farm Hospital)	Dartford, Kent	Erected 1902	767
Fever or Smallpox			
Joyce Green	Dartford, Kent	28 Dec. 1903	986
Orchard	Dartford, Kent	Erected 1902	664
Smallpox	The River Hospitals		—— 8,421
Long Reach Pier Buildings	Dartford, Kent	27 Feb. 1902	48
Long Reach Hospital	Dartford, Kent	27 Feb. 1902 (Hospital reconstructed 1928–29)	200 —— 248
Ophthalmia Neonatorum			
St. Margaret's	Leighton Road, Kentish Town, NW.5	16 Sept. 1918	60[3]

[1] A summary of M A B hospital beds follows at the end of this list.
[2] This number included 125 beds for the post-encephalitis unit.
[3] This number included 18 beds for marasmus or zymotic enteritis cases.

Document VI—continued

Institution	Location	Date of Opening	Number of Beds
B. INSTITUTION FOR VENEREAL DISEASES			
Sheffield St. Hospital	Kingsway, WC.2	21 June 1920	52
C. INSTITUTIONS FOR TUBERCULOSIS			
King George V Sanatorium	Near Godalming, Surrey	8 June 1922	232
Pinewood	Wokingham, Berks.	7 July 1919	160
Colindale Hospital	Colindale Ave., Hendon, NW.9	1 Jan. 1920	349
Grove Park Hospital	Lee, SE.12	9 Feb. 1926	322
St. George's Home	Milman's Street, Chelsea, SW.10	14 May 1914	50
St. Luke's Hospital	Lowestoft, Suffolk	9 May 1922	205
Princess Mary's Hospital for Children	Margate, Kent	26 June 1898	271
High Wood Hospital for Children	Brentwood, Essex	26 July 1904	370
Millfield	Rustington, Sussex	6 April 1904	98
			—— 2,057[1]
D. LABORATORIES			
Antitoxin Establishment (with stables)	Belmont, Sutton, Surrey	May 1907	—
Northern Group Research and Pathological Laboratory	North-Eastern Hospital, South Tottenham, N.15		—
Southern Group Research and Pathological Laboratory	Park Hospital, Lewisham, S.E.13	May 1927	—
E. CHILDREN'S INSTITUTIONS			
Queen Mary's Hospital for Children	Carshalton, Surrey	29 Jan. 1909	900
The Downs Hospital for Children	Sutton, Surrey	26 Feb. 1903	360
St. Anne's Convalescent Home	Herne Bay, Kent	26 Dec. 1897	150

[1] In addition to this total of tuberculosis beds, there were another 560 at Queen Mary's Hospital and 100 at the Northern Hospital.

Document VI—continued

Institution	Location	Date of Opening	Number of Beds	
Goldie Leigh Homes (ringworm and other skin diseases)	Abbey Wood, SE.2	1 Nov. 1914	218	
White Oak (ophthalmia and interstitial keratitis)	Swanley Junction, Kent	20 March 1903	364	
			——	1,992
F. MENTAL HOSPITALS				
Tooting Bec	Tooting Bec Road, SW.17	19 Jan. 1903	2,230	
Leavesden	Abbot's Langley, Watford, Herts.	October 1870	2,159	
Caterham	Caterham, Surrey	October 1870	2,068	
Fountain	Tooting Grove, SW.17	October 1893	670	
Training Colony				
(i) Imbeciles	Darenth, Nr. Dartford, Kent	November 1878	1,614	
(ii) Feeble-minded			646	
			——	9,387
Colony for Sane Epileptics (men and boys)	Silver Street, Edmonton, N.18	December 1916		355
G. AMBULANCE STATIONS				
Brook	Shooter's Hill, SE.18	18 Aug. 1896	—	
Eastern	Brooksby's Walk, E.9	20 June 1885	—	
North-Western	Lawn Road, NW.3	1 Sept. 1897	—	
South-Eastern	New Cross Road, SE.14	1 Oct. 1883	—	
South-Western	Landor Rd., SW.9	2 May 1898	—	
Western	Seagrave Rd., SW.6	9 July 1884	—	
Mechanical Transport Department	Carnwath Rd., SW.6	April 1902	—	
Wharves and Steamers				
North Wharf	Blackwall, E.14	January 1884	9	
South Wharf	Rotherhithe, SE.16	December 1883	24	
West Wharf	Fulham, SW.6	February 1885	—	
5 Ambulance Steamers	—	May 1884 to March 1902	178	
			——	211
H. TRAINING SHIP				
'Exmouth'	Gray's Essex	March 1876	700	
Ship's Infirmary	Gray's, Essex	August 1905	34	
			——	734

Document VI—continued

Institution	Location	Date of Opening	Number of Beds
I. INSTITUTIONS FOR CASUAL POOR			
9 Casual Wards	Various parts of the Metropolis	Transferred to the M A B 1 April 1912	758
The Hostel	Little Gray's Inn Lane, EC.1	20 July 1923	76 ——— 834
Homeless Poor 'Night Office'	Under Charing Cross Railway Bridge, WC.2 (formerly near Waterloo Pier)	16 Dec. 1921 (30 Oct. 1912)	— —
J. ADMINISTRATIVE DEPARTMENTS			
Head Office of the M A B	Victoria Embankment, EC.4	March 1900	—
Engineer-in-Chief's Department	Sheffield St., WC.2	September 1914	—
Central Stores	Peckham Rye, SE.15	September 1908	—

SUMMARY OF M A B HOSPITAL BEDS AT THE TIME OF THEIR TRANSFER TO THE LCC IN 1930

Institutions for the Treatment of:	Number of Units	Number of Beds
'Fever'[1]	14	8,421
Smallpox	2	248
Ophthalmia Neonatorum	1	60
Venereal Diseases	1	52
Tuberculosis	9	2,057
Sick Children	5	1,992
The Mentally Disordered and Feeble-Minded	5	9,387
Sane Epileptics	1	355
Totals:	38	22,572

[1] The comprehensive term 'fever' included such diseases as scarlet fever, typhoid fever, typhus, plague and cholera.

M A B Fever and Smallpox Hospitals

ARCHITECTURAL NOTES ON TWO M A B FEVER HOSPITALS, MODELS OF WHICH WERE EXHIBITED IN THE SOCIAL SCIENCE SECTION OF THE INTERNATIONAL EXHIBITION HELD IN PARIS IN 1900.

1. *NORTH-EASTERN (TEMPORARY) FEVER HOSPITAL:* St. Ann's Road, South Tottenham, London (later St. Ann's General Hospital).

Architects: Messrs. A. and C. Harston, FRIBA, of 15 Leadenhall Street, London.

Accommodation: 500 patients and necessary staff.

Original Cost: £54,446, plus £12,000 for the site (about 28 acres).

Date of Opening: October 1892. Built in six weeks when scarlet fever was epidemic in London.

Architectural Details (see figure 1):

Materials. The boiler house and chimney shaft, steam coal store and heating room were constructed in brickwork. The remainder of the buildings were of wood upon brick piers, raised upon concrete platforms which extended about six feet beyond the walls. The floors were of double thickness with a layer of felt between; the walls were of timber framing, filled and weather-boarded outside and match-lined inside; and the roofs were match-lined, boarded and covered with galvanized corrugated iron.

Lay-out, Dimensions, etc. The principal buildings were connected by covered ways, with which were combined brick ducts for the reception of the water, gas and steam pipes. The ducts formed a quadrangle and their total length was 2,120 feet.

Each of the *ward huts* contained a ward 120 feet by 24 feet, sanitary room, bathroom, scullery, pantry, and linen closet; the isolation huts had each two wards 24 feet square, with similar subsidiary rooms; and the sick nurses' hut and isolation nurses' hut each had six separate bedrooms, a scullery, bathroom, etc. Bed space was as follows: linear wall space, 12 feet; floor area, 144 square feet; cubic space, 1,656 cubic feet.

The *ventilation* of the wards and dormitories was effected by means of inlets near floor level, covered with perforated zinc inside and protected by flaps externally. A ventilating panel ran along the centre of the ceiling, and a raised ridge capping permitted the escape of vitiated air. The windows throughout were filled with double hung sashes, with deep fillet at sill, permitting the sash to be raised without draught.

Heating. All the buildings were warmed by steam pipes or radiators worked by the central boilers, which also supplied steam to the kitchen and laundry and to the bath water heaters, which were situated in the basement of the two receiving rooms.

Lighting. The buildings were lit by gas throughout.

(The North-Eastern Hospital was reconstructed as a permanent hospital in 1898 at a cost of £126,850. Other buildings were added later, e.g. a laundry in 1900 at a cost of £10,251.)

2. *THE BROOK (PERMANENT) FEVER HOSPITAL:* Shooter's Hill Road, Woolwich.

Architect: Mr. T. W. Aldwinckle, FRIBA, of 1 Victoria Street, Westminster, London.

Accommodation: 488 beds, distributed as follows: scarlet fever, 352; typhoid fever and diphtheria, 112; 'isolation wards' for serious smallpox cases, 24. *Staff employed:* 325.

Original Cost: £301,456, plus £16,200 for the site (about 29 acres).

Date of Opening: August 1896.

Description (as given in a pamphlet prepared by the M A B for visitors to the Paris International Exhibition of 1900, see figure 1):

'*Site*. The hospital and administrative buildings occupy a site 200 feet above sea level which falls rapidly to the south, thus enabling the buildings to be arranged in terraces, sheltered from the north and east winds.

'The *administrative buildings* and *nurses' home* are entirely separate and distinct from the patients' wards, and have a separate entrance from the public roadway. The patients' pavilions are two-storeyed, with an open space, varying from 4 to 8 feet in height, under the ground floor.

'The following are the *spaces allowed per bed* in the wards, all wards being 13 feet high:

	Scarlet Fever	Typhoid Fever and Diphtheria
Linear wall space	12 feet	15 feet
Floor area	156 square feet	195 square feet
Cubic space	2,028 cubic feet	2,535 cubic feet

'Attached to each ward is a separation ward, bathroom, duty-room (for nurses' use), a linen store and larder, and w.c. turrets. Also, on the ground floor, a w.c. and lavatory for the nurses. The ward floors are of polished teak. The wards are warmed by means of (a) open ventilating fireplaces and (b) low pressure hot-water apparatus, the latter being supplementary to the former, as the principal reliance is placed on the open fireplaces as being the best means of warming a hospital ward.

'The wards, duty rooms, bathrooms, and ward corridors are kept at the same temperature, so as to avoid draughts by the opening of doors in the wards.

'*Ventilation*. The inlet ventilation of the wards comprises external fresh air admitted through the ward stoves and through radiator cases attached to the external walls, the air in each case being thus warmed; also by valvular gratings in the external walls at the floor line. Most important of all, there are the windows (one to each bed) on opposite sides of the ward. The ordinary double-hung sashes are supplemented by hopper-hung fanlights; and these means of admitting fresh external air into the ward are the most valuable of all inlet ventilation in this climate, where on about 300 to 330 days in the year it is possible to open the windows of a hospital ward without injury to the patients—a simple fact which renders mechanical ventilation entirely unsuitable in this country.

'There are two means of exhaust ventilation to each ward in addition to the open windows, viz. (a) open fireplaces, and (b) vertical shafts. There are four open fireplaces to each ward, and these form, undoubtedly, the most effective means of exhaust ventilation. It is, however, prudent to supplement these by vertical shafts. These are 14 inches square internally and lined with salt-glazed bricks with rounded internal angles. There are three to each ward, and an upward current is generated in each shaft by means of a copper steam coil. Two connexions with each shaft are made in each ward—one at the floor line, and one at the ceiling line—and valvular gratings are provided in each opening, so regulated by hand gearing that when the upper one is open the lower one is closed, and vice versa.

'*Lighting*. All the buildings are lighted by electricity.

'*Water Supply*. The water is first received from a public supply company into a water-tower and being somewhat hard is, before use, passed through a water-softening apparatus.

'*Equipment*. Fire alarms, fire-extinguishing appliances, telephones, and all modern hospital appliances have been provided; and the hospital is considered one of the most perfect of infectious disease hospitals.'

TABLE A

SMALLPOX IN LONDON, 1838–1900: ANNUAL MORTALITY

Year	Estimated Population (mid-year)	Total Smallpox Deaths	Rate per million (annual)	Rate per million (annual average: 5 years)
1838	1,766,169	3,817	2,161	—
1839	1,802,751	634	352	—
1840	1,840,091	1,235	671	—
1841	1,878,205	1,053	561	—
1842	1,917,108	360	188	787
1843	1,954,041	438	224	399
1844	2,033,816	1,804	887	506
1845	2,073,298	909	438	460
1846	2,113,535	257	122	372
1847	2,202,673	955	434	421
1848	2,244,837	1,620	722	521
1849	2,287,302	521	228	389
1850	2,330,054	499	214	344
1851	2,373,081	1,062	448	409
1852	2,416,367	1,159	480	418
1853	2,459,899	211	86	291
1854	2,503,662	694	277	301
1855	2,547,639	1,039	408	340
1856	2,591,815	531	205	291
1857	2,636,174	156	59	207
1858	2,680,700	242	90	208
1859	2,725,374	1,158	425	237
1860	2,770,181	898	324	221
1861	2,815,101	217	77	195
1862	2,860,117	366	128	209
1863	2,905,210	1,996	687	328
1864	2,950,361	547	185	280
1865	2,995,551	640	214	258
1866	3,040,761	1,391	457	334
1867	3,085,971	1,345	436	396
1868	3,131,160	597	191	297
1869	3,176,308	275	87	277
1870	3,221,394	973	302	295
1871	3,267,251	7,912	2,421	688
1872	3,319,736	1,786	537	708

TABLE A—*continued*

Year	Estimated Population (mid-year)	Total Smallpox Deaths	Rate per million (annual)	Rate per million (annual average: 5 years)
1873	3,373,065	113	33	676
1874	3,427,250	57	16	661
1875	3,482,306	46	12	602
1876	3,538,246	736	207	161
1877	3,595,085	2,551	709	194
1878	3,652,837	1,417	387	266
1879	3,711,517	450	120	287
1880	3,771,139	471	124	309
1881	3,824,980	2,367	617	391
1882	3,862,956	430	110	271
1883	3,901,309	136	34	201
1884	3,940,042	1,236	307	238
1885	3,979,160	1,419	347	283
1886	4,018,666	24	5	160
1887	4,058,565	9	2	139
1888	4,098,860	9	2	132
1889	4,139,555	—	—	71
1890	4,180,654	4	1	2
1891	4,223,720	8	2	1·4
1892	4,269,634	41	10	3
1893	4,312,263	206	48	12
1894	4,351,501	89	22	16
1895	4,387,248	55	13	18
1896	4,419,411	9	2	18
1897	4,447,907	16	4	17
1898	4,472,664	1	0·2	7·6
1899	4,493,617	3	0·6	3·8
1900	4,510,711	4	0·8	1·4

Source: Returns of the Registrar-General.

M A B SMALLPOX HOSPITALS, 1870–1900[1]
Annual Admissions, Deaths, Case Fatality Rates, and London Rates of Mortality from Smallpox.

Year	Admissions			Deaths			Hospital Case Fatality Rates %[2]	London Mortality Rates per 1,000 est. popn.
	Small-pox	Other Diseases	Totals	Small-pox	Other Diseases	Totals	Small-pox	Small-pox
1870–71	582	—	582	97	—	97	20·81	—
1871–72	13,139	6	13,145	2,460	—	2,460	18·95	2·42
1872–73	2,359	3	2,362	467	I	468	17·84	0·54
1873–74	174	17	191	35	—	35	} 17·02	0·03
1874	112	8	120	10	—	10		0·02
1875	89	22	111	22	—	22		0·01
1876	2,134	16	2,150	372	I	373	21·64	0·21
1877	6,516	104	6,620	1,214	4	1,218	17·92	0·71
1878	4,558	96	4,654	824	9	833	17·99	0·39
1879	1,628	60	1,688	273	5	278	15·69	0·12
1880	1,982	50	2,032	286	2	288	15·95	0·12
1881	8,551	120	8,671	1,417	14	1,431	16·61	0·62
1882	1,799	55	1,854	260	3	263	12·96	0·11
1883	598	28	626	93	—	93	16·06	0·03
1884	6,363	204	6,567	940	3	943	15·98	0·31
1885	6,146	198	6,344	1,052	3	1,055	15.80	0.35
1886	99	33	132	22	2	24	} 14·28	0·01
1887	56	3	59	3	—	3		0·00
1888	62	5	67	8	—	8		0·00
1889	5	—	5	—	—	—		—
1890	22	5	27	3	—	3		0·00
1891	63	I	64	8	—	8		0·00
1892	325	23	348	35	—	35	11·29	0·01
1893	2,376	118	2,494	180	2	182	7·64	0·05
1894	1,117	120	1,237	102	7	109	8·87	0·02
1895	941	81	1,022	64	I	65	6·36	0·01
1896	190	41	231	9	I	10	4·01	0·00
1897	70	26	96	13	I	14	18·44	0·00
1898	5	9	14	—	—	—	—	0·00
1899	18	18	36	3	—	3	20·69	0·00
1900	66	19	85	3	—	3	4·30	0·00
Totals (1870–1900)[1]	62,145	1,489	63,634	10,257	59	10,334	ann. av. 16·53	

[1] Annual statistics for M A B Smallpox Hospitals for the twentieth century (1901–1929) are given in Table C, following.

[2] Case fatality rates were calculated according to the Registrar-General's formula, i.e. by dividing the deaths, multiplied by 100, by half the sum of the admissions, discharges and deaths for the year.

Sources: M A B Annual Reports and Registrar-General's Annual Summaries.

TABLE C
M A B SMALLPOX HOSPITALS, 1901–1929
Annual Admissions, Deaths and Case Fatality Rates.

Year	Admissions			Deaths			Hospital Case Fatality Rates %
	Smallpox	Other Diseases	Totals	Smallpox	Other Diseases	Totals	Smallpox
Totals							ann. av.
1870–1900[1]	62,145	1,489	63,634	10,275	59	10,334	16·53
1901	1,743	107	1,850	257	3	260	14·74
1902	7,916	608	8,524	1,337	5	1,342	16·89
1903	355	80	435	12	1	13	3·38
1904	449	64	513	27	—	27	6·01
1905	53	34	87	8	1	9	
1906	27	6	33	—	—	—	
1907	2	13	15	—	1	1	
1908	1	3	4	—	—	—	
1909	15	13	28	2	—	2	
1910	5	5	10	—	—	—	12·22
1911	70	21	91	11	—	11	
1912	5	5	10	1	—	1	
1913	1	8	9	—	—	—	
1914	1	7	8	—	—	—	
1915	11	1	12	2	—	2	
1916	1	4	5	—	—	—	
1917	—	3	3	—	—	—	
1918	45	8	53	—	—	—	9·70
1919	25	6	31	4	—	4	
1920	50	4	54	7	—	7	
1921	2	—	2	—	—	—	
1922	72	—	72	23	—	23	31·94
1923	13	—	13	2	—	2	15·38
1924	5	—	5	—	—	—	—
1925	11	—	11	1	—	1	9·09
1926	5	—	5	1	—	1	20·00
1927	9	—	9	3	—	3	33·33
1928	288	51	339	2	—	2	—
1929	3,031	211	3,242	9	1	10	0·31
Totals 1901–1929	14,211	1,262	15,473	1,709	12	1,721	—
Combined Totals 1870–1929	76,356	2,751	79,107	11,984	71	12,055	—

[1] Annual statistics for the period 1870–1900 are given in preceding Table B.
Source: M A B Annual Reports for the years indicated.

M A B FEVER HOSPITALS, 1871–1900[1]
Annual Admissions, Deaths, Case Fatality Rates and London Rates of Mortality from the Diseases treated.

Year	Admissions						Deaths		
	Scarlet Fever	Diphtheria[3]	Typhus	Enteric Fever	Other Diseases	Totals	Scarlet Fever	Diphtheria[3]	Typhus
1871 {15[2]	—	—	—	—	—	—	—	—	—
1872 } mths.	108	—	134	279	343	864	11	—	30
1873	92	—	401	381	271	1,145	6	—	91
1874	804	—	536	435	359	2,134	89	—	106
1875	1,182	—	65	299	269	1,815	160	—	16
1876	671	—	139	288	294	1,392	90	—	28
1877	479	—	170	372	186	1,207	54	—	36
1878	679	—	168	484	233	1,564	91	—	47
1879	1,469	—	48	385	196	2,098	211	—	11
1880	1,949	—	28	248	239	2,464	242	—	6
1881	1,477	—	219	415	211	2,322	168	—	34
1882	1,850	—	148	515	354	2,867	189	—	27
1883	1,920	—	45	486	269	2,720	234	—	11
1884	1,845	—	29	493	180	2,547	234	—	5
1885	1,353	—	53	220	229	1,855	130	—	7
1886	1,780	—	10	333	74	2,197	151	—	4
1887	5,900	—	35	441	161	6,537	489	—	4
1888	4,408	99	1	450	194	5,152	501	46	—
1889	4,518	772	23	290	219	5,772	366	275	6
1890	6,537	942	16	498	341	8,334	510	316	5
1891	5,262	1,312	18	755	462	7,809	357	397	1
1892	13,093	2,009	19	430	725	16,276	839	583	2
1893	14,548	2,848	2	544	732	18,674	901	865	1
1894	11,598	3,666	6	534	863	16,667	717	1,035	1
1895	11,271	3,635	3	661	1,277	16,847	591	820	—
1896	15,982	4,508	9	600	1,174	22,273	666	948	2
1897	15,113	5,673	2	664	1,417	22,869	619	987	—
1898	12,125	6,566	9	869	1,488	21,057	514	991	1
1899	13,290	8,676	11	1,535	1,582	25,094	353	1,182	—
1900	10,343	7,873	4	1,728	1,706	21,654	313	988	1
Totals 1871–1900[1]	161,646	48,529	2,351	15,632	16,048	244,206	9,796	9,433	483

[1] Annual statistics for M A B Fever Hospitals for the twentieth century (1901–1929) are given in Table E, following.

[2] From 1 December 1870 to 30 September 1871, the M A B Fever Hospitals were used for smallpox cases only.

Deaths			Hospital Case Fatality Rates %[4]				London Mortality Rates per 1,000			
Enteric Fever	Other Diseases	Totals	Scarlet Fever	Diph-theria[3]	Typhus	Enteric Fever	Scarlet Fever	Diph-theria[3]	Typhus	Enteric Fever
—	—	—	—	—	—	—	0·58	0·11	0·12	0·27
57	70	168	10·78	—	23·62	21·96	0·28	0·08	0·05	0·24
56	58	211	6·55	—	23·15	15·13	0·19	0·09	0·08	0·27
63	84	342	12·15	—	19·62	14·87	0·77	0·12	0·09	0·26
78	54	308	13·69	—	23·35	24·68	1·06	0·17	0·04	0·23
59	71	248	12·13	—	19·31	20·34	0·65	0·11	0·04	0·22
79	33	202	12·10	—	23·07	22·93	0·44	0·09	0·04	0·25
100	40	278	14·34	—	26·25	20·26	0·49	0·15	0·04	0·28
74	39	335	15·27	—	21·56	19·73	0·72	0·15	0·02	0·23
43	37	328	12·30	—	20·68	15·63	0·82	0·14	0·02	0·19
86	46	334	11·10	—	16·95	21·47	0·55	0·17	0·02	0·25
104	60	380	10·37	—	16·92	20·71	0·52	0·22	0·01	0·25
74	66	385	12·38	—	21·15	15·64	0·51	0·24	0·01	0·25
98	55	392	12·27	—	20·00	18·82	0·36	0·24	0·01	0·23
36	46	219	9·47	—	12·17	15·82	0·18	0·23	0·01	0·15
47	22	224	9·04	—	42·10	14·85	0·17	0·21	0·00	0·15
61	59	613	9·54	—	11·59	14·59	0·36	0·23	0·00	0·15
72	60	679	9·89	59·35	—	14·64	0·30	0·32	0·00	0·17
41	48	736	8·85	40·74	31·57	15·15	0·19	0·39	0·00	0·13
93	81	1,005	7·86	33·55	25·66	19·68	0·21	0·33	0·00	0·15
106	102	963	6·67	30·63	5·88	14·52	0·14	0·32	0·00	0·13
65	140	1,629	7·28	29·35	9·76	13·20	0·27	0·46	0·00	0·10
110	105	1,982	6·11	30·42	50·00	20·54	0·37	0·76	0·00	0·16
96	150	1,999	5·92	29·29	16·67	18·13	0·22	0·62	0·00	0·15
119	142	1,672	5·45	22·85	—	18·17	0·19	0·54	0·00	0·14
96	109	1,821	4·29	21·20	25·00	15·84	0·21	0·60	0·00	0·13
124	140	1,870	4·07	17·69	—	18·64	0·18	0·51	0·00	0·12
143	147	1,796	4·12	15·37	11·11	17·73	0·13	0·39	0·00	0·13
240	160	1,935	2·65	13·95	—	16·47	0·09	0·43	0·00	0·17
245	167	1,714	2·97	12·27	22·22	14·09	0·08	0·34	0·00	0·16
2,665	2,391	24,768	6·07 ann. av.	19·68 ann. av.	20·54 ann. av.	18·44 ann. av.	—	—	—	—

[3] M A B Fever Hospitals began to admit diphtheria cases on 23 October 1888. The practice of antitoxin ~~se~~rum in the treatment of diphtheria began in 1894.

[4] Hospital case fatality rates in M A B hospitals were calculated according to the Registrar-General's ~~fo~~rmula, i.e. by dividing the deaths, multiplied by 100, by half the sum of the admissions, discharges and ~~de~~aths for the year.

Sources: M A B Annual Reports and Registrar-General's Annual Summaries.

TABLE E
M A B FEVER HOSPITALS 1901–1929[1]

Annual Admissions, Deaths, Case Fatality Rates, and Metropolitan Rates of Mortality from some of the Diseases treated.

Year	Admissions											
	Diphtheria	*Diphtheria (bacteriological)*	*Enteric Fever*	*Measles*[2]	*Scarlet Fever*	*Typhus*	*Whooping-Cough*[2]	*Other Diseases*[3]	*Total Admissions*	*Diphtheria*	*Diphtheria (bacteriological)*	*Enteric Fever*
Totals 1871–1900[1]	48,529	—	15,632	—	161,646	2,351	—	16,048	244,206	9,433	—	2,665
1901	7,622	—	1,129	—	14,539	13	—	2,365	25,668	849	—	175
1902	6,520	—	1,420	—	14,503	—	—	2,108	24,551	739	—	218
1903	5,072	—	967	—	10,345	19	—	1,913	18,316	504	—	145
1904	4,687	—	750	—	11,155	3	—	1,993	18,588	469	—	115
1905	4,148	—	586	—	16,958	5	—	2,157	23,854	347	—	82
1906	5,218	—	698	—	17,933	4	—	2,151	26,004	445	—	108
1907	5,744	—	541	—	22,764	3	—	3,117	32,169	544	—	72
1908	5,230	—	509	—	19,629	2	—	2,597	27,967	507	—	80
1909	4,393	210	331	—	15,384	4	—	2,324	22,646	432	3	45
1910	3,634	222	509	297	8,782	3	64	1,727	15,238	281	2	77
1911	5,034	356	360	3,144	8,818	—	1,184	2,242	21,138	428	7	54
1912	4,844	375	222	4,314	9,883	2	1,731	1,930	23,301	331	4	42
1913	5,076	399	238	3,400	15,010	4	1,044	2,575	27,746	330	2	37
1914	6,591	522	316	770	22,006	—	736	2,598	33,539	540	2	54
1915	6,776	475	269	1,260	15,197	3	114	3,761	27,855	576	4	40
1916	7,201	494	202	1,171	7,646	1	734	3,243	20,692	517	8	27
1917	6,791	600	172	2,951	5,294	—	391	4,047	20,246	485	8	30
1918	6,634	392	130	1,345	6,078	1	276	2,577	17,433	557	2	18
1919	7,184	557	136	751	11,010	—	146	2,178	21,962	635	6	14
1920	10,636	1,043	109	526	20,821	—	103	2,678	35,916	890	11	0
1921	12,432	937	111	393	29,806	—	156	4,024	47,859	1,071	12	20
1922	11,737	1,015	77	1,483	15,279	—	208	3,513	33,312	1,115	15	10
1923	7,522	838	110	1,767	8,730	—	528	3,590	23,085	570	9	13
1924	7,569	619	159	4,694	9,715	—	1,077	4,409	28,242	516	3	11
1925	9,247	1,004	137	1,902	10,508	—	1,488	4,666	28,952	458	4	13
1926	10,527	1,108	178	2,959	10,653	—	775	4,203	30,403	510	14	3
1927	9,155	1,165	109	2,350	11,470	—	1,888	4,267	30,404	370	11	6
1928	8,981	1,037	230	7,307	13,065	—	1,455	4,725	36,800	335	9	7
1929	9,009	881	141	2,322	13,596	—	2,967	5,515	34,431	312	10	18
Totals 1901–1929	205,214	14,249	10,846	45,106	396,577	67	17,065	89,193	778,317	15,663	146	1,544
Combined Totals 1871–1929	253,743	14,249	26,478	45,106	558,223	2,418	17,065	105,241	1,022,523	25,096	146	4,213

[1] Annual statistics and notes applicable to the period 1871–1900 are given in preceding Table D.
[2] Measles and Whooping-Cough became legally admissible to M A B Fever Hospitals in 1911–12.

Measles²	Scarlet Fever	Typhus	Whooping-Cough²	Other Diseases³	Total Deaths	Diphtheria	Enteric Fever	Measles²	Scarlet Fever	Typhus	Whooping-Cough²	Diphtheria	Measles	Scarlet Fever	Whooping-Cough²
	Deaths					Hospital Case Fatality Rates %						London Mortality Rates, per 1,000			
—	9,796	403	—	2,391	24,768	ann. av. 19·68	ann. av. 18·44	—	ann. av. 6·07	ann. av. 20·54	—	—	—	—	—
—	542	4	—	167	1,737	11·1	14·2	—	3·8	30·8	—	0·30	—	0·13	—
—	512	—	—	178	1,647	11·0	15·5	—	3·4	—	—	0·25	—	0·12	—
—	333	4	—	166	1,152	9·7	15·4	—	3·1	21·0	—	0·16	—	0·08	—
—	364	—	—	183	1,131	10·0	14·6	—	3·4	—	—	0·16	—	0·08	—
—	536	—	—	147	1,112	8·3	13·1	—	3·3	—	—	0·12	—	0·12	—
—	521	—	—	163	1,237	8·8	16·0	—	2·9	—	—	0·15	—	0·11	—
—	622	—	—	167	1,405	9·6	13·1	—	2·8	—	—	0·17	—	0·14	—
—	520	—	—	148	1,255	9·7	16·3	—	2·6	—	—	0·15	—	0·11	—
—	371	—	—	184	1,035	9·4	11·9	—	2·3	—	—	0·13	—	0·08	—
38	213	—	1	89	701	7·8	15·8	15·8	2·3	—	2·2	0·09	0·41	0·04	0·28
438	167	—	144	125	1,363	8·4	14·3	13·9	1·9	—	13·2	0·14	0·57	0·04	0·23
414	154	2	146	135	1,228	6·2	17·8	10·4	1·6	100·0	8·5	0·10	0·40	0·04	0·22
428	176	—	137	133	1,243	6·2	16·2	11·3	1·2	—	12·8	0·09	0·34	0·04	0·17
70	304	—	87	154	1,211	7·9	17·1	9·3	1·4	—	10·8	0·16	0·31	0·07	0·20
132	329	2	14	257	1,360	8·4	16·7	10·3	2·0	66·7	11·0	0·16	0·50	0·07	0·25
97	152	—	71	158	1,030	6·8	13·1	8·9	1·8	—	9·9	0·14	0·19	0·03	0·19
348	98	—	50	178	1,197	6·7	17·3	11·7	1·9	—	13·4	0·14	0·49	0·02	0·14
187	111	—	55	206	1,136	7·7	13·4	13·2	1·8	—	17·5	0·16	0·41	0·03	0·42
49	152	—	15	152	1,023	9·3	10·4	6·7	1·5	—	10·7	0·18	0·08	0·03	0·05
63	214	—	12	149	1,345	8·6	5·2	11·4	1·1	—	11·5	0·22	0·22	0·05	0·17
31	304	—	8	139	1,585	8·8	18·2	8·4	1·0	—	5·2	0·25	0·05	0·06	0·12
141	301	—	14	146	1,742	8·7	13·2	9·4	1·8	—	7·3	0·25	0·35	0·07	0·25
114	115	—	76	96	993	6·8	12·3	7·7	1·2	—	14·6	0·13	0·08	0·02	0·09
451	125	—	97	147	1,350	7·0	7·8	9·0	1·3	—	10·3	0·12	0·29	0·03	0·11
121	111	—	219	135	1,061	5·0	8·4	7·6	1·1	—	13·4	0·11	0·08	0·02	0·19
223	88	—	59	139	1,036	4·9	1·6	6·8	0·8	—	9·2	0·12	0·20	0·02	0·05
123	64	—	217	129	920	4·0	5·7	6·7	0·6	—	10·9	0·08	0·12	0·01	0·10
561	81	—	122	172	1,287	3·7	3·0	7·1	0·6	—	9·3	0·09	0·30	0·02	0·09
141	74	—	485	183	1,223	3·6	13·3	7·1	0·6	—	15·3	0·08	0·04	0·02	0·30
4,170	7,654	12	2,029	4,539	35,749	—	—	—	—	—	—	—	—	—	—
4,170	17,450	495	2,029	6,930	60,527	—	—	—	—	—	—	—	—	—	—

³ 'Other Diseases' included: cerebro-spinal meningitis, zymotic enteritis, encephalitis lethargica, poliomyelitis, as well s cases of 'mistaken diagnosis'.

Sources: M A B Annual Reports and Registrar-General's Annual Summaries for the years indicated.

TABLE F

PRINCIPAL DISEASES TREATED IN THE M A B ISOLATION HOSPITALS, 1871–1900[1]

(A) Admissions; (B) Hospital Case Fatality Rates; (C) London Rates of Mortality for quinquennial periods.

Quinquennium	Scarlet Fever (Annual Averages)			Diphtheria[2] (Annual Averages)			Typhus (Annual Averages)			Enteric Fever (Annual Averages)			Smallpox (Annual Averages)		
	A No.	B per cent	C per 1,000	A No.	B per cent	C per 1,000	A No.	B per cent	C per 1,000	A No.	B per cent	C per 1,000	A No.	B[3] per cent	C per 1,000
1871–75	514	10·16	0·68	—	—	0·13	267	21·12	0·08	328	18·03	0·25	3,240	14·68	0·59
1876–80	1,049	13·23	0·62	—	—	0·13	111	22·17	0·03	355	19·78	0·23	3,364	17·84	0·31
1881–85	1,689	11·12	0·42	—	—	0·22	99	17·44	0·01	426	18·50	0·23	4,691	15·48	0·28
1886–90	4,629	9·04	0·25	—	—	0·30	17	22·18	0·00	402	15·78	0·15	49	14·28	0·00
1891–95	11,554	6·29	0·24	2,694	28·51	0·52	10	16·46	0·00	585	16·91	0·14	964	9·69	0·02
1896–1900[1]	13,371	3·62	0·14	6,659	16·10	0·45	7	11·67	0·00	1,079	16·55	0·14	70	9·49	0·00

[1] For comparable statistics for the period 1901–1929 see Table G following. *Annual* statistics for the quinquennia shown above (1871–1900) are shown in preceding Table B (smallpox hospitals) and Table D (fever hospitals).

[2] Diphtheria was first treated in M A B fever hospitals in October 1888.

[3] *Smallpox case fatality rates* per cent in M A B hospitals during the six major epidemics in London of virulent smallpox were as follows:

Smallpox Epidemic Periods	1870–72	1876–78	1881	1884–85	1893–94	1901–02
Case Fatality Rates %	18·8	18·2	16·5	15·9	8·0	16·8

Sources: M A B Annual Reports and Registrar-General's Annual Summaries for the years indicated.

TABLE G

PRINCIPAL DISEASES TREATED IN THE M A B ISOLATION HOSPITALS, 1901–1929[1]

Admissions, Hospital Case Fatality Rates and London Rates of Mortality expressed as annual averages for quinquennial periods.

Quinquennium	Admissions (Annual Averages)						Hospital Case Fatality Rates % (Annual Averages)						London Mortality Rates per 1,000 (Annual Averages)			
	Diphtheria[2]	Enteric Fever	Measles	Scarlet Fever	Small-pox	Whooping-Cough	Diphtheria	Enteric Fever	Measles	Scarlet Fever	Small-pox	Whooping-Cough	Diphtheria	Measles	Scarlet Fever	Whooping-Cough
1901–05[1]	5,610	970	—	13,500	2,103	—	10·02	14·56	—	3·40	9·53	—	0·20	—	0·10	—
1906–10	4,844	518	—	16,898	10	—	9·06	14·62	—	2·58	12·22	—	0·14	—	0·10	—
1911–15	5,664	281	2,578	14,183	18	962	7·42	16·42	11·40	1·62	10·96	11·26	0·13	0·42	0·05	0·21
1916–20	7,689	150	1,349	10,170	24	330	7·82	11·88	10·38	1·62	9·70	12·60	0·17	0·27	0·03	0·19
1921–25	9,901	119	2,048	14,808	21	691	7·26	11·98	8·42	1·28	11·8	10·16	0·17	0·17	0·04	0·15
1926–29 (4 years)	9,418	165	3,735	12,196	844	1,771	4·05	5·90	6·93	0·65	0·95[3]	11·17	0·10	0·17	0·02	0·11

[1] For comparable statistics for the first thirty years (1871–1900) see preceding Table F. *Annual* statistics for the quinquennia shown above (1901–29) are shown in preceding Table C (smallpox hospitals) and Table E (fever hospitals).

[2] These diphtheria admission figures exclude doubtful and negative cases.

[3] During the epidemic period 1928–29 there were only 11 hospital deaths out of a total of 3,319 admissions, mostly suffering from the sub-toxic type of smallpox. (For M A B hospital mortality rates during earlier smallpox epidemics see preceding Table F, note 3.)

Sources: M A B Annual Reports and the Registrar-General's Annual Returns for the years indicated.

AGE AND SEX DISTRIBUTION OF SCARLET FEVER ADMISSIONS
AND DEATHS, 1871 TO 1891[1] (42,111 cases)

Age Group	Scarlet Fever Patients: 1871–91[1]								
	Males			Females			Totals		
	Admissions	Deaths	Fatality Rate %	Admissions	Deaths	Fatality Rate %	Admissions	Deaths	Fatality Rate %
Under 5	6,057	1,245	20·5	6,020	1,162	19·3	12,077	2,407	19·9
5–9+	8,282	587	8·0	9,141	588	6·4	17,423	1,175	6·7
10–14+	3,188	112	3·5	3,806	126	3·3	6,994	238	3·4
15–19+	1,275	53	4·2	1,584	42	2·6	2,859	95	3·3
20–24+	573	19	3·3	855	30	3·5	1,428	49	3·4
25–29+	242	13	5·4	419	14	3·3	661	27	4·1
30–34+	151	9	6·0	220	12	5·4	371	21	5·7
35–39+	61	6	9·8	107	5	4·7	168	11	6·5
40–44+	36	5	13·9	35	1	2·9	71	6	8·4
45–49+	9	—	—	22	1	4·5	31	1	3·2
50–54+	11	1	9·1	10	—	—	21	1	4·8
55–59+	1	1	100·0	1	—	—	2	1	50·0
60 and over	1	—	—	4	1	25·0	5	1	20·0
Totals	19,887	2,051	10·3	22,224	1,982	8·9	42,111	4,033	9·6

[1] The period 1871–91 represents the two decades during which the M A B fever hospitals functioned as poor law institutions.

AGE AND SEX DISTRIBUTION OF SCARLET FEVER ADMISSIONS
AND DEATHS, 1892 to 1899[2] (107,020 cases)

Age Group	Scarlet Fever Patients: 1892–99[2]								
	Males			Females			Totals		
	Admissions	Deaths	Fatality Rate %	Admissions	Deaths	Fatality Rate %	Admissions	Deaths	Fatality Rate %
Under 5	16,039	1,843	11·5	15,966	1,754	11·0	32,005	3,597	11·2
5–9+	20,612	593	2·8	22,944	619	2·7	43,556	1,212	2·8
10–14+	9,343	116	1·2	10,336	105	1·0	19,679	221	1·1
15–19+	3,175	40	1·3	3,061	38	1·2	6,236	78	1·3
20–24+	1,241	17	1·4	1,515	22	1·5	2,756	39	1·4
25–29+	580	10	1·7	856	9	1·1	1,436	19	1·3
30–34+	289	8	2·8	465	7	1·5	754	15	2·0
35–39+	126	2	1·6	193	4	2·1	319	6	1·9
40–44+	62	4	} 7·2	95	3	} 2·6	157	7	} 4·7
45–49+	34	3		34	1		68	4	
50–54+	21	2		17	—		38	2	
55–59+	6	—		5	—		11	—	
60 and over	2	—		3	—		5	—	
Totals	51,530	2,638	5·1	55,490	2,562	4·6	107,020	5,200	4·9

[2] This period, 1892–99, represents the first eight years following the Public Health (London) Act, 1891, during which the M A B fever hospitals functioned as public health institutions.

TABLE H 2 A

AGE AND SEX DISTRIBUTION OF DIPHTHERIA ADMISSIONS AND DEATHS
1888 to 1894[1] (11,598 cases)

Age Group	Diphtheria Patients: 1888–94[1]								
	Males			Females			Totals		
	Admissions	Deaths	Fatality Rate %	Admissions	Deaths	Fatality Rate %	Admissions	Deaths	Fatality Rate %
Under 5	2,155	1,111	51·6	2,280	1,102	48·3	4,435	2,213	49·9
5–9 +	1,733	456	26·3	1,990	590	29·6	3,723	1,046	28·1
10–14 +	573	61	10·6	757	80	10·6	1,330	141	10·6
15–19 +	305	16	5·2	477	18	3·8	782	34	4·3
20–24 +	188	9	4·8	355	16	4·5	543	25	4·6
25–29 +	119	9	7·6	235	10	4·3	354	19	5·4
30–34 +	70	2	2·9	113	7	6·2	183	9	4·9
35–39 +	44	3	6·8	66	2	3·0	110	5	4·5
40–44 +	28	3	⎫	34	3	⎫	62	6	⎫
45–49 +	11	—	⎪	23	4	⎪	34	4	⎪
50–54 +	11	4	⎬17·2	8	2	⎬17·5	19	6	⎬17·4
55–59 +	6	2	⎪	9	1	⎪	15	3	⎪
60 and over	2	1	⎭	6	4	⎭	8	5	⎭
Totals	5,245	1,677	32·0	6,353	1,839	28·0	11,598	3,516	30·3

[1] During the period 1888–94 diphtheria was treated in the M A B fever hospitals, but antitoxin serum was not generally used.

TABLE H 2 B

AGE AND SEX DISTRIBUTION OF DIPHTHERIA ADMISSIONS
AND DEATHS, 1895 to 1899[2] (29,055 cases)

Age Group	Diphtheria Patients: 1895–99[2]								
	Males			Females			Totals		
	Admissions	Deaths	Fatality Rate %	Admissions	Deaths	Fatality Rate %	Admissions	Deaths	Fatality Rate %
Under 5	6,011	1,536	25·6	5,952	1,511	25·4	11,963	3,047	25·5
5–9 +	4,769	695	14·6	5,809	889	15·3	10,578	1,584	15·0
10–14 +	1,547	92	5·9	1,970	120	6·1	3,517	212	6·0
15–19 +	482	17	3·5	702	20	2·8	1,184	37	3·1
20–24 +	247	7	2·8	433	6	1·4	680	13	1·9
25–29 +	143	4	2·8	331	4	1·2	474	8	1·7
30–34 +	109	5	4·6	221	9	4·1	330	14	4·2
35–39 +	48	1	2·1	114	3	2·6	162	4	2·5
40–44 +	25	—	⎫	57	2	⎫	82	2	⎫
45–49 +	13	1	⎪	25	—	⎪	38	1	⎪
50–54 +	7	1	⎬7·5	13	2	⎬5·3	20	3	⎬6·0
55–59 +	3	1	⎪	11	—	⎪	14	1	⎪
60 and over	5	1	⎭	8	2	⎭	13	3	⎭
Totals	13,409	2,361	17·6	15,646	2,568	16·4	29,055	4,929	17·0

[2] The period 1895–99 represents the first five years during which antitoxin serum was practised in the M A B fever hospitals for the treatment of diphtheria.

TABLE H 3
AGE AND SEX DISTRIBUTION OF ENTERIC FEVER ADMISSIONS AND DEATHS, 1871 to 1899[1] (13,552 cases)

Age Group	Enteric Fever Patients: 1871–99[1]								
	Males			Females			Totals		
	Admissions	Deaths	Fatality Rate %	Admissions	Deaths	Fatality Rate %	Admissions	Deaths	Fatality Rate %
Under 5	227	26	11·5	199	24	12·1	426	50	11·7
5–9+	916	77	8·4	854	71	8·3	1,770	148	8·4
10–14+	1,621	161	9·9	1,370	207	15·1	2,991	368	12·3
15–19+	1,509	223	14·8	1,320	254	19·2	2,829	477	16·9
20–24+	1,057	235	22·2	963	173	18·0	2,020	408	20·2
25–29+	846	206	24·3	669	140	20·9	1,515	346	22·8
30–34+	489	140	28·7	411	82	20·0	900	222	24·7
35–39+	262	71	27·1	275	66	24·0	537	137	25·5
40–44+	150	43	28·6	136	33	24·3	286	76	26·6
45–49+	70	31	44·3	88	23	26·1	158	54	34·2
50–54+	32	13	⎫	38	8	⎫	70	21	⎫
55–59+	15	7	⎬43·1	14	8	⎬32·3	29	15	⎬37·5
60 and over	11	5	⎭	10	4	⎭	21	9	⎭
Totals	7,205	1,238	17·2	6,347	1,093	17·2	13,552	2,331	17·2

[1] The period 1871–99 represents the 28 years from the opening of the M A B fever hospitals until the end of the nineteenth century, during which enteric fever was treated.

TABLE H 4
AGE AND SEX DISTRIBUTION OF TYPHUS ADMISSIONS AND DEATHS, 1871 to 1899[2] (2,200 cases)

Age Group	Typhus Patients: 1871–99[2]								
	Males			Females			Totals		
	Admissions	Deaths	Fatality Rate %	Admissions	Deaths	Fatality Rate %	Admissions	Deaths	Fatality Rate %
Under 5	40	1	2·5	49	1	2·0	89	2	2·2
5–9+	108	1	0·9	139	—	—	247	1	0·4
10–14+	173	5	2·9	210	11	5·2	383	16	4·2
15–19+	168	10	6·0	200	18	9·0	368	28	7·6
20–24+	126	28	22·2	127	22	17·3	253	50	19·8
25–29+	77	21	27·3	85	15	17·6	162	36	22·2
30–34+	78	26	33·3	86	22	25·6	164	48	29·3
35–39+	57	26	45·6	76	21	27·6	133	47	35·3
40–44+	75	46	61·3	95	35	36·8	170	81	47·6
45–49+	43	21	48·8	55	21	38·2	98	42	42·9
50–54+	23	16	69·6	39	21	53·8	62	37	59·7
55–59+	14	9	64·3	18	15	83·3	32	24	75·0
60 and over	17	13	76·5	22	15	68·2	39	28	71·8
Totals	999	223	22·3	1,201	217	18·1	2,200	440	20·0

[2] The period 1871–99 represents the 28 years from the opening of the M A B fever hospitals until the end of the nineteenth century, during which typhus was treated.

ADMISSIONS, DEATHS AND LONDON NOTIFICATIONS
OF DISEASES TREATED IN THE M A B HOSPITALS IN 1929[1]

Admissible Diseases	Admissions	Hospital Deaths	Notifications in London[2]
Cerebro-spinal meningitis	11	6	123
Diphtheria	9,890	322	11,880
Encephalitis lethargica	9	1	93
Enteric (or Typhoid) Fever	141	18	358
Measles[3]	2,322	141	—
Ophthalmia neonatorum	224 (babies) 135 (women)	10 (babies)	728
Poliomyelitis	11	—	65
Puerperal pyrexia and fever	226	18	773
Scarlet Fever	13,596	74	15,928
Smallpox	3,031[4]	9 (3 toxic and 6 sub-toxic)	1,909
Whooping-cough[3]	2,967	485	—

[1] 1929 was the last complete year of the Asylums Board's administration.
[2] Estimated population 4·43 millions.
[3] *Measles* was notifiable only in the Port of London (1 case); *Whooping-cough* was notifiable in Holborn (160 cases), Wandsworth (1,518 cases), and in Greenwich (471 cases).
[4] *Smallpox admissions* included cases from outside London by special arrangement.
Source: M A B Annual Report for 1929.

LENGTH OF STAY OF PATIENTS IN M A B INFECTIOUS DISEASE
HOSPITALS IN 1900 and 1929

Disease	Average length of stay (days)								
	Cerebro-spinal Fever	Diph-theria	Encephalitis lethargica	Enteric (or Typhoid) Fever	Measles	Puerperal Pyrexia and Puerperal Fever	Scarlet Fever	Small-pox	Whoop-ing-Cough
1900: Acute Hospital only	—	59	—	59	—	—	69	35	—
Combined Period in Acute and Convalescent Hospitals	—	76	—	—	—	—	80	not recorded	—
1929: Acute Hospital only	61	56	68	53	30	30	52	not recorded	63
Combined Period in Acute and Convalescent Hospitals	—	78	—	—	83	—	58	not recorded	90

Sources: M A B Annual Reports for 1900 and 1929.

TABLE L
TWENTIETH-CENTURY SMALLPOX EPIDEMICS IN LONDON
M A B Admissions and Deaths and London Notifications and Deaths.

Epidemic Years[1]	M A B Smallpox Admissions[2]	M A B Smallpox Deaths		Notifications of Smallpox in London	Deaths from Smallpox in London	Population of London (millions)
		No.	Case Rate %			
1901[3]	1,743	257	14·74	1,700	229	4·54
1902[3]	7,916	1,337	16·89	7,796	1,314	4·58
1929[4]	3,031	9	0·31	1,909	6	4·43

[1] For nineteenth-century smallpox statistics see preceding Tables A, B and F.

[2] These admissions included patients from peripheral areas and poor law children from industrial schools outside London.

[3] During the 1901–2 epidemic, smallpox was mainly of the toxic type.

[4] During the 1929 outbreak, smallpox was, with few exceptions, of the sub-toxic type. The epidemic died down about 1931.

Sources: M A B Annual Reports and the Registrar-General's Annual Returns for the years indicated.

Graph A

Incidence of Scarlet Fever and Diphtheria per 1,000 of the population of
London during the years 1913–1929

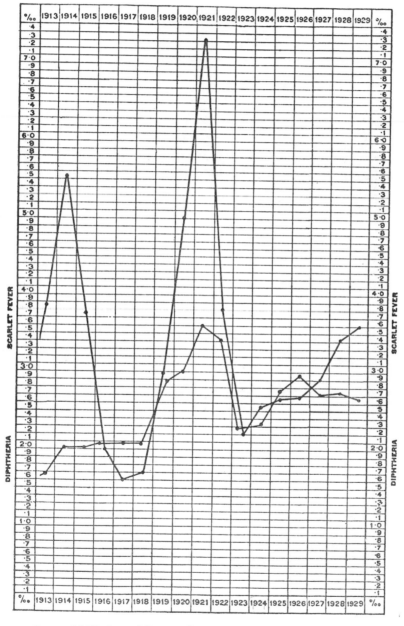

Source: MAB Annual Report for 1929–30.

Graph B

Scarlet Fever, Diphtheria, and Enteric Fever in London:
Case Mortality per cent during the seventeen years 1913–1929

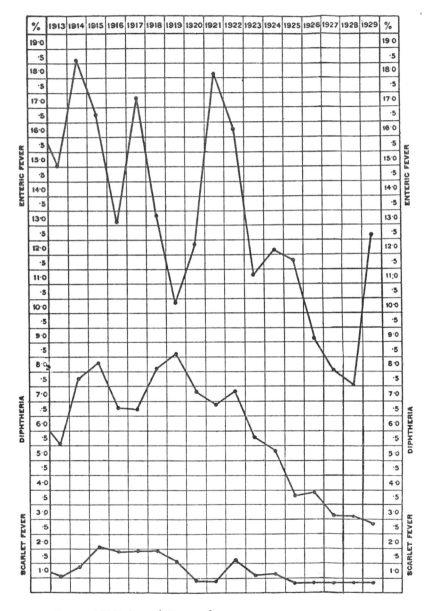

Source: MAB Annual Report for 1929–30.

Showing the course of Smallpox in London, 1902 (the last epidemic year of major smallpox)

I.   The mean number of smallpox patients remaining under treatment each week in the MAB hospitals;

II. The number of cases notified in the Metropolis each week (uncorrected for errors of diagnosis);

III. The number of cases admitted into the MAB hospitals each week (uncorrected for errors of diagnosis).

Estimated population of the Metropolis (to nearest 10,000): 4,580,000

Total number of smallpox cases admitted to the MAB hospitals: 7,916

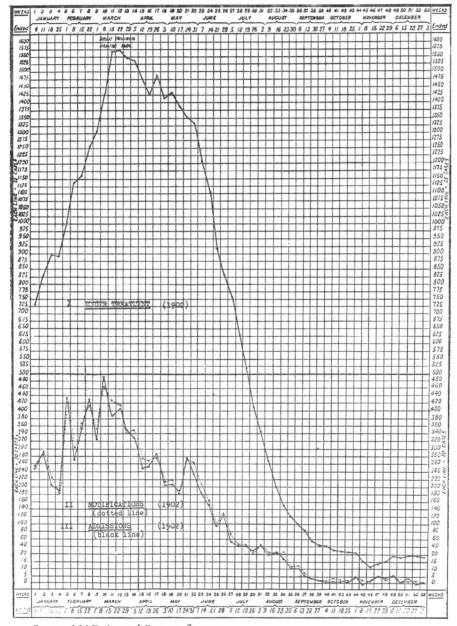

Source: MAB Annual Report for 1902.

Charts A, B, C & D
Age Distribution of M A B Smallpox during the Epidemic Years 1893, 1902, 1928 and 1929

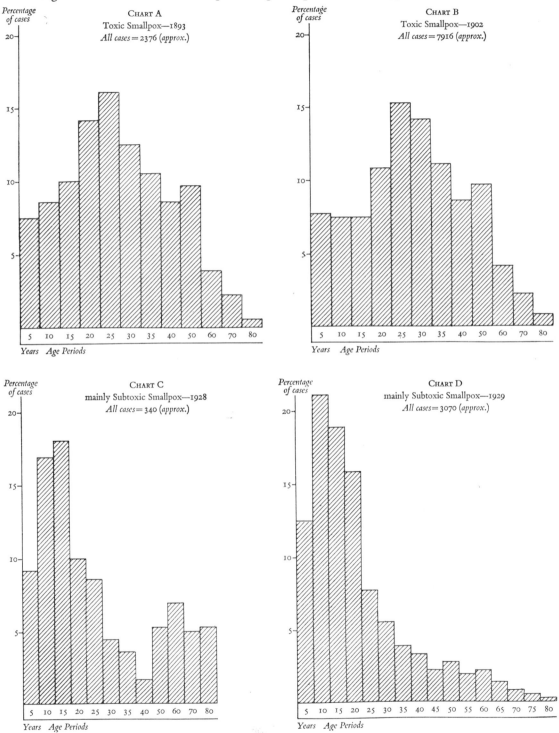

M A B Mental Institutions

TABLE A

M A B MENTAL INSTITUTIONS, 1870-1899, LUNACY ACTS CASES

Admissions, Discharges, Deaths and numbers resident (aggregate figures for the period).

	Leavesden Asylum			Caterham Asylum			Darenth Asylum for Adults			Darenth Asylum for Children			Totals		
	Males	Females	Totals	Males	Females	Totals	Males	Females	Totals	Males	Females	Totals	Males	Females	Totals
Admitted from parishes and unions	4,261	4,111	8,372	4,204	3,820	8,024	777	1,222	1,999	1,799	1,189	2,988	11,041	10,342	21,383
Re-admissions	55	22	77	38	32	70	2	9	11	56	44	100	151	107	258
Transfers	194	243	437	129	204	333	516	484	1,000	230	211	441	1,069	1,142	2,211
Totals:	4,510	4,376	8,886	4,371	4,056	8,427	1,295	1,715	3,010	2,085	1,444	3,529	12,261	11,591	23,852
Discharged:															
Not certified	—	—	—	—	—	—	—	—	—	—	—	—	—	—	—
Not insane	13	8	21	6	2	8	8	14	22	—	—	—	27	24	51
Recovered	254	131	385	251	187	438	30	21	51	50	57	107	585	396	981
Relieved	246	169	415	278	167	445	118	123	241	170	120	290	812	579	1,391
Not improved	331	306	637	218	191	409	96	123	219	178	87	265	823	707	1,530
Transfers	46	34	80	87	48	135	85	93	178	561	495	1,056	779	670	1,449
Died	2,723	2,640	5,363	2,600	2,387	4,987	527	769	1,296	495	358	853	6,345	6,154	12,499
Total discharged and died	3,613	3,288	6,901	3,440	2,982	6,422	864	1,143	2,007	1,454	1,117	2,571	9,371	8,530	17,901
Remaining	897	1,088	1,985	931	1,074	2,005	431	572	1,003	631	327	958	2,890	3,061	5,951
Average numbers resident	838	1,050	1,888	851	1,060	1,911	349	493	842	409	258	667	2,447	2,861	5,308

1 This table was included in a pamphlet produced by the M A B for the International Exhibition in Paris (Social Science Section) in 1900. The statistics are, however, of limited interest inasmuch as they do not indicate how many patients were subnormal and how many were insane or demented. All M A B patients at this time were intended to be harmless, incurable 'imbeciles'. For a classification of M A B patients according to mental disorder, see Tables G (a) and (b) following.

DIETARY TABLE FOR PATIENTS IN THE ADULT 'IMBECILE ASYLUMS' AT LEAVESDEN, CATERHAM AND DARENTH (as revised in 1887)

| | BREAKFAST — Males | | | BREAKFAST — Females | | | DINNER — Males | | Irish Stew (Fresh Meat cooked) | Irish Stew (Dumpling) | | | | DINNER — Females (Description of Food similar to Males) | | Irish Stew (Fresh Meat cooked) | Irish Stew (Dumpling) | | | | TEA — Males | | | TEA — Females | | |
	Bread (Ozs.)	Butter or Margarine (Oz.)	Cocoa (Pt.)	Bread (Ozs.)	Butter or Margarine (Oz.)	Tea (Pt.)	Pie (containing 4 ozs. uncooked fresh Meat) (Ozs.)	Fresh Meat (Ozs.)	(Ozs.)	(Ozs.)	Potatoes, Greens or Other Vegetables (Ozs.)	Bread (Ozs.)	Beer (Pt.)	Pie (containing 4 ozs. uncooked fresh Meat) (Ozs.)	Fresh Meat (Ozs.)	(Ozs.)	(Ozs.)	Potatoes, Greens or Other Vegetables (Ozs.)	Bread (Ozs.)	Beer (Pt.)	Bread (Ozs.)	Butter or Margarine (Oz.)	Tea (Pt.)	Bread (Ozs.)	Butter or Margarine (Oz.)	Tea (Pt.)
Sunday	6	½	1	5	½	1	—	5	—	—	10	4	½	—	4	—	—	9	4	½	6	½	1	5	½	1
Monday	6	½	1	5	½	1	—	5	—	—	10	4	½	—	4	—	—	9	4	½	6	½	1	5	½	1
Tuesday	6	½	1	5	½	1	13	—	—	—	9	—	½	13	—	—	—	8	—	½	6	½	1	5	½	1
Wednesday	6	½	1	5	½	1	—	—	3	4	12	4	½	—	—	3	3	12	4	½	6	½	1	5	½	1
Thursday	6	½	1	5	½	1	—	5	—	—	10	4	½	—	4	—	—	9	4	½	6	½	1	5	½	1
Friday	6	½	1	5	½	1	—	5	—	—	10	4	½	—	4	—	—	9	4	½	6	½	1	5	½	1
Saturday	6	½	1	5	½	1	13	—	—	—	9	—	½	13	—	—	—	8	—	½	6	½	1	5	½	1

Notes:

Male and female patients 'laboriously employed' were allowed 4 oz. of bread, 1 oz. of cheese and half-pint of beer at 11 a.m.

The infirmary diet, in the absence of special orders, was the same as the above, with the exception of dinner, which consisted of 5 oz. of cooked mutton daily (or 10 oz. fish in lieu), with vegetables, etc. as on Sunday.

Formulae for Preparation of Foods.

TEA	Quantity of each ingredient to 10 pints	COCOA	Quantity of each ingredient to 10 pints	IRISH STEW	Quantity of each ingredient per ration	MEAT PIE	Quantity of each ingredient per ration
Tea	1½ ozs.	Cocoa	3 ozs.	Meat	4½ ozs.	Meat	4 ozs.
Sugar	5 ozs.	Sugar	5 ozs.	Flour	2 ozs.	Flour	5 ozs.
Milk	1 pint	Milk	1 pint	Suet	¼ oz.	Dripping	¼ oz.

Source: LGB Orders to the M A B, 1887.

TABLE C

M A B MENTAL INSTITUTIONS, 1870–1929. LUNACY ACTS CASES

Admissions, Discharges, Deaths, and Rates of Recovery and Death (annual figures from 1900).

Year	Admisions			Discharges (including Transfers)								
				Recovered			Relieved			Not improved		
	M	F	Totals	M	F	Totals	M	F	Totals	M	F	Totals
1870–1899	12,261	11,591	23,852	612	420	1,032	812	579	1,391	823	707	1,530
1900	175	209	384	10	8	18	14	6	20	24	27	51
1901	218	219	437	5	1	6	1	3	4	15	21	36
1902	246	207	453	4	2	6	10	3	13	26	24	50
1903	588	637	1,225	8	7	15	13	15	28	22	22	44
1904	395	375	770	9	10	19	14	9	23	16	36	52
1905	351	335	686	8	15	23	23	19	42	38	48	86
1906	426	448	874	11	6	17	21	6	27	41	32	73
1907	415	417	832	16	7	23	5	5	10	57	45	102
1908	475	497	972	3	4	7	3	2	5	44	44	88
1909	403	381	784	12	8	20	9	2	11	77	64	141
1910	478	435	913	10	8	18	2	2	4	52	47	99
1911	527	511	1,038	8	—	8	4	6	10	56	53	109
1912	406	449	855	6	5	11	11	15	26	55	49	104
1913	449	494	943	8	4	12	13	8	21	71	73	144
1914	525	555	1,080	3	2	5	9	11	20	52	47	99
1915	426	500	926	4	7	11	47	40	87	60	51	111
1916	595	794	1,389	7	3	10	37	33	70	93	72	165
1917	426	508	934	16	3	19	36	23	59	58	60	118
1918	379	515	894	13	9	22	24	17	41	52	81	133
1919	363	557	920	4	7	11	24	13	37	53	60	113
1920	452	423	875	22	4	26	14	18	32	57	73	130
1921	402	376	778	17	7	24	21	20	41	48	67	115
1922	261	431	692	aggregated discharges[1]			79	115	194			
1923	314	384	698				58	84	142			
1924	233	246	479				64	68	132			
1925	210	387	597				48	68	116			
1926	156	213	369				43	75	118			
1927	148	167	315				42	42	84			
1928	182	117	299				40	36	76			
1929	127	111	238				57	52	109			
Totals: 1870–1929	23,012	23,489	46,501	aggregated discharges:			4,303	3,744	8,047			

[1] Discharges were not classified after 1921.

TABLE C—continued

Deaths			Remaining on Registers December 31 in each year			Average Daily Number Resident			Percentage of 'Recoveries' on number of Admissions	Percentage of Deaths on average number Resident	Year
M	F	Totals	M	F	Totals	M	F	Totals			
6,345	6,154	12,499	—	—	—	—	—	—			
235	284	519	2,782	2,945	5,727	2,836	2,995	5,831	4·7	8·9	1900
170	172	342	2,809	2,967	5,776	2,769	2,919	5,688	1·3	6·0	1901
156	164	320	2,857	2,981	5,838	2,853	2,972	5,825	1·3	5·5	1902
233	223	456	3,170	3,351	6,521	3,097	3,271	6,368	1·2	7·2	1903
272	283	555	3,254	3,388	6,642	3,312	3,385	6,697	2·5	8·3	1904
306	281	587	3,230	3,360	6,590	3,245	3,370	6,615	3·3	8·9	1905
334	335	669	3,249	3,429	6,678	3,236	3,396	6,632	1·7	10·1	1906
306	356	662	3,280	3,433	6,713	3,273	3,431	6,704	2·2	9·9	1907
331	314	645	3,374	3,566	6,940	3,385	3,394	6,879	0·3	9·4	1908
343	365	708	3,336	3,508	6,844	3,370	3,537	6,907	2·0	10·3	1909
320	274	594	3,430	3,612	7,042	3,328	3,515	6,843	2·0	8·7	1910
321	362	683	3,568	3,702	7,270	3,474	3,674	7,148	0·8	9·6	1911
335	378	713	3,567	3,704	7,271	3,568	3,701	7,269	1·3	9·8	1912
336	403	739	3,588	3,710	7,298	3,593	3,669	7,262	1·3	10·2	1913
373	450	823	3,676	3,755	7,431	3,642	3,736	7,378	0·5	11·2	1914
476	536	1,012	3,515	3,622	7,137	3,591	3,654	7,245	1·2	14·0	1915
570	594	1,164	3,403	3,714	7,117	3,462	3,728	7,190	0·7	16·2	1916
714	665	1,379	3,005	3,471	6,476	3,154	3,564	6,718	2·0	20·5	1917
902	744	1,646	2,393	3,135	5,528	2,719	3,367	6,086	2·5	27·0	1918
369	472	841	2,306	3,140	5,446	2,327	3,069	5,396	1·2	15·6	1919
228	366	594	2,437	3,102	5,539	2,426	3,128	5,554	2·6	10·7	1920
270	408	678	2,483	2,976	5,459	2,431	3,026	5,457	2·6	12·4	1921
310	422	732	2,355	2,870	5,225	2,395	2,894	5,289	'Recoveries'	13·2	1922
221	294	515	2,390	2,876	5,266	2,366	2,864	5,230	(if any)	10·0	1923
245	284	529	2,314	2,770	5,084	2,328	2,826	5,154	not	10·2	1924
216	276	492	2,262	2,817	5,079	2,287	2,765	5,052	recorded	10·0	1925
184	232	416	2,191	2,723	4,914	2,220	2,745	4,965	separately after 1921	8·4	1926
160	257	417	2,137	2,591	4,728	2,165	2,621	4,786		8·8	1927
161	182	343	2,118	2,490	4,608	2,103	2,519	4,622		7·4	1928
139	172	311	2,049	2,377	4,426 [2]	2,073	2,403	4,476		7·0	1929
5,881	16,702	32,583									

[2] These 4,426 patients remaining at the end of the Board's last year are classified according to mental disorder in Table G (b) following.

Sources: M A B Annual Reports for the years indicated.

TABLE D
M A B MENTAL INSTITUTIONS, 1919–1929
UNCERTIFIED AND MENTAL DEFICIENCY ACTS CASES
Admissions, Deaths and Discharges.

	Year	Feeble-Minded Patients (Uncertified)	Mental Deficiency Acts Cases	Sane Epileptics	Senile Dements[1] (Uncertified)	Totals
Admissions	1919	128	522	84	—	734
	1920	87	588	70	—	745
	1921	121	382	367	—	870
	1922	95	406	141	—	642
	1923	86	377	162	—	625
	1924	91	376	162	—	629
	1925	114	470	208	427	1,219
	1926	103	379	238	499	1,219
	1927	81	326	285	618	1,310
	1928	86	242	242	521	1,091
	1929	111	262	181	356	910
	Totals:	1,103	4,330	2,140	2,421	9,994
Discharges (including Transfers to other (non-M A B) Institutions)	1919	60	28	86	—	174
	1920	33	66	50	—	149
	1921	62	74	107	—	243
	1922	61	134	94	—	289
	1923	46	62	81	—	189
	1924	69	145	101	—	315
	1925	74	109	175	17	375
	1926	68	186	211	31	496
	1927	80	176	257	75	588
	1928	71	187	249	53	560
	1929	106	155	236	26	523
	Totals:	730	1,322	1,647	202	3,901
Deaths	1919	13	25	7	—	45
	1920	7	45	4	—	56
	1921	7	77	11	—	95
	1922	10	73	10	—	93
	1923	9	95	27	—	131
	1924	7	75	12	—	94
	1925	8	75	30	53	166
	1926	7	62	30	195	294
	1927	14	66	31	349	460
	1928	7	78	15	330	430
	1929	5	78	17	350	450
	Totals:	94	749	194	1,277	2,314

[1] Before 1925 senile dements were included among Lunacy Acts cases.

	Year	Feeble-Minded Patients (Uncertified)	Mental Deficiency Acts Cases	Sane Epileptics	Senile Dements (Uncertified)	Totals
	1918	665	236	267	—	1,168
	1919	720	703	259	—	1,682
	1920	767	1,181	274	—	2,222
	1921	819	1,412	523	—	2,754
Remaining	1922	843	1,611	560	—	3,014
at end of	1923	874	1,831	614	—	3,319
Year	1924	889	1,987	663	—	3,539
	1925	921	2,273	666	357	4,217
	1926	949	2,404	663	630	4,646
	1927	936	2,489	660	824	4,909
	1928	944	2,466	638	962	5,010
	1929	944	2,495	566	942	4,947

Sources: Annual returns of the superintendents of M A B mental institutions.

TABLE E
M A B MENTAL INSTITUTIONS
Principal Statistics for Selected Years Between 1889 and 1929.

	1889	1899	1919	1929
Number of Units	3	3[2]	6	6
Normal number of Beds	5,520	5,983	8,964	9,742
Number of Patients[1] (daily average)	5,492	5,952	7,560	9,218
Patient-Costs[3] (weekly average): 'Maintenance' (mainly food)[4]	3/9½d.	3/9½d.	6/9d.	5/11d.
Total Cost	8/8d.	9/10d.	21/1d.	22/1d.
Resident Staff (daily average)	not recorded	595	1,270	2,321

[1] All cases—certified and uncertified.

[2] In 1899, the Tooting Bec Asylum was in course of erection with 750 projected beds.

[3] For further details of M A B expenditure in the mental institutions, see Appendix IV, Tables D and E.

[4] For dietary, see preceding Table B.

Sources: M A B Annual Reports for the years indicated.

TABLE F
CURRICULUM AND ANALYSIS OF CHILDREN'S PERFORMANCE AT THE M A B DARENTH SCHOOL FOR THE MENTALLY DEFECTIVE IN 1890
(468 children: 300 boys and 168 girls)

	Classes							Total
	1	2	3	4	5¹	6	7	
SPEECH								
Make no attempt	—	—	—	—	—	I	39	40
Make a few articulate sounds	—	—	—	—	—	—	31	31
Speak indistinctly	3	10	16	25	—	25	20	99
Speak fairly	8	37	35	27	—	43	39	189
Speak well	50	6	—	—	—	—	—	56
READING								
Know no words or letters	—	—	—	3	30	6	69	108
Know a few letters	—	—	—	21	11	35	30	97
Know a few words at sight	—	—	—	—	4	15	—	19
Know all the letters	—	—	—	17	12	11	22	62
Know easy words and spell them	—	20	51	10	7	—	—	88
Read fairly	50	33	—	1	—	—	—	84
Read fluently	11	—	—	—	—	—	—	11
WRITING								
Do nothing but scribble	—	—	—	1	30	12	75	118
Form strokes on a slate	—	—	—	26	20	25	15	86
Form letters on a slate	—	32	46	25	11	30	23	167
Form letters in copy-books	—	4	2	—	3	—	—	9
Write easy words in copy-books	18	15	3	—	—	—	—	36
Write fairly	18	2	—	—	—	—	—	20
Write well	25	—	—	—	—	—	—	25
COUNTING AND TABLES								
Cannot count at all	—	—	—	—	40	—	60	100
Count to 10	—	—	—	3	19	40	50	112
Count to 50 and repeat to 3 × 12	—	—	15	34	3	27	—	79
Count to 100, to 6 × 12 and all questions	20	31	36	15	2	—	—	104
Count to 1,000, to 12 × 12 and all questions	23	22	—	—	—	—	—	45
The above, and money tables	18	—	—	—	—	—	—	18
ARITHMETIC								
Cannot recognize objects or numbers	—	—	—	3	30	10	75	118
Recognize objects and numbers to 5	—	—	8	18	20	50	14	110
Recognize objects and numbers to 20	—	—	40	22	10	7	—	79
Recognize and work addition sums	—	37	3	8	4	—	—	52
Work easy sums in simple rules	44	16	—	1	—	—	—	61

TABLE F—*continued*

	Classes							Total
	I	2	3	4	5[1]	6	7	
ARITHMETIC								
Work all simple and compound money sums	14	—	—	—	—	—	—	14
Beyond the above	3	—	—	—	—	—	—	3
CLOCK LESSON								
Know neither hours nor minutes	—	—	—	40	60	67	—	167
Know some of the hours	—	14	37	12	2	—	—	65
Know all the hours	—	30	14	—	2	—	—	46
Know the hours and quarters	29	5	—	—	—	—	—	34
Know the above and 5 minutes	12	5	—	—	—	—	—	17
Can tell the time to a minute	20	4	—	—	—	—	—	24
SHOP LESSON								
Know no coins or weights	—	—	—	30	45	55	—	130
Know a few coins	—	—	45	25	10	12	—	92
Know a few coins and weights	—	20	6	6	9	—	—	41
Know all coins and some weights	31	13	—	—	—	—	—	44
Know all coins and weights	20	20	—	—	—	—	—	40
Coins, weights and calculate fairly	10	—	—	—	—	—	—	10
COLOUR LESSON								
Recognize no colours	—	—	1	6	35	10	65	117
Know the colour 'red'	—	—	—	20	20	10	23	73
Know one or two simple colours	—	—	—	10	—	30	20	60
Know all simple colours	—	20	38	10	4	17	21	110
Know all simple and compound shades	48	26	12	6	5	—	—	95
Know and can match compound shades	13	17	—	—	—	—	—	30
KINDERGARTEN DRAWING								
No knowledge of drawing at all	—	—	—	25	50	30	120	225
Can make straight lines	—	—	13	20	2	18	9	62
Can form outlines	31	26	26	15	8	9	—	115
Can draw objects	30	27	12	2	4	—	—	75

[1] Class 5 in Speech comprised 64 deaf and dumb children who were taught to speak and read on fingers.

Source: 1890 Annual Report of the Medical Superintendent of the Darenth Schools for Imbecile Children. (The method of analysis was devised by the Board's Statistical Committee in 1887.)

TABLE G (a)

M A B PATIENTS CLASSIFIED ACCORDING TO MENTAL DISORDER IN
(a) 1889 and (b) 1929

(a) *Form of Mental Disorder:* December **1889**	*M*	*F*	*Totals*
1. Mania	2	13	15
2. Mania, chronic	17	113	130
3. Mania and Epilepsy	7	6	13
4. Melancholy	60	105	165
5. General Paresis	35	12	47
6. Dementia	694	753	1,447
7. Dementia and Paralysis	98	123	221
8. Dementia and Epilepsy	207	281	488
9. Senile Dementia	114	152	266
10. Idiocy	71	92	163
11. Imbecility	805	797	1,602
12. Imbecility with Epilepsy	151	248	399
13. Of weak mind	25	33	58
Totals:	2,286	2,728	5,014

Sources: Reports of Medical Superintendents of M A B Imbecile Asylums for 1889.

TABLE G (b)

(b) *Form of Mental Disorder: December* **1929**	*M*	*F*	*Total*
Congenital or infantile mental deficiency (idiocy or imbecility):			
1. Intellectual—with epilepsy	329	352	681
without epilepsy	1,152	879	2,031
2. Moral	—	—	—
Insanity occurring later in life:			
1. Insanity with Epilepsy	19	1	20
2. General Paralysis of the Insane	1	2	3
3. Insanity with grosser brain lesions	19	7	26
4. Acute delirium	—	—	—
5. Confusional insanity	9	8	17
6. Stupor	—	—	—
7. Primary Dementia	41	67	108
8. Mania—Recent	—	—	—
Chronic	4	48	52
Recurrent	—	—	—
9. Melancholia—Recent	—	3	3
Chronic	19	38	57
10. Alternating Insanity	—	10	10
11. Delusional Insanity—systematized	8	45	53
non-systematized	38	43	81
12. Volitional Insanity—impulse	—	—	—
obsession	—	—	—
doubt	—	—	—
13. Moral Insanity	—	—	—
14. Dementia—Senile	250	599	849
Secondary	160	275	435
Totals:	2,049	2,377	4,426
Prospect of mental recovery:			
Favourable	—	—	—
Doubtful	—	—	—
Unfavourable	2,049	2,377	4,426

Source: M A B Annual Report for 1929–30.

APPENDIX IV

M A B Finance

NOTE ON THE METROPOLITAN COMMON POOR FUND
FROM WHICH THE HOSPITAL SERVICES OF THE M A B WERE FINANCED

The Metropolitan Common Poor Fund was established in 1867 under the Metropolitan Poor Act of that year (30 & 31 Vict. c. 6). Its purpose was to equalize over the whole of London poor relief expenditure incurred in connexion with the maintenance of the 'insane', fever and smallpox patients in the 'asylums' provided under the 1867 Act, as well as of pauper school children, the casual poor, and 'pauper lunatics' in existing mental institutions. The Act also provided that the Fund should bear the cost of salaries of all officers employed by the metropolitan boards of guardians and managers of district schools, as well as by the poor law authorities created under the Act—the dispensary committees and the 'asylum' managers. Expenditure on all medicines and surgical appliances supplied to the rate-aided sick poor was likewise made a charge on the Fund, as also were fees for birth and death registration and for vaccination (see sections 61–72 of the Metropolitan Poor Act, 1867, summarized in Appendix I, Document II).

The Fund was raised by contributions from the boards of guardians of the parishes and unions of the metropolis in proportion to the rateable value of the property each comprised. Originally, the Fund was administered by the Poor Law Board and subsequently by its successors, the Local Government Board and the Ministry of Health. The 1867 Act decreed that the Poor Law Board should appoint a Receiver, whose salary was to be paid from the Fund, and that it should assess, and issue precepts for, the amounts payable by each board of guardians. The poor law authorities were empowered under the Act to claim repayment from the Fund in respect of expenditure incurred on the items cited above.

In practice, each board of guardians prepared every half-year a statement of its expenditure during the preceding six months, under headings stipulated by the central authority, and submitted a claim in respect of these items to the Receiver of the Fund. The claims were checked and audited and each board was credited with the amount as certified by the District Auditor. At the same time, each board of guardians was debited with the amount of its contribution to the Fund. The difference between the two amounts in each case represented the sum due to, or from, each board of guardians, and a net charge was levied or a net grant paid, as the case might be, by the Receiver.

By the Metropolitan Poor Amendment Act, 1869 (32 & 33 Vict. c. 63), the cost of maintenance of pauper boys on training ships, and the cost of maintenance and instruction of orphan and deserted children boarded out by the guardians, were also made chargeable upon the Fund.

The Metropolitan Poor Amendment Act, 1870 (33 & 34 Vict. c. 18), enlarged the operation of the Fund to include the cost of maintenance of adult paupers in workhouses, infirmaries and sick asylums to the extent of 5d. per head per day. Repayment in respect of resident officers' rations was also allowed under this Act (12s. per week for principal officers and 7s. per week for others). These provisions operated as a bribe to the guardians of metropolitan unions to promote indoor treatment as against domiciliary or dispensary treatment.

The Elementary Education Act, 1873 (36 & 37 Vict. c. 86), provided that school fees paid by guardians for outdoor pauper children should be recovered from the Fund.

The Poor Law Act, 1879 (42 & 43 Vict. c. 54 s. 16), laid down that expenses incurred by the M A B in providing ambulances under the Act should be chargeable to the Fund to the extent sanctioned by the Local Government Board.

Under the Poor Law Act of 1889 (52 & 53 Vict. c. 56 s. 3) and the Public Health (London)

Act of 1891 (54 & 55 Vict. c. 76 s. 80), the maintenance of non-pauper patients in M A B infectious disease hospitals became a charge on the Fund. The former enactment limited the claims on the Fund for this purpose to the cost of those non-destitute patients from whom the local guardians were unable to recover payment, while the latter statute, by omitting all reference to the recovery of non-paupers' charges, cast upon the Fund the maintenance costs of *all* patients in M A B fever and smallpox hospitals, irrespective of ability to pay.

The M A B did not draw upon the Fund directly, but, in accordance with the 1867 Metropolitan Poor Act, divided certain 'common charges' proportionally among the metropolitan poor law districts and levied precepts periodically upon parochial boards on the basis of the rateable value of each district. Until 1916, these charges were recoverable by the guardians from the Fund. Under the Local Government (Emergency Provisions) Act of 1916 (6 & 7 Geo. 5 c. 12 s. 7), a more direct system of financing the M A B services was provided which by-passed the Metropolitan Common Poor Fund. Instead of contributing to, and claiming from, the Fund in respect of M A B expenditure, guardians made payments direct to the account of the Metropolitan Asylum District so that the total of M A B expenditure was covered and each locality contributed proportionally according to its rateable value.

In 1921, owing to financial difficulties in some parts of London due to a substantial increase in the cost of poor relief, a readjustment of the financial burden between the metropolitan boroughs was demanded and the Minister of Health (Sir Alfred Mond) convened a conference of London local authorities on 17 October 1921 to consider the matter. The outcome of this conference was agreement on the following recommendations:

(i) that the capitation grant for indoor poor should be increased from 5d. to 1s. 3d. per person per day as from 1 October 1921;

(ii) that expenditure on outdoor relief throughout London should be equalized through the Metropolitan Common Poor Fund as from the same date;

(iii) that guardians be authorized by the Minister of Health, as might be necessary, to borrow on overdraft or to raise loans to an amount and at a rate of interest to be sanctioned by him, the interest payable being allowed as a charge upon the Metropolitan Common Poor Fund; and

(iv) that the Ministry of Health should make regulations prescribing scales of relief and other conditions governing the charge on the Fund under the above arrangement.

Effect was given to this agreement by the Local Authorities (Financial Provisions) Act, 1921 (11 & 12 Geo. 5 c. 67). The Act provided *inter alia* for the repayment of expenditure on out-relief, but no repayment was to be made in respect of relief in excess of a scale or in contravention of conditions to be prescribed by regulations of the Minister of Health. The powers conferred on the Minister were to be in addition to any other powers possessed by him of making orders and regulations respecting the grant of out-relief. No repayment was to be made from the Fund where the Minister was satisfied that proper investigation had not been made within reasonable time of granting out-relief (Section 1). It was recognized when this Act was passed that the placing of out-relief on the Fund involved an entirely new departure in policy and would probably result in changes in the practice of individual boards of guardians in granting relief. The fact that for over fifty years the application of the Fund had been limited (except for the salaries of non-institutional officers) to indoor relief indicated that the policy of Parliament had been to discourage out-relief and it was thought to be likely that the placing of the cost of out-relief on the Fund would be an inducement to the guardians to give outdoor rather than indoor relief, and also that relief in future might be so dispensed as to involve London in a much heavier total burden. Doubts were also expressed concerning the feasibility of effective control by the measures proposed. In accordance with the provisions of the Act, the Minister of Health issued regulations known as the Metropolitan Common Poor Fund (Outdoor Relief) Regulations, 1922, which prescribed the limits beyond which outdoor relief should not be charged on the Fund. These regulations and the scale known as the Mond scale were in force for twelve months to September 1922.

Further temporary legislation became necessary with the expiry of the Act of 1921. The Local Authorities (Emergency Provisions) Act, 1923 (13 & 14 Geo. 5 c. 6), which operated from October 1922, continued in force the provisions of the Act of 1921 with regard to the daily rate charged on the Fund in respect of indoor poor, and to the charging of out-relief, but with important alterations in the latter case. The provisions in respect of the Minister's power to prescribe scales and to disallow repayment were dropped, and in their place a rate to be charged on the Fund for out-relief was fixed at not exceeding 9d. per person per day. The Local Authorities (Emergency Provisions) Acts, 1924 and 1926 (14 & 15 Geo. 5 c. 29 and 16 & 17 Geo. 5 c. 10) continued the Act of 1923 for successive periods of two years until 1 April 1928. While these temporary measures tended to equalize the cost of relief over London, they in no way centralized the control of the expenditure, except for the short-lived attempt in 1922, and left the granting of relief in the hands of independent boards of guardians with widely differing policies, particularly in the important matter of the granting of out-relief. During the year prior to the coming into operation of the temporary Acts (the year ended September 1921) the total amount charged on the Fund was £3,531,039, while for the year ended March, 1927, the amount charged was £6,364,416.

It was clearly necessary to make some further provision for equalizing the cost of relief after the expiry of the temporary Acts on 31 March 1928, and it was indicated in the King's Speech at the opening of the Session that a measure would be introduced dealing with the law relating to the Metropolitan Common Poor Fund. It appeared that no one would be content with a mere continuation of the current arrangements. On the one hand, certain boards were pressing for more assistance from the Fund, while others, in view of the heavy calls made upon them, were seeking a reduction of the amounts charged on the Fund, and it was admittedly difficult to justify a continuation of the arrangement under which a common fund of some £6 million was drawn upon by a number of independent bodies with no sort of centralized control.

Various suggestions were made for meeting the criticisms which had been directed against the working of the Fund, none of which was free from difficulty. One was that the Minister should resume the powers which he had under the Act of 1921 to prescribe regulations relating to out-relief and to disallow claims on the Fund in certain circumstances. The Minister pointed out that the Fund was purely a London one and should be dealt with by representatives of London rather than by the Minister who dealt with the country as a whole, and who in any case from his position would be exposed to criticism however impartially he exercised his judgment in a matter which might become the subject of party controversy. The LCC considered the subject and rejected the idea that the Council should administer the Fund, as they were 'strongly of opinion that there would be no advantage in transferring the Fund to the Council in anticipation of a reform of the Poor Law'. A further proposal was made to the Minister, by a conference representing the paying boroughs, that an *ad hoc* commission should be nominated by him to control the Fund. The Minister, however, was not prepared at that time to set up a new authority in London.

While the whole question was under consideration the possibility of the Metropolitan Asylums Board controlling the Fund was discussed between the Minister of Health and the Chairman of the Board. It was pointed out that the Board was a central London body on which every board of guardians was represented by members knowledgeable and experienced in problems of relief. The invitation to administer the Fund, however, was not accepted with alacrity and the hope was expressed that, if the duty were imposed on the Board, it would be accompanied by adequate powers to enable the Board to carry it out.

These were embodied in the Local Authorities (Emergency Provisions) Act, 1928 (18 & 19 Geo. 5 c. 9), which extended the material provisions of the Local Authorities (Emergency Provisions) Act, 1923, as amended by the Acts of 1924 and 1926 and the consolidating Poor Law Act, 1927 (17 & 18 Geo. 5 c. 14).

Section 2 of the 1928 Act laid down that metropolitan boards of guardians were to submit to the Metropolitan Asylums Board half-yearly estimates of the expenditure they proposed to incur in respect of which repayments were to be made out of the Fund. The Metropolitan Asylums Board had full powers to approve or reduce these estimates as they thought fit and to furnish the District Auditor with a copy of such estimates as approved. The District Auditor, in granting to the boards of guardians the certificate required by section 202 of the Poor Law Act, 1927, was obliged to exclude from the certificate any amount which the Metropolitan Asylums Board decided to disallow. The Act did not provide for the administration of relief on uniform principles throughout London but sought to impose some check on the amounts which boards of guardians might draw from the Fund. Any expenditure in excess of the sums sanctioned as chargeable on the Fund had to be raised in the poor law district concerned. During the debate on the second reading of the Bill the new principle of control was unanimously accepted.

On 19 May 1928, the Metropolitan Asylums Board appointed a committee of eleven of its members to consider the estimates submitted by the boards of guardians under the provisions of the Act and to conduct such negotiations as might be called for. During the ensuing year the Metropolitan Asylums Board reduced by 12 per cent the estimated claims on the Fund which amounted to over £6 million, the economies recommended being chiefly in respect of outdoor relief. Thus began—and ended—the Board's brief term as administrator of the Metropolitan Common Poor Fund. The Local Government Act, 1929 (19 Geo. 5 c. 17 s. 121, ninth schedule, Part I, No. 8) provided that the temporary legislation affecting the charges on the Common Poor Fund should cease on 1 April 1929. Thereafter the cost of the relief of the metropolitan poor was spread over the County of London through the County rate.

TABLE A (I)
SUMMARIZED ANALYSIS OF CAPITAL EXPENDITURE OF THE M A B, 1867–1930[1]

	£	Percentage of Total
A. Institutions and Services for Infectious Patients:		
Fever, Smallpox, etc.	3,620,325	46·65
Tuberculosis	1,007,712	12·99
Ambulance Services	355,329	4·58
Laboratories	26,619	0·34
Total:	£5,009,985	64·56%
B. Institutions for Mental and Epileptic Patients	1,872,956	24·14
C. Institutions for Children and Training Ship	674,154	8·69
D. Casual Wards	57,951	0·75
E. Administrative Buildings	144,653	1·86
Total of Capital Expenditure:	£7,759,699	100·00%

[1] Capital expenditure in respect of each separate institution and service is shown in Table A (II), following.

Source: M A B Financial Records.

TABLE A (II)
M A B CAPITAL EXPENDITURE FOR SEPARATE INSTITUTIONS AND SERVICES, 1867–1930
(for date of opening of each institution see Appendix I, Document VI)

A. INFECTIOUS DISEASE INSTITUTIONS AND SERVICES

	£	£
(a) *Fever*		
Eastern Hospital	366,047	
North-Eastern Hospital	178,893	
North-Western Hospital	197,660	
Western Hospital	237,083	
South-Western Hospital	175,319	
Grove Hospital	283,299	
South-Eastern Hospital	282,561	
Park Hospital	283,402	
Brook Hospital	325,204	
Northern Hospital	198,177	
		2,527,645
(b) *Smallpox*		
Southern Hospital (formerly Gore Farm)	399,361	
Hospital Ships and Shore Buildings	656,347	
		1,055,708
(c) *Ophthalmia Neonatorum*		
St. Margaret's Hospital		24,864
(d) *Venereal Diseases*		
Sheffield Street Hospital		12,108
(e) *Tuberculosis*		
Pinewood Hospital	40,312	
King George V Sanatorium	232,807	
Colindale Hospital	182,393	
St. Luke's Hospital	76,274	
Princess Mary's Hospital	81,924	
High Wood Hospital	111,778	
Millfield Hospital	28,573	
Grove Park Hospital	248,612	
Copthorne (site)	5,039	
		1,007,712
Total for all Infectious Disease Institutions:		4,628,037
(f) *Land Ambulance Service*		
Eastern Hospital Station	4,089	
North-Western Hospital Station	20,986	

TABLE A (II)—*continued*

	£	£
Western Hospital Station	5,483	
South-Western Hospital Station	20,616	
South-Eastern Hospital Station	3,946	
Brook Hospital Station	16,898	
Mead Works	45,799	
Southern Hospital Repair Shop (equipment only)	298	
Vehicles	128,844	
		246,959

(g) *River Ambulance Service*

Wharves, Steamers, etc.		108,370

(h) *Laboratories*

Belmont Antitoxin Establishment	12,048	
Research and Pathological Laboratories	14,571	
		26,619

A. Total for all Infectious Disease Institutions and Services:	5,009,985

B. Mental and Epileptic Institutions

Leavesden Hospital	287,596	
Caterham Hospital	272,277	
Tooting Bec Hospital	629,152	
Fountain Hospital	150,301	
Darenth Training Colony	392,432	
Edmonton Epileptic Colony	11,365	
Belmont Institution	129,833	

B. Total for all Mental and Epileptic Institutions:	1,872,956

C. Children's Institutions
   (a) *Hospitals*

Queen Mary's Hospital	325,696	
The Downs Hospital	119,856	
St. Anne's Home	16,037	
White Oak Hospital	136,917	
The Clinic (contents only)	455	
	598,961	

   (b) *Training Ship*

Exmouth I and Shore Buildings	75,193	

C. Total for Children's Institutions:	674,154

TABLE A (II)—*continued*

		£	£
D. CASUAL WARDS			
	Hackney	26,503	
	Poplar	6,613	
	The Hostel (contents only)	511	
	Chelsea	6,910	
	St. Pancras	9,451	
	Southwark	7,963	
	D. Total for Casual Wards:		57,951
E. M A B ADMINISTRATIVE OFFICES AND STORES			
	Offices of the Board	123,336	
	Central Stores	21,317	
	E. Total for Administrative Buildings:		144,653

TOTAL M A B CAPITAL EXPENDITURE FROM 1867 to 1930: £7,759,699

TABLE B
CAPITAL COSTS OF THE EARLIEST M A B HOSPITALS BUILT BETWEEN 1869 and 1878
(Leavesden, Caterham, Hampstead, Homerton, Stockwell, Fulham and Deptford).

Hospital	Acreage of site (to nearest acre)	Cost of Land	Cost of Building, including Drainage, Walls, Gasworks, Farm Buildings, etc.	Architects' and Surveyors' charges and salary of Clerk of Works	Engineering Works, Fixtures, and Fittings	Laying out Grounds and making Roads	Furniture, Bedding and Clothing	Solicitors' Charges, Printing, Insurances, and all other Charges	Total Cost of each Hospital	Cost per Bed for each Hospital	Number for which each Hospital was originally certified
		£	£	£	£	£	£	£	£	£	
Leavesden Asylum	80	8,651	121,674	5,108	16,162	3,008	16,235	1,526	172,364	86	1,995
Caterham Asylum	72	5,846	133,832	5,439	15,503	3,320	17,424	1,640	183,004	89	2,052
Hampstead Hospital (North-Western)	8	15,544	20,511	344	1,884	902	2,482	150	41,817	139	300
Homerton Hospitals (Eastern) (2 units)	8	11,812	53,788	3,560	7,431	722	6,745	1,007	85,065	281	200 (Fever) 102 (Smallpox)
Stockwell Hospitals (South-Western) (2 units)	7	15,075	56,480	2,876	8,275	1,662	7,065	1,497	92,930	339	172 (Fever) 102 (Smallpox)
Fulham Hospital (Western)	6	10,000	41,364	1,223	3,227	300	1,617	189	57,920	241	240
Deptford Hospital (South-Eastern)	9	10,000	45,317	1,081	3,311	565	2,173	60	62,507	189	330
Totals:		£76,928	£472,966	£19,631	£55,793	£10,479	£53,741	£6,069	£695,607	—	—

Sources: M A B Financial Records for the years indicated.

TABLE C

M A B ANNUAL REVENUE RAISED BY PRECEPTS ON THE METROPOLITAN POOR LAW AUTHORITIES IN SELECTED YEARS BETWEEN 1871 and 1929

Year	Rateable Value of the Metropolitan Asylum District at 30 Sept. of each year	Produce of 1d. rate in the £ on the rateable value at 30 Sept. of each year	Precepts					
			Amount in the £ worked out as a metropolitan rate[1]			Amount raised[1]		
			Common charges[2]	Direct charges[2]	Totals	Common charges[2]	Direct charges[2]	Totals
	£	£	d.	d.	d.	£	£	£
1871	19,812,058	82,550	1·20	0·38	1·58	99,199	31,400	130,599
1876	23,035,324	95,980	1·50	0·55	2·05	138,209	51,980	190,189
1881	25,012,087	104,217	1·75	0·77	2·52	182,380	81,400	263,780
1886	29,289,747	122,040	3·00	0·50	3·50	366,122	61,600	427,722
1891	31,362,718	130,677	2·12	0·71	2·83	277,699	99,600	377,299
1896	35,608,442	148,368	3·25	0·83	4·08	460,340	114,800	575,140
1901	39,678,072	165,325	4·62	0·83	5·45	719,466	133,000	852,466
1906	43,376,568	180,736	5·39	0·74	6·13	934,221	127,700	1,061,921
1911	44,565,025	185,687	4·50	0·65	5·15	839,570	121,000	960,570
1914	45,024,837	187,604	5·25	0·73	5·98	982,860	138,100	1,120,960
1921	48,613,149	202,555	Charges combined after 1916[3]		14·25	Charges combined after 1916[3]		2,886,406
1929	57,383,912	235,853			8·00			1,886,826

[1] The rates in the £ of the precepts raised were calculated on the basis of the rateable values in force at the time the half-yearly estimates of expenditure were approved and adopted by the M A B, i.e. about March and July respectively of each year.

[2] The Metropolitan Poor Law Act of 1867 decreed that certain items of M A B expenditure should be charged direct to separate poor law districts, while others were to be equalized, on a basis of rateable value, among all the constituent poor law districts.

[3] In accordance with the Local Government (Emergency Provisions) Act, 1916, the direct and common charges were combined after March 1916 and the total proportionally assessed on all constituent parishes and unions.

Sources: M A B Financial Records for the years indicated.

TABLE D

ANALYSIS OF M A B REVENUE EXPENDITURE AT FIVE DECENNIAL PERIODS IN THE HISTORY OF THE BOARD, 1889, 1899, 1909, 1919 and 1929

Institution, Service or General (Central) Account	Year	Average Daily Number of Patients	'Maintenance' of Patients (mainly food, clothing, and funerals) charged separately to Parishes and Unions according to Number of Patients	Common Charges assessed on rateable values of constituent Metropolitan					
				Salaries and Wages	Staff Provisions and Uniforms	Buildings and Establishment (including furniture, heating, lighting and cleaning)	Rates, Taxes, Insurances, Rents (e.g. for moorings, etc.)	Drugs, Medical and Surgical Appliances	Office Expenses: Stationery, Postage, Telephones Advertising etc.
			(1)	(2)	(3)	(4)	(5)	(6)	(7)
			£	£	£	£	£	£	£
1. Infectious Disease Hospitals (fever and smallpox: V.D. from 1916)	1889	926	12,560	23,272	14,225	33,619	6,706	562	1,226
	1899	4,116	58,975	82,370	63,981	89,960	18,462	2,557	5,190
	1909	4,100	46,439	108,503	60,580	97,564	36,181	8,055	2,671
	1919	2,518	69,482	142,163	66,553	104,667	27,987	10,327	2,146
	1929	5,038	99,103	348,793	95,386	166,696	63,206	21,884	3,729
2. Mental Institutions	1889	5,492	53,892	20,179	11,701	24,120	3,628	599	1,094
	1899	5,952	59,147	24,948	18,380	37,350	5,562	620	1,180
	1909	6,911	61,948	51,726	21,680	43,348	10,723	1,001	1,016
	1919	7,560	117,828	123,007	26,788	77,966	13,993	2,363	1,600
	1929	9,218	137,982	266,613	28,878	110,984	26,163	3,149	1,838
3. Sick Children's Institutions (from 1899)	1899	157	1,832	1,610	839	1,641	328	67	85
	1909	1,962	18,245	20,031	9,955	18,107	5,804	935	726
	1919	1,638	32,813	47,552	18,401	31,360	13,157	3,299	686
	1929	1,724	29,895	80,482	19,225	40,010	16,375	5,979	933
4. T.B. Sanatoria (from 1912)	1919	297	13,825	11,012	3,323	5,677	2,027	1,018	203
	1929	1,967	52,575	92,962	20,249	51,245	11,258	4,989	1,650
5. Path. Laboratories, Research and Production of Antitoxin (other than amounts charged to separate institutions)	1899			559				2,411	
	1909			881					
	1919			516					
	1929			569				1,518	
TOTALS FOR INSTITUTIONS FOR THE SICK AND MENTALLY DISORDERED (with each head of annual expenditure expressed as a Percentage of the Total Cost of Patients in these institutions: items 1–5)	1889	6,418	£66,452 (31·84%)	£43,451 (20·83%)	£25,926 (12·43%)	£57,739 (27·67%)	£10,334 (5·00%)	£1,161 (0·57%)	£2,320 (1·13%)
	1899	10,225	£119,954 (24·04%)	£109,487 (21·94%)	£83,200 (16·68%)	£128,951 (25·84%)	£24,352 (4·89%)	£5,655 (1·13%)	£6,455 (1·29%)
	1909	12,973	£126,632 (18·17%)	£181,141 (25·99%)	£92,215 (13·23%)	£159,019 (22·82%)	£52,708 (7·56%)	£9,991 (1·43%)	£4,413 (0·63%)
	1919	12,013	£233,948 (23·54%)	£324,250 (32·63%)	£115,065 (11·58%)	£219,670 (22·10%)	£57,164 (5·75%)	£17,007 (1·71%)	£4,635 (0·47%)
	1929	17,947	£319,555 (15·75%)	£789,419 (38·91%)	£163,738 (8·07%)	£368,935 (18·19%)	£117,002 (5·77%)	£37,549 (1·85%)	£8,150 (0·40%)

TABLE D—*continued*

oor law districts			*TOTALS*								*Year*
Travelling Expenses, Running Expenses of Ambulances, and Sundry Expenses	*'Special' Expenditure (of a capital or semi-capital nature) and General Expenditure*	*Receipts on Farm, Industrial, and Ambulance Accounts (Deduct)*	*Net Total 'Common' Charges (Cols. 2–8)*	*Gross Total 'Common' Charges (incl. 'Special' Expenditure: Col. 9) less Receipts (Col. 10)*	*Combined Total of Gross 'Common' Charges (Col. 12) and 'Maintenance' Charges (Col. 1)*	*Totals for each separate Service etc., expressed as Percentage of Grand Total (see Col. 13 overleaf)*					
(8)	(9)	(10)	(11)	(12)	(13)	1889	1899	1909	1919	1929	
£	£	£	£	£	£	%	%	%	%	%	
281	—	—	79,891	79,891	92,451	28·08					1889
1,367	14,210	—	263,887	278,097	337,072		43·96				1899
1,356	40,787	−3,819	314,910	351,878	398,317			36·96			1909
5,344	6,929	−3,610	359,187	362,506	431,988				29·71		1919
20,420	103,711	−10,950	720,114	812,875	911,978					38·21	1929
794	—	—	62,115	62,115	116,007	35·23					1889
1,063	3,735	—	89,103	92,838	151,985		19·82				1899
1,085	12,420	−5,705	130,579	137,294	199,242			18·49			1909
2,224	15,294	−8,519	247,941	254,716	372,544				25·62		1919
25,340	50,698	−13,289	462,965	500,374	638,356					26·75	1929
124	380	—	4,694	5,074	6,906		0·90				1899
1,200	22,311	−295	56,758	78,774	97,019			9·00			1909
3,418	1,783	−879	117,873	118,777	151,590				10·42		1919
11,174	20,190	−2,603	174,178	191,765	221,660					9·29	1929
122	227	−298	23,382	23,311	37,136				2·55		1919
2,840	18,342	−1,693	185,193	201,842	254,417					10·66	1929
			2,970	2,970	2,970		0·39				1899
	1,473		881	2,354	2,354			0·22			1909
			516	516	516				0·04		1919
	115		2,117	2,232	2,232					0·09	1929
£1,075 (0·53%)	—	—	£142,006	£142,006	£208,458 (100·00%)	63·31%					1889
£2,554 (0·51%)	£18,325 (3·68%)	—	£360,654	£378,979	£498,933 (100·00%)		65·07%				1899
£3,641 (0·52%)	£76,991 (11·05%)	£−9,819 (−1·40%)	£503,128	£570,300	£696,932 (100·00%)			64·67%			1909
£11,108 (1·12%)	£24,233 (2·44%)	£−13,306 (−1·34%)	£748,899	£759,826	£993,774 (100·00%)				68·34%		1919
£59,774 (2·95%)	£193,056 (9·52%)	£−28,535 (−1·41%)	£1,544,567	£1,709,088	£2,028,643 (100·00%)					85·00%	1929

Continued overleaf

TABLE D—*continued*

ANALYSIS OF M A B REVENUE EXPENDITURE AT FIVE DECENNIAL PERIODS IN THE HISTORY OF THE BOARD, 1889, 1899, 1909, 1919 and 1929

Institution, Service or General (Central) Account	Year	Average Daily Number of Patients	'Maintenance' of Patients (mainly food, clothing, and funerals) charged separately to Parishes and Unions according to Number of Patients	Salaries and Wages	Staff Provisions and Uniforms	Buildings and Establishment (including furniture, heating, lighting and cleaning)	Rates, Taxes, Insurances, Rents (e.g. for moorings, etc.)	Drugs, Medical and Surgical Appliances	Office Expenses: Stationery, Postage, Telephones, Advertising, etc.
			(1)	(2)	(3)	(4)	(5)	(6)	(7)
			£	£	£	£	£	£	£
6. Ambulance Services: a. Land b. River	1889a			2,378	1,115	3,431	412	—	76
	1889b			2,057	42	992	1,110	—	12
	1899a			10,722	4,031	2,033	1,133	—	202
	1899b			3,011	348	895	1,521	3	37
	1909a			12,236	4,305	5,955	1,808	—	140
	1909b			2,558	596	1,227	1,104	3	13
	1919a			18,139	6,885	3,957	1,831	—	220
	1919b			3,781	755	1,891	1,205	4	21
	1929a			41,362	785	5,695	3,320	—	229
	1929b			6,744	891	2,567	1,836	10	25
7. Training Ship	1889	579	7,694	3,300	2,910	3,822	358	29	229
	1899	561	8,154	3,344	1,940	4,211	353	93	185
	1909	616	6,771	3,707	1,547	3,925	640	48	155
	1919	622	16,876	8,113	2,019	7,483	722	385	322
	1929	540	12,198	14,921	1,250	6,947	793	160	219
8. Children's Remand Homes (1902–1910)	1909	72	542	793	421	421	423	1	33
9. Casual Wards (from 1912)	1919	59	441	3,837	56	1,423	2,916	8	26
	1929	746	7,323	18,942	212	6,750	3,001	65	186
10. Head Office and other (Central) Admin. Depts.	1889			4,263	—	—	1,231	—	3,358
	1899			10,531	35	305	2,158	—	5,380
	1909			21,581	168	1,029	518	—	3,963
	1919			30,412	80	1,299	1,022	—	5,046
	1929			67,002	82	1,941	4,476	—	8,502
11. Special Administrative Costs: Loan Charges, Legal Expenses and Superannuation and Workmen's Compensation Payments	1889 1899 1909 1919 1929								
12. Notification of Inf. Diseases (fees to Local Authorities: from 1890)	1899 1909 1919 1929								
COMBINED TOTALS OF M A B ANNUAL EXPENDITURE (Items 1–12 above)	1889	6,997	£ 74,146	£ 55,449	£ 29,993	£ 65,984	£ 13,445	£ 1,190	£ 5,995
	1899	10,786	128,108	137,095	89,554	136,395	29,517	5,751	12,259
	1909	13,589	133,945	222,016	99,252	171,576	57,201	10,043	8,717
	1919	12,694	251,265	388,532	124,860	235,723	64,860	17,404	10,270
	1929	19,233	339,076	938,390	166,958	392,835	130,428	37,784	17,311

Source: M A B Financial Records.

TABLE D—*continued*

poor law districts			*TOTALS*								*Year*
Travelling Expenses, Running Expenses of Ambulances, and Sundry Expenses	*'Special' Expenditure (of a capital or semi-capital nature) and General Expenditure*	*Receipts on Farm, Industrial, and Ambulance Accounts (Deduct)*	*Net Total 'Common' Charges (Cols. 2–8)*	*Gross Total 'Common' Charges incl. 'Special' Expenditure (Col. 9) less Receipts (Col. 10)*	*Combined Total of Gross 'Common' Charges (Col. 12) and 'Maintenance' Charges (Col. 1)*	*Totals for each separate Service etc., expressed as Percentage of Grand Total (Col. 13)*					
(8)	(9)	(10)	(11)	(12)	(13)	1889	1899	1909	1919	1929	
£	£	£	£	£	£	%	%	%	%	%	
1,135	—	—	8,547	8,547	8,547	2·60					1889
12	—	—	4,225	4,225	4,225	1·29					
4,219	34	—	22,340	22,374	22,374		2·92				1899
35	529	—	5,850	6,379	6,379		0·83				
3,410	2,928	−793	27,854	29,989	29,989			2·78			1909
25	866	—	5,526	6,392	6,392			0·59			
16,797	3,584	−6,829	47,829	44,584	44,584				3·07		1919
38	1,467	−4	7,695	9,158	9,158				0·63		
20,606	23,219	−27,497	71,997	67,719	67,719					2·84	1929
141	263	−14	12,214	12,463	12,463					0·52	
164	—	—	10,812	10,812	18,506	5·62					1889
192	4,705	—	10,318	15,023	23,177		3·02				1899
337	950	—	10,359	11,309	18,080			1·68			1909
566	1,402	−10	19,610	21,002	37,878				2·60		1919
1,135	2,944	−102	25,425	28,267	40,465					1·69	1929
26	116	—	2,118	2,234	2,776			0·26			1909
115	9,010	−176	8,381	17,215	17,656				1·21		1919
17,645	3,052	−406	46,801	49,447	56,770					2·38	1929
641	—	—	9,493	9,493	9,493	2·83					1889
513	47	—	18,922	18,969	18,969		2·48				1899
400	1,968	—	27,659	29,627	29,627			2·75			1909
419	—	—	38,278	38,278	38,278				2·63		1919
1,862	1,571	−14	83,865	85,422	85,422					3·58	1929
	80,054			80,054	80,054	24·35					1889
	192,665			192,665	192,665		25·12				1899
	290,435			290,435	290,435			26·94			1909
	311,610			311,610	311,610				21·43		1919
	90,324			90,324	90,324					3·79	1929
	4,287			4,287	4,287		0·56				1899
	3,541			3,541	3,541			0·33			1909
	1,300			1,300	1,300				0·09		1919
	4,797			4,797	4,797					0·20	1929
£3,027	£80,054	£—	£175,083	£255,137	£329,283	100·00 %	%	%	%	%	1889
7,513	220,592	—	418,084	638,676	766,784		100·00				1899
7,839	377,795	−10,612	576,644	943,827	1,077,772			100·00			1909
29,043	352,606	−20,325	870,692	1,202,973	1,454,238				100·00		1919
101,163	319,226	−56,568	1,784,869	2,047,527	2,386,603					100·00	1929

TABLE E

WEEKLY COST OF PATIENTS IN M A B INFECTIOUS DISEASE AND MENTAL HOSPITALS IN SELECTED YEARS BETWEEN 1886 and 1929

Year	Fever Hospitals			Smallpox Hospitals			Mental Hospitals		
	'Maintenance' Charges[1]	Other Charges[2]	Total	'Maintenance' Charges[1]	Other Charges[2,4]	Total[4]	'Maintenance' Charges[1]	Other Charges[2]	Total
1886[3]	6/5d.	32/-	38/5d.	13/5d.	—	—	3/11d.	4/5d.	8/4d.
1889	5/6½d.	40/7½d.	46/2d.	8/2d.	—	—	3/9½d.	4/10½d.	8/8d.
1894	5/7d.	25/3½d.	30/10½d.	7/-	67/1d.	74/1d.	3/10½d.	5/7d.	9/5½d.
1899	5/7d.	23/1d.	28/8d.	7/-	—	—	3/9½d.	6/0½d.	9/10d.
1904	4/11½d.	33/0½d.	38/-	11/10d.	41/9½d.	53/7½d.	3/10d.	7/4d.	11/2d.
				(for the year 1902)					
1909	4/4d.	27/9d.	32/1d.	9/-	—	—	3/5d.	6/11d.	10/4d.
1914	4/6½d.	24/10d.	29/4½d.	8/-	—	—	3/2½d.	7/9d.	10/11½d
1919	9/6d.	44/-	53/6d.	8/9d.	—	—	6/9d.	14/4d.	21/1d.
1924	7/2d.	60/9½d.	67/11½d.	7/2½d.	—	—	5/3d.	18/11½d.	24/2½d.
1929	7/10d.	51/8d.	59/6d.	6/6½d.	51/2½d.	57/9d.	5/11d.	16/2d.	22/1d.
				(for the year 1928)					

[1] 'Maintenance' or 'direct' charges related mainly to patients' food and clothing while in hospital and to funeral expenses. These were charged separately to the respective unions and parishes from which the patients were sent.

[2] 'Other' or 'common' charges comprised all items of hospital expenditure other than patients' 'maintenance', and were met by contributions from the metropolitan boards of guardians, assessed in proportion to the rateable value of each constituent poor law district.

[3] 1886 was the first year in which hospital expenditure in the various M A B institutions was recorded on a uniform basis.

[4] Where the daily average number of smallpox patients was statistically insignificant, 'other charges' and totals have been omitted from this table. Average smallpox patient-costs have been included for epidemic years, which are near enough for comparisons of costs to be made with those at the other institutions.

Sources: M A B Statements of Expenditure for the years indicated.

TABLE F

COST OF THE 1884–85 SMALLPOX EPIDEMIC IN LONDON
DURING WHICH SOME 11,000 CASES WERE TREATED IN THE M A B HOSPITALS

	£	£
Floating Hospitals:		
Maintenance and Administrative Costs for 1884 and 1885	68,631	
Less average normal cost of maintaining the ships for two years when without patients	24,000	
		44,631
Darenth (1,000-bed) Convalescent Camp Hospital (temporary):		
Maintenance and Administrative Costs (two years)		81,112
Plaistow Hospital (100 beds):		
Rent (18 months) for temporary hire and maintenance of patients		8,882
River Ambulance Service:		
Maintenance for two years		16,860
M A B London Hospitals:		
Maintenance and Administrative Costs (two years)	171,760	
Less one-half (since hospitals were also used for fever cases)[1]	85,880	
		85,880[2]
Land Ambulance Service:		
Maintenance for two years	26,400	
Less one-quarter for cases other than smallpox[3]	6,600	
		19,800

Total Cost of treating 11,060 smallpox patients: £257,165

Average cost per patient: £23   5   0

---

[1] At the beginning of the epidemic three-fourths of all the patients admitted into the M A B hospitals in London were suffering from smallpox, but convalescents were at an early stage transferred to the ships; *mild* cases were soon afterwards removed from their homes to the wharves. Eventually, almost *all cases* were so treated, and the London hospitals then admitted fever cases only. The total cost of the hospitals in these circumstances was £171,760.

[2] This sum (£85,880) includes £20,000 spent on clothes given to every patient on discharge to replace the clothes worn at the time of admission, which were destroyed.

[3] Three-fourths of the patients removed by the M A B Land Ambulance Service were suffering from smallpox.

Sources: M A B Annual Reports (Finance and Ambulance Committees).

TABLE G
WEEKLY COST OF SICK CHILDREN IN M A B HOSPITAL-SCHOOLS AND HOMES IN 1909, 1919 and 1929

	HOSPITAL-SCHOOLS FOR INFECTIOUS EYE DISEASES			HOSPITAL-SCHOOLS FOR INFECTIOUS SKIN DISEASES		
Year	Average Daily Number of Children	Cost of 'Maintenance' (Food and Clothing) per child per week	Total Cost[1] per child per week	Average Daily Number of Children	Cost of 'Maintenance' (Food and Clothing) per child per week	Total Cost[1] per child per week
1909	572	3/6d.	15/11d.	353	3/3d.	13/11d.
1919	250	7/7d.	33/3d.	231	5/6½d.	28/–
1929	295	7/–	38/2½d.	150	5/3d.	44/10d.

HOSPITALS AND HOMES FOR THE SICK AND CONVALESCENT

	QUEEN MARY'S HOSPITAL[2]			OTHER M A B INSTITUTIONS FOR SICK CHILDREN		
1909	502	4/2d.	18/4d.	363	3/8d.	12/11d.
1919	738	8/9d.	37/7½d.	419	7/7d.	25/1d.
1929	818	6/5d.	44/11d.	461	7/–	36/6d.

[1] Figures for total cost exclude loan charges, rent and central expenditure. For analysis of total annual expenditure of Sick Children's Institutions see preceding Table D (item 3).

[2] Costs for Queen Mary's Hospital (known on opening in 1909 as The Children's Infirmary) are given separately from the average of the Board's other institutions for sick children on account of its greater size and other differentiating characteristics.

Sources: M A B Financial Records.

TABLE H
COST OF TUBERCULOSIS PATIENTS[1] (OTHER THAN POOR LAW) IN M A B INSTITUTIONS IN 1915, 1922 and 1929

Year	Average daily number of Tuberculosis Patients	Average weekly cost per Patient	Total annual current expenditure (gross) on Tuberculosis Institutions[2]	Rate in £ to meet net annual expenditure on Tuberculosis Institutions[3]	Rate in £ to meet total M A B annual expenditure
1915	335	28/–	£30,621	0·2d.	9d.
1922	1,197	60/3d.	£218,788	1·1d.	13d.
1929	1,967	43/10d.	£254,417	1·2d.	8d.

[1] Tuberculosis patients suffering from all forms of the disease are included, adults and children.

[2] Inclusive of rates, taxes and semi-capital expenditure, which have been excluded from calculation of patient-costs. For analysis of revenue expenditure in M A B tuberculosis institutions, see preceding Table D (item 4).

[3] Exchequer grants taken into account.

Sources: M A B Financial Records for years indicated.

TABLE J
M A B MEDICAL OFFICERS' RATES OF REMUNERATION IN
1870, 1890, 1910 and 1925

	Medical Officers' Annual Salary Scales							
	1870		1890		1910		1925	
	Min. £	Max. £	Min. £	Max. £	Min. £	Max. £	Min. £	Max. £
MEDICAL SUPERINTENDENTS[1] *Type of Hospital:*								
Fever and Smallpox	350	450	350	500	400	700	900	1,150
Tuberculosis	—	—	—		—	—	770	1,050
Children's	—	—	—	—	500	700	770	1,250
Mental	—	500	450	600	600	800	850	1,250
ASSISTANT MEDICAL OFFICERS[2] *Fever, Smallpox, TB, and Children's Hospitals:*								
Senior	120	—	250	300	250	300	650[2]	750[2]
Second	—	—	180	200	180	240	550[2]	600[2]
Junior	—	—	150	170	—	—	500[2]	—
Mental Hospitals:								
Senior	150	—	150	200	250	300	650[2]	800[2]
Second	—	—	130	—	180	200	560[2]	650[2]
Junior	—	—	—	—	150	170	500[2]	560[2]

[1] Medical Superintendents' emoluments included a furnished house.

[2] AMOs' emoluments included board, lodging and laundry, except in 1925, by which time £130 p.a. was being deducted for these items.

Sources: M A B Financial Records and Board Minutes.

TABLE K
M A B NURSING STAFF RATES OF PAY[1]
DURING THREE DECENNIAL PERIODS[2] BETWEEN 1870 and 1929

	Nurses' Annual Salary Scales					
	1870–79		1900–09		1920–29	
	Min. £	Max. £	Min. £	Max. £	Min. £	Max. £
Fever and Smallpox, Tuberculosis and Children's Hospitals						
Matron[3]	75	120	100	150	160	340[3]
Superintendent Nurse/Sister	36	42	42	46	110	130
Charge Nurse/Ward Sister	27	—	36	40	80	95
Staff Nurse	—	—	30	34	60	70
Assistant Nurse: Class I	—	—	24	28	42	48
Class II	—	—	20	24	32	34
Assistant Nurse	20	—	—	—	29	31
Senior Probationer	—	—	—	—	42	48
Probationer	—	—	10	18	30	34
Mental Hospitals						
Female:						
Matron[3]	150	200[3]	100	150	240	340[3]
Superintendent Nurse	—	—	42	46	151	182½
Chief Charge Nurse/Ward Sister	30	40	33	43	96	128
Charge Attendant/Staff Nurse	—	—	25	31	94	114
Attendant	15	25	18	25	—	—
Probationer	—	—	—	—	83	104
Male:						
Inspector/Senior Head Attendant	60	80	70	100	200	217
Head Nurse/Head Attendant	40	60	52	62	160	192
Chief Charge Nurse/Attendant	—	—	34	40	130	156
Staff Nurse	—	—	—	—	114	150
Attendant	25	30	26	32	—	—
Probationer	—	—	—	—	104	130

[1] Rates shown are cash emoluments, in addition to which nursing staff in the non-mental hospitals were provided with board, residence and laundry. In the mental hospitals, uniforms only were provided. Matrons were allowed (except where otherwise stated) board, residence (or an unfurnished house) and laundry.

[2] Changes in rates of pay were not always made simultaneously for all grades and all institutions. The highest rate in the decennial period is given.

[3] Matrons' rates of pay varied with the size of institution. By 1920 there were 5 grades for institutions ranging from 48 beds (tuberculous children) to 2,260 beds (mental). During the 1870–79 period, matrons in mental hospitals received higher pay in lieu of board.

Sources: M A B Financial Records and Board Minutes.

Maps of the Metropolitan Asylum District

Bibliography

BIBLIOGRAPHY

[Place of publication of works and reports listed: London, unless otherwise stated.]

I. OFFICIAL PUBLICATIONS—*Periodical Reports*. (Reports on special topics are listed under subject headings.)

*Metropolitan Asylums Board**
  Annual Reports, 1886–1930
  Circulars, 1903–13
  Minutes, 1867–1930
  Statistical Committee Reports, 1886–99
Poor Law Commissioners
  Annual Reports, 1835–47
Poor Law Board
  Annual Reports, 1848–71
Local Government Board
  Annual Reports, 1872–1919
Commissioners in Lunacy
  Twenty-fifth Report (1871) and subsequent reports: entries relating to the Metropolitan District Asylums
Ministry of Health
  Annual Reports, 1919–35
Medical Officers of the Committee of Council on Health
  Annual Reports, 1859–71
Medical Officers of the Privy Council and Local Government Board
  Annual Reports (New Series), 1874–1919
Chief Medical Officers of the Ministry of Health
  Annual Reports, 1920–35
Registrar-General
  Annual Reports, 1837/38–1930
  Annual Summaries of Births, Deaths and Causes of Death in London, 1840–69
  Annual Summaries of Births, Deaths and Causes of Death in London and Other Great Towns, 1870–1912
  Quarterly Returns, including Annual Tables, 1913–30

II. AUTOBIOGRAPHIES, BIOGRAPHIES, DIARIES AND MEMOIRS

Cook, Sir Edward, *The Life of Florence Nightingale* (2 vols.), 1913.
Elliot, H. S. R. (ed.), *The Letters of John Stuart Mill* (2 vols.), 1910.
Feiling, K., 1910. *The Life of Neville Chamberlain*, 1946.
Finer, S. E., *The Life and Times of Sir Edwin Chadwick*, 1952.

 * Most M A B reports are available at the British Museum, the Greater London County Record Office, the Royal Society of Medicine, the London School of Hygiene and Tropical Medicine, and the Oxford Radcliffe Library. Some may be found at the Wellcome Institute of the History of Medicine.

Gathorne-Hardy, A. E. (ed.), *Gathorne-Hardy, First Earl of Cranbrook: a Memoir* (2 vols.), 1910.

Gwynn, S. and Tuckwell, G., *The Life of the Rt. Hon. Sir Charles W. Dilke* (2 vols.), 1917.

Hammond, J. L. and Barbara, *James Stansfeld—A Victorian Champion of Sex Equality*, 1932.

Haw, G., *From Workhouse to Westminster: the Life of Will Crooks, MP*, 1907.

Hill, G. B., *The Life of Sir Rowland Hill* (2 vols.), 1880.

Lambert, Royston, *Sir John Simon, 1816–1904, and English Social Administration*, 1963.

Liveing, S., *A Nineteenth-Century Teacher: John Henry Bridges, MB, FRCP*, 1926.

Mill, John Stuart, *Autobiography*, 1873 (World's Classics ed. 1926).

Long, Viscount, *Memories*, 1923.

Preston-Thomas, H., *The Work and Play of a Government Inspector*, 1909.

Rogers, J., *Reminiscences of a Workhouse Medical Officer* (ed. by J. T. Rogers), 1889.

Simey, T. S. and M., *Charles Booth, Social Scientist*, 1960.

Twining, L., *Recollections of My Life and Work*, 1893.

Woodham-Smith, C., *Florence Nightingale, 1820–1910*, 1951 (Penguin Books, 1955).

III. GOVERNMENT

(a) *Central Control*

Bagehot, W., *The English Constitution* (Nelson edn.), 1872.

Barnard, C. T., *The Functions of the Executive*, Harvard, 1956.

Brebner, J. B., 'Laissez-faire and State Intervention', *Journal of Economic History*, viii, 1948.

Kelsall, R. K., *Higher Civil Servants in Britain*, 1955.

Lowell, A. L., *The Government of England* (2 vols.), New York, 1918.

MacDonagh, O. O. G. M., 'The Nineteenth-Century Revolution in Government: A Re-appraisal', *Historical Journal*, i, 1958.

MacDonagh, O. O. G. M., 'Delegated Legislation and Administrative Discretions in the Fifties: A Particular Study', *Victorian Studies*, ii, 1958.

Parris, H., 'The Nineteenth-Century Revolution in Government: A Re-appraisal re-appraised', *Historical Journal*, iii, 1960.

Simon, Sir John, *English Sanitary Institutions*, 2nd Edn., 1897.

Smellie, K. B., *One Hundred Years of English Government*, 1937.

Thomas, M. W., 'The Origins of Administrative Centralization', *Current Legal Problems* (1950), iii.

Trail, H., *Central Government*, 1881.

Webb, S. and B., *English Poor Law History: vols. 7–9 of English Local Government: 9 vols.*, 1906–29.

Wheare, K. C., *The Civil Service in the Constitution*, 1954.

Willis, J., *The Parliamentary Powers of English Government Departments*, Cambridge, Mass., 1933.

Willson, F. M. G., 'Ministries and Boards', *Public Administration*, xxxiii (1955).

Reports on General Legislative Powers of Central Departments:
    Royal Commission on Poor Law, 1909, *Report*, part iv, chap. i, pp. 119 ff;
    Royal Commission on Local Government, 1925–30; *Minutes of Evidence*, vol. i, pp. 240 ff., pp. 407 ff.

(b) *Local Government* (general)

Ashley, P., *English Local Government*, 1905.

Cannan, E., *The History of Local Rates in England*, 1927.

Glen, A. and Jenkin, A. F., *The Law of Public Health and Local Government* (2 vols.), 11th edn. 1895.

Laski, H. J., et al. (eds.), *A Century of Municipal Progress*, 1935.

Smellie, K. B., *A History of Local Government*, 1946.

Smith, J. Toulmin, *What is Bureaucracy and What is Local Self-Government?*, 1955.

Stewart, A. P. and Jenkins, E., *The Medical and Legal Aspects of Sanitary Reform*, 1867.

Vine, J. S., *English Municipal Institutions*, 1879.

Webb, S. and B., *English Local Government* (9 vols.), 1906–29.

Report of the Ministry of Reconstruction Local Government Committee on the Transfer of Functions of the Poor Law Authorities in England and Wales, 1918 (Cmd. 8917).

Reports and Minutes of Evidence of the Royal Commission on Local Government, 1925–30.

(c) *Local Government in London*

Firth, J., *Municipal London*, 1876.

Firth, J. and Simpson, E. R., *London Government under the Local Government Act, 1888*, 1889.

Gibbon, Sir I. G., and Bell, R. W., *History of the London County Council*, 1939.

Jephson, H., *Sanitary Evolution of London*, 1907.

Rendle, W., *London Vestries and their Sanitary Work*, 1865.

Rendle, W., *Fever in London and its Social and Sanitary Lessons*, 1866.

Robson, W. A., *The Government and Misgovernment of London*, 1939.

Report of the Select Committee on Metropolitan Local Government, 1867.

Report and Minutes of Evidence of the Royal Commission on the Local Government of Greater London, 1921–23 (Cmd. 1830).

IV. HISTORIES OF MEDICINE AND PUBLIC HEALTH

Brockington, C. Fraser, *A Short History of Public Health*, 1956.

Frazer, W. M., *The History of English Public Health, 1834–1939*, 1950.

Greenwood, M., *Some British Pioneers of Social Medicine*, 1948.

Lloyd, Wyndham E. B., *A Hundred Years of Medicine*, 1936.

Richardson, Sir B. W., *The Health of Nations: a review of the works of Edwin Chadwick* (2 vols.), 1887.

Simon, Sir John, *English Sanitary Institutions* (2nd edn., 1897).

Singer, C., *A Short History of Medicine*, Oxford, 1928.

Still, G. F., *The History of Paediatrics* 1931.

Walker, K., *The Story of Medicine*, 1954.

Williams, J. H. Harley, *A Century of Public Health in Britain, 1832–1929*, 1932.

V. Hospitals (general)

Abel-Smith, B., *The Hospitals, 1800–1948*, 1964.

Acton Society Trust, *Hospitals and the State: Hospital Organization and Administration under the National Health Service:*
1. *Background and Blueprint*, 1955
2. *The Impact of the Change*, 1956
3. *Groups, Regions and Committees:*
   Part I, *Hospital Management Committees*, 1957
4. Part II, *Regional Hospital Boards*, 1957
5. *The Central Control of the Service*, 1958
6. *Creative Leadership in a State Service*, 1959

Aikin, John, *Thoughts on Hospitals*, 1771.

Bristowe, J. S., and Holmes, T., *The Hospitals of the United Kingdom*, HMSO, 1864.

Burdett, H. C., *Hospitals and Asylums of the World* (4 vols.), 1891–93 (vol. 4 is a comprehensive bibliography on general hospitals).

Dainton, C., *The Story of England's Hospitals*, 1961.

Langdon-Davies, J., *Westminster Hospital—Two Centuries of Voluntary Service, 1719–1948*, 1952.

London County Council, *Municipal Hospitals, Clinics and Dispensaries*, 1933 (Part II of Joint Survey of Medical and Surgical Services).

London County Council, *The LCC Hospitals: A Retrospect*, 1949 (LCC Publication No. 3657).

McInnes, E. M., *St. Thomas' Hospital*, 1963.

Nightingale, Florence, *Notes on Hospitals*, 3rd edn., 1863.

Nuffield Provincial Hospitals Trust, *The Hospital Surveys*, Oxford, 1946.

Nuffield Provincial Hospitals Trust, *Studies in the Functions and Design of Hospitals*, 1955.

Oppert, F., *Hospitals, Infirmaries and Dispensaries*, 1883.

Pinker, R., *English Hospital Statistics, 1861–1938*, 1966.

Poynter, F. N. L. (ed.), *The Evolution of Hospitals in Britain*, 1964.

Ross, J. S., *The National Health Service in Great Britain*, 1952 (Chapter 17).

Sheffield City Libraries, *The Sheffield Hospitals*, 1959.

Titmuss, R. M., *Problems of Social Policy*, 1950 (Chapters V, XI, XXII, XXIII and XXIV).

Titmuss, R. M., *Essays on 'The Welfare State'*, 1958 (Chapter 7: 'The Hospital and its Patients').

Reports of the House of Lords Select Committee on Metropolitan Hospitals, 1890–93 (First Report, HMSO, 1890; Second Report, HMSO, 1891; Third Report, HMSO, 1893).

Interim Report on the Future Provision of Medical and Allied Services, Cmd. 693, 1920 (the Dawson Report).

Voluntary Hospitals Committee (Final Report), Cmd. 1335, 1921 (the Cave Committee).

Ministry of Health, Voluntary Hospitals Commission (Interim Report), 1923 (Chairman, Lord Onslow).

Report of the Voluntary Hospitals Commission (Sankey Commission), British Hospitals Association, 1937.

Draft Interim Report of the Medical Planning Commission, 1942.

Report of the Committee on the Internal Administration of Hospitals (Bradbeer Report), 1954.

VI. INFECTIOUS DISEASES AND INFECTIOUS DISEASE HOSPITALS

Bascombe, E., *History of Epidemic Pestilence from the Earliest Ages*, 1851.

Blacklock, J. W. S., 'The Epidemiology of Tuberculosis', *British Medical Journal*, i, 707; 1947.

Bradley, W. H., 'Notifiable Infectious Diseases: A Re-Assessment', *Royal Society of Health Journal*, vol. 79, No. 4 (July–August), 1959.

Brownlee, J., 'The History of the Birth and Death Rates in England and Wales . . . from 1570 to the present time', *Public Health*, 211–22, 228–38; 1916.

Budd, W., *Typhoid Fever*, 1873.

Buer, M. A., *Health, Wealth and Population in the Early Days of the Industrial Revolution*, 1926.

Burnet, Sir MacFarlane, *Virus as Organism*, Harvard, 1946.

Burnet, Sir MacFarlane, *The Natural History of Infectious Diseases*, 1953.

Burnet, Sir MacFarlane, *Viruses and Man*, 1955.

Burdett, H. C., *Cottage Hospitals, General, Fever and Convalescent*, 1896.

Colnat, Albert, *Les Epidemies et l'Histoire*, Paris, 1937.

Crawford, R., *Plague and Pestilence in Literature and Art*, 1914.

Creighton, C., *A History of Epidemics in Great Britain*, vol. i, 1891; vol. ii, 1894.

Crookshank, F. M., *The History and Pathology of Vaccination* (2 vols.), 1889.

Cummins, S. L., *Tuberculosis in History*, 1949.

Dixon, C. W., *Smallpox*, 1962.

Drew, J., *Man, Microbe and Malady*, 1940.

Edwards, E. J., 'The German Vaccination Commission', *Trans. Epidemiological Society of London*, 5, 27, 1885–86.

Gale, A. H., *Epidemic Diseases*, 1959.

Goodall, E. W. A., *A Short History of the Epidemic Diseases*, 1934.

Graunt, J., *Observations on Bills of Mortality*, 1665.

Greenhow, T. M., *Cholera*, 1832.

Greenhow, E. H., *Diphtheria*, 1860.

Greenwood, L. H., *Epidemics and Crowd Diseases*, 1935.

Gregory, G., *Some Account of the Hospital for Smallpox and Vaccination at Battle Bridge, St. Pancras*, 1830.

Guy, W. A., 'Two Hundred and Fifty Years of Smallpox in London', *Journal of the Statistical Society*, 45, 399–443, 1882.

Hare, Ronald, *Pomp and Pestilence: Infectious Disease, Its Origins and Conquest*, 1954.

Jenner, Sir William, *Lectures and Essays on Fevers and Diphtheria, 1847–79*, 1893.

Kennett-Barrington, Sir Vincent, *Floating Hospitals for Infectious Cases*, 1883.

Kennett-Barrington, Sir Vincent, *Hospital and Ambulance Organization of the Metropolis during Epidemics*, 1884.

Kennett-Barrington, Sir Vincent, *Hospital and Ambulance Organization of the Metropolitan Asylums Board*, 1893.

Laidlaw, Sir Patrick, *Virus Diseases and Viruses*, 1938.

Ledingham, J. C. G. and Arkwright, J. A., *The Carrier Problem in Infectious Diseases*, 1912.

Miller, G., *The Adoption of Inoculation for Smallpox in England and France*, Philadelphia, 1957 (includes extensive bibliography).

Murchison, C., *A Treatise on the Continued Fevers of Great Britain*, 1862.

Ozanam, J. A. F., *Histoire médicale des Maladies épidemiques*, Paris, 1835.

Parsons, H. F., *The Pandemic of Influenza* (My. of H. Report), 1920.

Paul, J., *Clinical Epidemiology*, Chicago, 1958.

Philip, Sir Robert, *Collected Papers on Tuberculosis*, 1937.

Rolleston, J. A., *A History of the Acute Exanthemata*, 1937.

Smith, Theobald, *Parasitism and Disease*, Princeton, 1934.

Snow, John, *On the Mode of Communication of Cholera*, 1849.

Sutherland, Halliday (ed.), *The Control and Eradication of Tuberculosis*, Edinburgh, 1911.

Thomson, D., 'The Ebb and Flow of Infection', *Monthly Bulletin, Ministry of Health and PHLS*, 14, 106; 1955.

Torres, C. M., 'Further Studies on the Pathology of Alastrim and their significance in the Variola Alastrim Problem', *Proceedings of the Royal Society of Medicine*, 29, 1525, 1935.

Vaughan, V. C., *Epidemiology and Public Health* (3 vols.), 1922.

Winslow, C. E. A., *The Conquest of Epidemic Disease: A Chapter in the History of Ideas*, Princeton, 1944.

Report of the Select Committee appointed to examine the state of contagious fever in the metropolis, 1818 (BPP, 1818, vol. viii, 332).

Report of the House of Commons Select Committee on the M A B Hospital at Hampstead, 1875 (BPP, 1875, vol. x (363), 643).

Report of the Royal Commission on Smallpox and Fever Hospitals, 1882 (Cmd. 3314).

Reports of the Royal Commission on Vaccination, 1889–96 (Six reports).

Local Government Board, *Report on Sanatoria for Consumption and certain other aspects of the Tuberculosis Question*, by H. T. Bulstrode, 1908.

VII. MEDICAL EDUCATION (nineteenth century)

Beck, A., 'The British Medical Council and British Medical Education in the Nineteenth Century', *Bulletin of the History of Medicine*, xxx, 1956.

Newman, C., *The Evolution of Medical Education in the Nineteenth Century*, Oxford, 1957.

Lambert, R., *Sir John Simon, 1816–1904 and English Social Administration*, 1963 (Chapter XIX).

Report of the House of Commons Select Committee on Medical Education, 1834.

VIII. MENTAL DEFICIENCY AND MENTAL HOSPITALS

Barr, M. W., *Mental Defectives, their History, Treatment and Training*, 1904.

Beach, Fletcher, 'Mental Deficiency' (Presidential Address), *Journal of Mental Science*, 46, 623 *et seq.*, 1900.

Burdett, H. C., *Hospitals and Asylums of the World*, 1891–93. (Vol. 2 contains a bibliography on mental institutions.)

Duncan, P. M., *First Report of the Eastern Counties' Asylum for Idiots and Imbeciles*, Colchester, 1860.

Flugel, J. C., *A Hundred Years of Psychology*, 1933.

Fox, Dame Evelyn, 'Historical Survey of Modern Developments in Work for Mental Defectives', *Conference on Mental Welfare* (Central Association for Mental Welfare), 1934.

Gaskell, Samuel, 'Education of Idiots at Bicêtre', *Chambers Edinburgh Journal*, pp. 20, 71, 105, 1847.

Gaskell, Samuel, 'On the want of better provision for the labouring and middle classes when attacked or threatened with insanity', *Journal of Mental Science*, 6, 321 *et seq.*, 1860.

Gibson, J., *St. Lawrence's Hospital, Caterham, Surrey, 1870–1956*, Caterham [1957?].

Hodgkinson, Ruth G., 'Provision for Pauper Lunatics, 1834–1871', *Medical History*, vol. x, No. 2, 138–54, 1966.

Itard, J. M.-G., *The Wild Boy of Aveyron* (1798). Translated by Humphrey, G. & M., New York, 1932.

Jones, Kathleen, *Lunacy, Law and Conscience, 1744–1845*, 1955.

Jones, Kathleen, *Mental Health and Social Policy, 1845–1959*, 1960.

Lapage, C. P., *Feeble-Mindedness in Children of School Age*, 1920.

Maudsley, Henry, 'Middle-Class Hospitals for the Insane', *Journal of Mental Science*, 8, 356, 1862.

Mott, Sir F. W. (ed.), *London County Council Archives of Neurology and Psychiatry*, 1900–22.

Penrose, L. S., *The Biology of Mental Defect*, 1949.

Turner, F. D., 'Mental Deficiency' (Presidential Address), *Journal of Mental Science*, 79, 563 *et seq.*, 1933.

Walk, Alexander, '"On the State of Lunacy", 1859–1959', *Journal of Mental Science*, 105, 879–92, 1959.

Walk, Alexander, 'The History of Mental Nursing', *Journal of Mental Science*, 107, 1–17, 1961.

Walk, Alexander, 'Mental Hospitals', *The Evolution of Hospitals in Britain* (Poynter, F. N. L., ed.), 1964.

Webb, S. and B., *The Break-Up of the Poor Law* (Chapter VI, 'The Mentally Defective'), 1909.

Wellcome Historical Medical Library, *Psychiatry and Mental Health in Britain*, Exhibition Guide, No. 1, 1963.

Wormald, J. and S., *A Guide to the Mental Deficiency Act, 1913*, 1914.

Commissioners in Lunacy, 'The Condition, Character and Treatment of Lunatics in Workhouses', Supplement to *Twelfth Report*, 1859.

Commissioners in Lunacy, *Twenty-fifth* (1871) *and subsequent Reports:* entries relating to the Metropolitan District Asylums.

Report of the Royal (Radnor) Commission on the Care and Control of the Feeble-Minded, HMSO, 1908.

Report of the Royal (MacMillan) Commission on Lunacy and Mental Disorders, Cmd. 2700, 1926.

Report of the Mental Deficiency Committee (Wood Report), HMSO, 1929.

Report of the Departmental Committee on Sterilization (Brock Report), HMSO, 1934.

Report of the Royal (Percy) Commission on the Law relating to Mental Illness and Mental Deficiency, 1954–57, Cmd. 169, 1957.

IX. NURSING

Abel-Smith, B., *A History of the Nursing Profession,* 1960.

Burdett, H. C., *Nurses' Food, Work and Recreation.* The British Hospitals Association Pamphlet No. 13, 1890.

Cope, Sir Z., *A Hundred Years of Nursing,* 1955.

Murphy, D. G., *They did not pass by,* 1956.

Nightingale, Florence, *Notes on Nursing: What it is, and what it is not:* 2nd edn., 1860. (Reviewed by the *Lancet,* 11 February 1860, p. 144.)

Nightingale, Florence, 'Suggestions on the subject of providing training and organizing nurses for the sick poor in workhouse infirmaries': Appendix XVI to the *Report of the Committee appointed to consider the cubic space of Metropolitan Workhouses,* 7 February 1867 (BPP, 1867, vol. lx (H/C 185), 3786).

Nightingale, Florence, *On Trained Nursing for the Sick Poor,* The Metropolitan and National Nursing Association, 1876.

Nuffield Provincial Hospitals Trust, *The work of nurses in hospital wards: report of a job-analysis,* 1953.

Nursing, Royal College of, *Recruitment and Training of Nurses,* 1948.

Nursing, Royal College of, *The Social and Economic Conditions of the Nurse,* 1950 (Nursing Reconstruction Committee Report, Section IV).

Nutting, M. A. and Dock, L. L., *A History of Nursing. The Evolution of Nursing Systems from the Earliest Times to the Foundation of the First English and American Training Schools for Nurses,* 1907.

Pavey, A. E., *Story of the Growth of Nursing,* 3rd edn., 1951.

Seymer, L. R., *A General History of Nursing,* 1954.

Walk, Alexander, 'The History of Mental Nursing', *Journal of Mental Science,* 107, 1–17, 1961.

Nursing by Religious Communities:

Anson, P., *The Call of the Cloister* (with bibliography), SPCK, 4th edn., 1964.

Hutton, R. E., *St. Margaret's Convent, East Grinstead,* rev. ed. 1959.

Memoirs of a Sister of St. Saviour's, Mowbray's, 1903.

Towle, Eleanor A., *John Mason Neale, a Memoir,* 1906.

X. Relief of the Poor (nineteenth century)

(a) *Histories and Commentaries*

Ashrott, P. F., *The English Poor Law System*, 1888.

Ashrott, P. F. and Preston-Thomas, H., *The English Poor Law System: Past and Present*, 2nd edn., 1902.

Booth, Charles, *Poor Law Reform*, 1910.

Booth, Charles, *Comments on Proposals for the Reform of the Poor Law* (with Note by Sir Arthur Downes), 1911.

Chance, Sir W., *The Better Administration of the Poor Law*, 1895.

Chance, Sir W., *Poor Law Reform*, 1910.

Glen, R. C., *The Poor Law Orders* (annotated), 11th edn., 1898.

Leach, R. A., *The Evolution of Poor Law Administration*, 1924.

Mackay, Thomas, *History of the English Poor Law, 1834–1898*, 1904.

Ross, Elizabeth M., 'Women and Poor Law Administration, 1857–1910', London University MA thesis (unpublished), 1956.

Slater, Gilbert, *Poverty and the State*, 1930.

Webb, S. and B., *English Poor Law Policy*, 1910.

Webb, S. and B., *English Poor Law History: vols. 7–9 of English Local Government*, 9 vols., 1906–29.

(b) *Medical Relief*

Brand, Jeanne L., 'The Parish Doctor. England's Poor Law Medical Officers and Medical Reform, 1870–1900', *Bulletin of the History of Medicine*, xxxv, 97–122, 1961.

Chadwick, E., 'The Administration of Medical Relief to the Destitute Sick of the Metropolis', *Fraser's Magazine for Town and Country*, vol. lxxiv, No. ccccxli, pp. 353–65, 1866.

Cobb, Frances Power, *The Workhouse as Hospital*, 1861.

Griffin, R., *The Grievances of Poor Law Medical Officers*, Weymouth, 1858.

Hart, Ernest, 'The Condition of our State Hospitals', *Fortnightly Review*, III, pp. 218–21; December 1865.

Hart, Ernest, 'Metropolitan Infirmaries for the Pauper Sick', *Fortnightly Review*, IV, pp. 460–62; April 1866.

Hart, Ernest, *The Sick Poor in Workhouses*, 1894.

Hodgkinson, Ruth G., *The Origins of the National Health Service: The Medical Services of the New Poor Law, 1834–1871*. Wellcome Historical Medical Library, Historical Monograph Series No. 11, 1967.

Hodgkinson, Ruth G., 'The Poor Law Medical Officers of England', *Journal of the History of Medicine*, xi, pp. 299–338, 1956.

Lancet Sanitary Commission for investigating the State of Infirmaries of Workhouses, *Report of*, 1866.

Lloyd, Edmund, *The Requirements and Resources of the Sick Poor*, 1858.

McCurrich, H. J., *The Treatment of the Sick Poor of this Country*, 1929.

346

O'Neill, James E., 'Finding a Policy for the Sick Poor', *Victorian Studies*, vol. vii, No. 3; March 1964.

Rogers, J., *Reminiscences of a Workhouse Medical Officer* (ed. by J. E. T. Rogers), 1889.

Rumsey, H. W., *Medical Relief for the Labouring Classes*, 1837.

Twining, Louisa, *The Sick in Workhouses and how they are treated*, 1861.

(c) *Pauper Children*

British Association for the Advancement of Science, *Annual Report*, 1893, pp. 614–20: 'Report of a study of intelligence in 100,000 school children' [including London poor law children].

British Medical Journal, 'A Report of investigations in fourteen London schools' [by a committee appointed by the BMA to investigate the average development . . . of brain function among children in primary and poor law schools], II, p. 187 *et seq.*, 27 July 1889.

Chance, Sir W., *Children under the Poor Law*, 1897.

Monnington, W., and Lambert, F. J., *Criticism of the Report of the Departmental Committee on the Metropolitan Poor Law Schools*, 1896.

Mouat, F. J., *The Education and Training of the Children of the Poor*, 1880.

(d) *Official Reports relating to Poor Law Administration*

Report from H.M. Commissioners for enquiring into the Administration and Practical Operation of the Poor Laws, 1834 (Fellowes reprint, 1905).

Report of the Select Committee of 1854 'to enquire into the mode in which medical relief is administered in the unions of England and Wales', BPP, 1854, vol. xii, 431.

Report of the H/C Select Committee on Poor Relief, 1864, BPP, 1864, vol. ix, 187.

Report of the Committee appointed to consider the cubic space of Metropolitan Workhouses (the Watson Committee), 1867; BPP, 1867, vol. lx (H/C), 185, 3786.

Report of the Departmental Committee on Metropolitan Poor Law Schools, 1896; BPP, 1896, vol. xliii, 1 [Cmd. 8027; Cmd. 8032; and Cmd. 8033].

Report of the Local Government Board Departmental Committee on Workhouse Accounts, 1903; BPP, 1903, vol. xxvi, p. 567 [Cmd. 1440].

Reports of the Royal Commission on the Poor Law and the Relief of Distress, 1909 (Majority and Minority); BPP, 1909, vols. xxxvii–xliv.

[The Minority Report of the 1905–9 Poor Law Commission was published (without references) as S. and B. Webb, *The Break-Up of the Poor Law*, 1909; and *The Public Organization of the Labour Market, 1809*.

XI. STATE MEDICINE

Acton Society Trust, *Hospitals and the State*, (6 parts, 1955–59: see Section V, above).

Burdett, H. C., *Hospitals and the State*, 1881.

Chalmers, R. W., *Hospitals and the State*, 1928.

Bruce, M., *The Coming of the Welfare State*, 1961.

Brand, Jeanne L., *The British Medical Profession and State Intervention in Public Health, 1870–1911*, unpublished thesis for PhD degree, London University, 1953.

Eckstein, H., *The English Health Service*, Harvard, 1959.

Lambert, R., 'A Victorian National Health Service: State Vaccination', *Historical Journal*, v (1962).

Lindsey, Almont, *Socialized Medicine in England and Wales*, 1962.

MacNalty, Sir Arthur, *The History of State Medicine in England*, 1948.

Newsholme, Sir Arthur, *The Ministry of Health*, 1925.

Newsholme, Sir Arthur, *International Studies on the Relation between the Private and Official Practice of Medicine* (3 vols.), 1928–32.

Newsholme, Sir Arthur, *Medicine and the State*, 1932.

Newsholme, Sir Arthur, *Fifty Years in Public Health*, 1935.

Newsholme, Sir Arthur, *The Last Thirty Years in Public Health*, 1936.

Roberts, D., *The Victorian Origins of the Welfare State*, 1960.

Ross, J., *The National Health Service in Great Britain*, 1952.

Rumsey, H. W., *Essays on State Medicine*, 1856.

Rumsey, H. W., *State Medicine in Great Britain and Ireland*, 1867.

Simon, Sir John, *Public Health Reports* (edited in 2 vols. by E. Seaton), 1887.

Simon, Sir John, *English Sanitary Institutions*, 2nd edn., 1897.

Titmuss, R. M., *Problems of Social Policy*, 1950 (Chapters XI, XXII, XXIII, XXIV and XXV).

Titmuss, R. M., *Essays on 'The Welfare State'*, 1958 (Chapters 7, 8, 9 and 10).

Titmuss, R. M., 'Health', *Law and Opinion in England in the Twentieth Century* (M. Ginsberg, ed.), pp. 299–318, 1959.

Webb, S. and B., *The State and the Doctor*, 1910.

XII. Victorian England

Arnold, Matthew, *Culture and Anarchy*, 1862 (ed. J. D. Wilson, 1932).

Bagehot, Walter, *The English Constitution* (Nelson edn.), 1872.

Booth, Charles, *Life and Labour of the People in London* (17 vols.), 3rd edn., 1902–3.

Briggs, Asa, *Public Opinion and Public Health in the Age of Chadwick*, 1946.

Briggs, Asa, *Victorian People*, 1954.

Briggs, Asa, *The Age of Improvement*, 1959.

Butler, J. R. M., *A History of England, 1815–1918*, 1928.

Dicey, A. V., *Lectures on the Relation between Law and Public Opinion in England* [during the nineteenth century], 1905.

Elliott-Binns, L. E., *Religion in the Victorian Era*, 1936.

Ensor, R., *England, 1870–1914*, Oxford, 1936.

Goodwin, M., *Nineteenth Century Opinion*, 1951.

Hammond, J. L. and B., *The Bleak Age*, 1947.

MacGregor, O. R., 'Social Research and Social Policy in the Nineteenth Century', *British Journal of Sociology*, viii, 1957.

BIBLIOGRAPHY

Mill, John Stuart, *Autobiography*, 1873.

Seeley, Sir John, *Ecce Homo* 1866.

Thomson, D., *England in the Nineteenth Century, 1815–1914*, 1950.

Trevelyan, G. M., *British History in the Nineteenth Century and after, 1782–1919*, 2nd edn., 1937.

Woodward, E. L., *The Age of Reform, 1815–1870*, Oxford, 1938.

Young, G. M., *Victorian England, Portrait of an Age*, 1936.

Medical Supplement

CLASSIFIED LIST OF MEDICAL ARTICLES
appended to the
ANNUAL REPORTS OF THE METROPOLITAN ASYLUMS BOARD

MEDICAL SUPPLEMENT

Classified List of Medical Articles
in M A B Annual Reports[1]

[1] Most of these Reports are available at the British Museum, the Greater London County Record Office, the Royal Society of Medicine, the London School of Hygiene and Tropical Medicine, and the Oxford Radcliffe Library. Some of them may be found at the Wellcome Institute of the History of Medicine.

[2] The year under reference is the date of the M A B Annual Report in which the article appeared. Pagination is in brackets.

Section II: Tuberculosis

A. *Pulmonary or Medical Tuberculosis*

Subject	Author	Reference
Sedimentation of red blood cells in	G. I. Davies, MB, BS	1927–28 (313–20)
Treatment of, in childhood	F. G. Caley, MA, MB, DPH	1912 (276–80)
	C. E. Last, MRCS, LRCP	1912 (286–92)
Tuberculin treatment in early tuberculosis	Noel A. Coward, MB, ChB	1912 (281–83)

B. *Tuberculosis (Surgical)*

Subject	Author	Reference
After-care of children	W. T. Gordon Pugh, MD, BS	1922–23 (201–9)
Diagnosis of, in bones and joints	W. M. Oakden, BA, MB, BC, FRCS	1925–26 (300–4)
Glands of the neck	W. G. Sutcliffe, OBE, FRCS	1924–25 (313–16)
Hip joint, treatment of by traction; by suspension	W. T. Gordon Pugh, MD, BS	1926–27 (361–63)
Light and open air treatment	(i) W. T. Gordon Pugh, MD, BS	1925–26 (285–89)
	(ii) N. Gray Hill, MC, MRCS, LRCP	1925–26 (290–99)
With meningitis	J. K. Haworth, MD, MS	1923–24 (258–59)
Sodium morrhuate in treatment of,	E. J. Mawson, MB, ChB and L. S. Fry, MB, DPH	1923–24 (265–67)
Spinal caries, symptom of pain in,	W. P. Grieve, MD, ChB	1925–26 (305–8)

Section III: Mental Disorders

Subject	Author	Reference
Aesthetics and mental deficiency	E. B. Sherlock, MD, BSc, DPH	1928–29 (334–42)
Amentia, primary with physical abnormalities	G. Brown, MB, ChB, DPM and J. N. Jacobson, MRCS, LRCP, DPM	1927–28 (302–5)
Brain, a markedly undeveloped	P. M. Turnbull, MB, DPM and B. F. Home, LRCP	1925–26 (222–23)
Cardiac rarities at Tooting Bec Hospital	C. J. C. Earl, MRCP	1928–29 (348–51)
Cases of interest at Tooting Bec Hospital	E. H. Beresford, MRCS, LRCP	1927–28 (297–98)
Degeneration, stigmata of,	James Nicoll, MD, CM, DPH	1924–25 (257–60)
Dwarfism, pituitary	J. P. Park Inglish, MD, ChB	1925–26 (231–33)
Dysostosis, cleido-cranial	S. J. Laverty, MB, ChB	1924–25 (261–62)
Educational methods of Dr. Ovide Decroly	Rose Munday	1925–26 (229–30) 1926–27 (305–10)
Encephalitis lethargica, after effects of,	(i) Edna Mawson, MB, ChB	1922–23 (240–41)
	(ii) C. Glen, MB, ChB	1923–24 (202–13)
	(iii) W. T. Gordon Pugh, MD, BS	1924–25 (340–42)
	(iv) G. A. Borthwick, MD, DPH	1926–27 (148–67)
Endarteritis obliterans in a brain	R. M. Stewart, MD, ChB	1926–27 (291–94)
Epilepsy, luminal in treatment of,	A symposium	1924–25 (251–56)
Epileptic idiocy, the pathology of,	E. B. Sherlock, MD, BSc, DPH	1907 (335–60)

SECTION IV: SICK CHILDREN[1]

[1] See Section I for children suffering from acute infectious diseases; Section II A for children suffering from pulmonary tuberculosis; and Section II B for orthopaedic cases.

Index

An asterisk denotes a Metropolitan Asylums Board institution

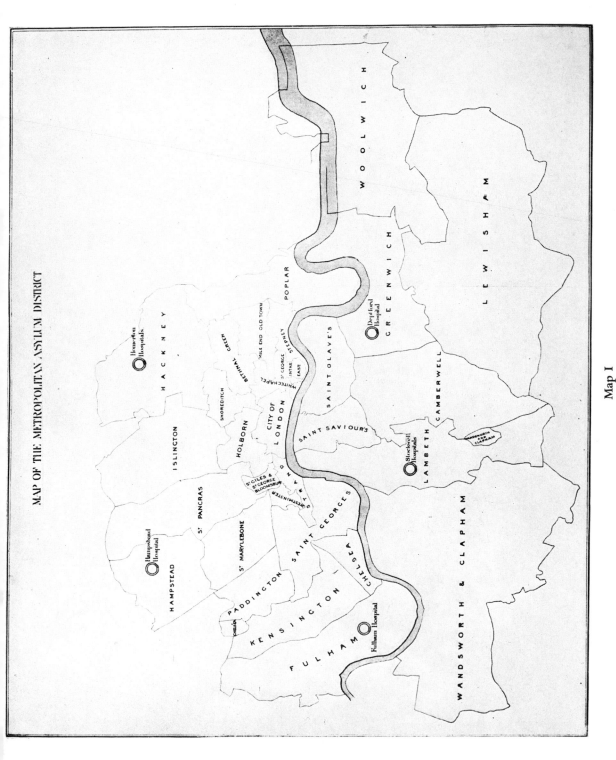

MAP OF THE METROPOLITAN ASYLUM DISTRICT

Map I

The Metropolitan Asylum District in 1877, showing the Poor Law districts and the position of the M. A. B hospitals for infectious diseases.

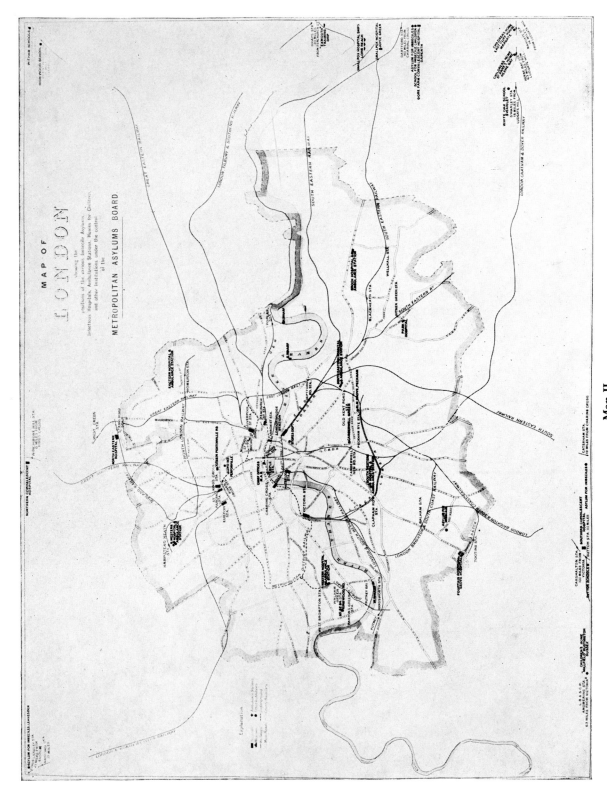

Map II

Institutions under the control of the Metropolitan Asylums Board in 1900.

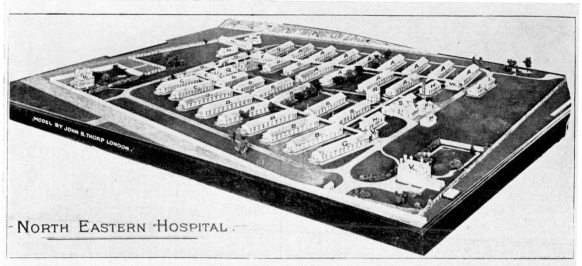

NORTH EASTERN HOSPITAL.

MODEL BY JOHN B. THORP LONDON.

REFERENCE.

A. FEMALES' WARDS
B. MALES' WARDS.
C. NURSES' DORMITORIES
D. SERVANTS' DORMITORIES
E. NURSES' MESS ROOM
F. SERVANTS' MESS ROOM

G. MALE STAFF QUARTERS
H. ISOLATION BLOCKS
I. SICK NURSES' BLOCK
J. ISOLATION NURSES' BLOCK
K. PATIENTS' CLOTHING
L. RECEIVING ROOM

M. MORTUARY
N. NURSES' DRESSING BLOCK
O. OFFICES
P. KITCHEN
Q. STORES
R. WATER TOWER

S. LAUNDRY
T. BOILER HOUSE
U. MEDICAL OFFICER'S HOUSE
V. ASST. MEDICAL OFFICERS' HOUSE
W. CHAPEL

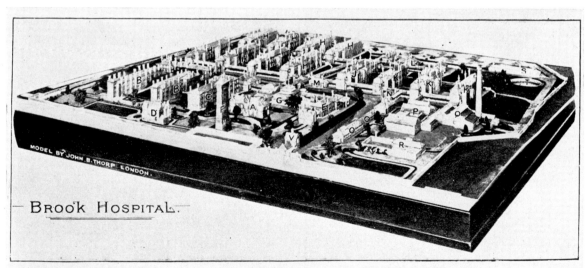

MODEL BY JOHN B. THORP LONDON.

BROOK HOSPITAL.

REFERENCE.

A. OFFICIAL BLOCK
B. NURSES' HOME
C. FEMALE SERVANTS' HOME
D. MEDICAL SUPERINTENDENT'S HOUSE
E. MALE SERVANTS' HOME

F. WATER TOWER
G. KITCHEN AND STORES
H. SCARLET FEVER PAVILIONS
J. ENTERIC FEVER PAVILIONS
K. DIPTHERIA PAVILIONS
L. ISOLATION WARDS

M. SCARLET FEVER RECEIVING WARDS
N. DIPTHERIA AND ENTERIC RECEIVING WARDS
O. DISCHARGE WARDS
P. LAUNDRY

Q. BOILER AND ENGINE HOUSE
R. MORTUARY
S. WORKSHOPS
T. RAIN WATER TANK
V. PORTER'S LODGE

Figure 1. Models of Metropolitan Asylums Board Fever Hospitals exhibited in the Social Science Section of the 1900 International Exhibition in Paris.

The North-Eastern Hospital, South Tottenham, London, N., was a temporary structure erected in six weeks in 1892. (It is now known as St. Ann's General Hospital.)
The Brook Hospital, Shooter's Hill, London, S.E., was opened in 1896.
Architectural details of these institutions are given in Appendix II.

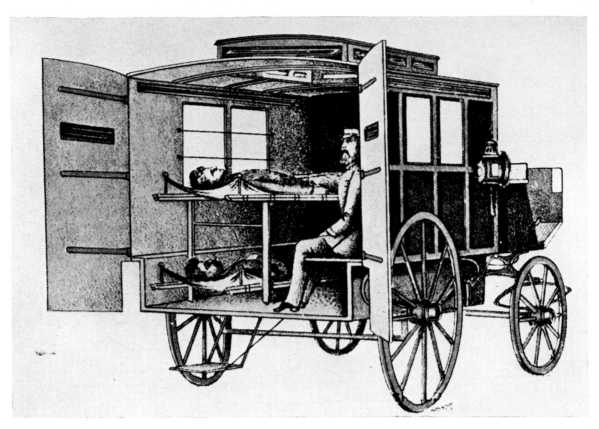

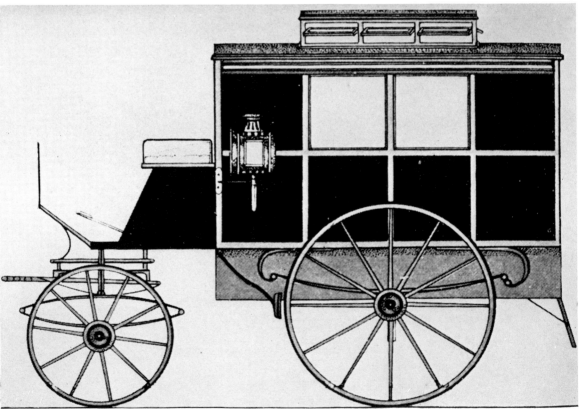

Figure 2. Metropolitan Asylums Board Horse Ambulance Carriage designed in 1883.
Above: rear view.   Below: side view.

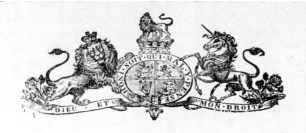

ANNO TRICESIMO

VICTORIÆ REGINÆ.

* *

C A P. VI.

An Act for the Establishment in the Metropolis of Asylums for the Sick, Insane, and other Classes of the Poor, and of Dispensaries; and for the Distribution over the Metropolis of Portions of the Charge for Poor Relief; and for other Purposes relating to Poor Relief in the Metropolis.   [29th *March* 1867.]

BE it enacted by the Queen's most Excellent Majesty, by and with the Advice and Consent of the Lords Spiritual and Temporal, and Commons, in this present Parliament assembled, and by the Authority of the same, as follows:

Preliminary.

1. This Act may be cited as The Metropolitan Poor Act, 1867.   Short Title.

2. In this Act—
The Term "the Poor Law Acts" means the Act of the Session   Interpretation of the Fourth and Fifth Years of King *William* the Fourth   tion of (Chapter Seventy-six) "for the Amendment and better Ad-   Terms.
P   " ministration

Figure 3. Metropolitan Poor Act, 1867.

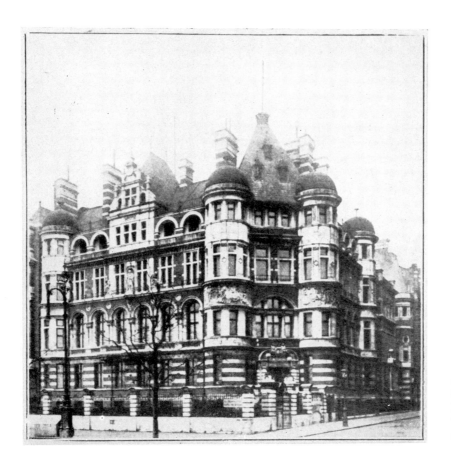

Figure 4. The head office of the Metropolitan Asylums Board at the corner of Victoria Embankment and Carmelite Street, London.

Figure 5. Coat-of-arms of the Metropolitan Asylums Board.

On the central white shield rests the St. George's cross, representing the red cross of medicine and ambulance work, and in the centre of the cross is the gold staff of Aesculapius, the heathen founder of the art of healing.

On the dexter side is an eagle, the bird of health and strength, wreathed with red and white roses, recalling the Wars of the Roses, which began in the Temple Gardens adjoining the head offices of the Metropolitan Asylums Board.

On the sinister side is a chained dragon symbolizing disease held in check.

Arising out of a celestial crown above the shield is a demi-figure of St. Luke, the Christian healer.

The motto on the scroll below the design may be translated: 'I learn to succor the wretched'.

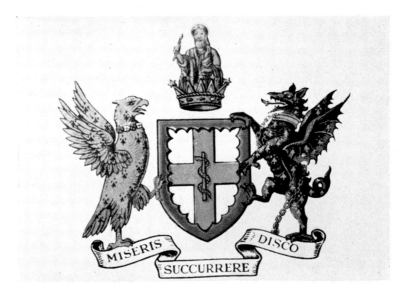

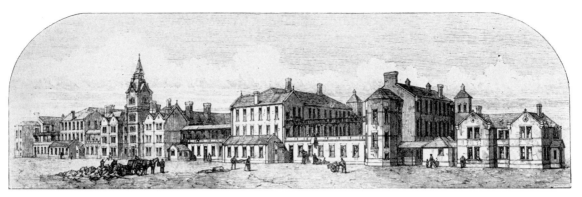

Figure 6, Poplar and Stepney Sick Asylum, for the reception of the pauper sick under the provisions of the Metropolitan Poor Act, 1867.

(From *Illustrated London News*, 1871, **59**, 537.)

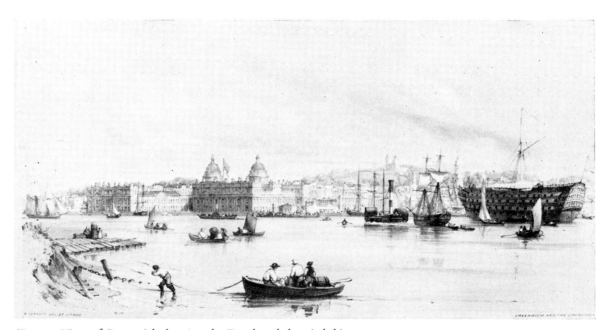

Figure 7. View of Greenwich showing the *Dreadnought* hospital ship.

(Lithograph in the Wellcome Institute of the History of Medicine, *c.* 1800. Reproduced by courtesy of the Wellcome Trustees.)

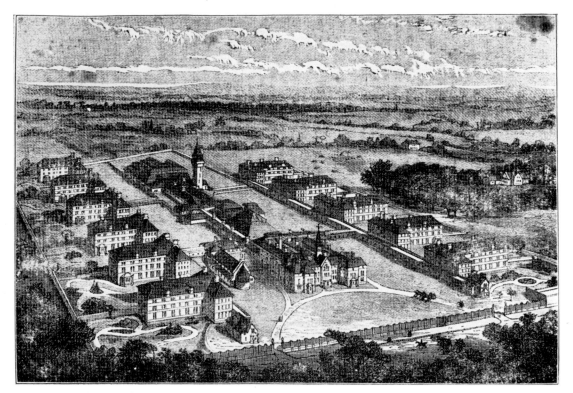

Figure 8. Caterham Asylum, 1870.

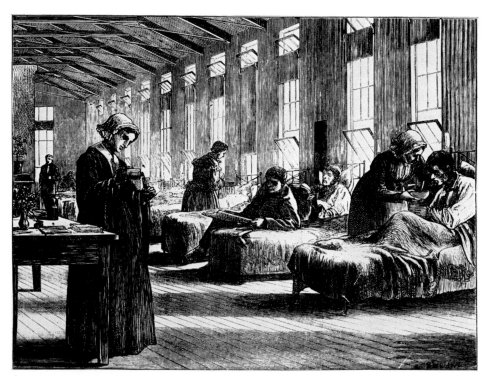

Figure 9. A ward in the Hampstead Smallpox Hospital.
(From *Illustrated London News*, 1871, **59**, 345.)